WHITE CELLS AND PLATELETS IN BLOOD TRANSFUSION

DEVELOPMENTS IN HEMATOLOGY AND IMMUNOLOGY

Lijnen, H.R., Collen, D. and Verstraete, M., eds: Synthetic Substrates in Clinical Blood Coagulation Assays. 1980. ISBN 90-247-2409-0

Smit Sibinga, C.Th., Das, P.C. and Forfar, J.O., eds: Paediatrics and Blood Transfusion. 1982. ISBN 90-247-2619-0

Fabris, N., ed: Immunology and Ageing. 1982. ISBN 90-247-2640-9

Hornstra, G.: Dietary Fats, Prostanoids and Arterial Thrombosis. 1982. ISBN 90-247-2667-0

Smit Sibinga, C.Th., Das, P.C. and Loghem, van J.J., eds: Blood Transfusion and Problems of Bleeding. 1982. ISBN 90-247-3058-9

Dormandy, J., ed: Red Cell Deformability and Filterability. 1983. ISBN 0-89838-578-4

Smit Sibinga, C.Th., Das, P.C. and Taswell, H.F., eds: Quality Assurance in Blood Banking and Its Clinical Impact. 1984. ISBN 0-89838-618-7

Besselaar, A.M.H.P. van den, Gralnick, H.R. and Lewis, S.M., eds: Thromboplastin Calibration and Oral Anticoagulant Control. 1984. ISBN 0-89838-637-3

Fondu, P. and Thijs, O., eds: Haemostatic Failure in Liver Disease. 1984. ISBN 0-89838-640-3

Smit Sibinga, C.Th., Das, P.C. and Opelz, G., eds: Transplantation and Blood Transfusion. 1984. ISBN 0-89838-686-1

Schmid-Schönbein, H., Wurzinger, L.J. and Zimmerman, R.E., eds: Enzyme Activation in Blood-Perfused Artificial Organs. 1985. ISBN 0-89838-704-3

Dormandy, J., ed: Blood Filtration and Blood Cell Deformability. 1985. ISBN 0-89838-714-0

Smit Sibinga, C.Th., Das, P.C. and Seidl, S., eds: Plasma Fractionation and Blood Transfusion. 1985. ISBN 0-89838-761-2

Dawids, S. and Bantjes, A., eds: Blood Compatible Materials and their Testing. 1986. ISBN 0-89838-813-9

Smit Sibinga, C.Th., Das, P.C. and Greenwalt, T.J., eds: Future Developments in Blood Banking. 1986. ISBN 0-89838-824-4

Berlin, A., Dean, J., Draper, M.H., Smith, E.M.B. and Spreafico, F., eds: Immunotoxicology. 1987. ISBN 0-89838-843-0

Ottenhoff, T. and De Vries, R.: Recognition of *M. leprae* antigens. 1987. ISBN 0-89838-887-2

Smit Sibinga, C.Th., Das, P.C. and Engelfriet, C.P., eds: White cells and platelets in blood transfusion. 1987. ISBN 0-89838-976-3

White cells and platelets in blood transfusion

Proceedings of the Eleventh Annual Symposium on Blood Transfusion, Groningen 1986, organized by the Red Cross Blood Bank Groningen-Drenthe

edited by

C.Th. SMIT SIBINGA and P.C. DAS

Red Cross Blood Bank Groningen-Drenthe
The Netherlands

C.P. ENGELFRIET

Central Laboratory of the Netherlands Red Cross
Amsterdam, The Netherlands

1987 **MARTINUS NIJHOFF PUBLISHING**
a member of the KLUWER ACADEMIC PUBLISHERS GROUP
BOSTON / DORDRECHT / LANCASTER

Distributors

for the United States and Canada: Kluwer Academic Publishers, P.O. Box 358, Accord Station, Hingham, MA 02018-0358, USA
for the UK and Ireland: Kluwer Academic Publishers, MTP Press Limited, Falcon House, Queen Square, Lancaster LA1 1RN, UK
for all other countries: Kluwer Academic Publishers Group, Distribution Center, P.O. Box 322, 3300 AH Dordrecht, The Netherlands

Library of Congress Cataloging in Publication Data

Symposium on Blood Transfusion (11th : 1986 : Groningen, Netherlands)
White cells and platelets in blood transfusion.

(Developments in hematology and immunology ; 19)
Includes bibliographies.
1. Blood platelets--Transfusion--Congresses.
2. Leucocytes--Congresses. I. Smit Sibinga, C. Th.
II. Das, P. C. III. Engelfriet, C. P. IV. Stichting Rode Kruis Bloedbank Groningen/Drente. V. Title.
VI. Series. [DNLM: 1. Blood Platelets--congresses.
2. Blood Transfusion--congresses. 3. Leukocytes--congresses. W1 DE997VZK v.19 / WB 356 S989w 1986]
RM177.S96 1986 615'.39 87-7301

ISBN 0-89838-976-3
ISBN 90-247-2432-5 (series)

PRINTED IN THE NETHERLANDS

TRAVENOL

Acknowledgement

This publication has been made possible through the support of Travenol, which is gratefully acknowledged.

CONTENTS

B. Absence of cells

III. Production aspects

IV. Laboratory aspects

MODERATORS AND SPEAKERS

Moderators

C.P. Engelfriet (chairman) – Central Laboratory of the Netherlands Red Cross, Amsterdam, NL

J.C. Chermann – Institute Pasteur, Paris, F

P.C. Das – Red Cross Blood Bank Groningen-Drenthe, Groningen, NL

M.R. Halie – Dept. of Internal Medicine, University of Groningen, Groningen, NL

M. Körbling – Ruprechts Karls University, Heidelberg, FRG

S.B. Moore – Mayo Clinic Blood Bank and Transfusion Service, Rochester, MI, USA

S. Murphy – Thomas Jefferson University, Philadelphia, PA, USA

Speakers

F.G. Arnaud – MRC Medical Cryobiology Group, Cambridge, UK

J.M. Beelen – Blood Group Laboratory, University of Groningen, Groningen, NL

A.E.G. Kr. von dem Borne – Central Laboratory of the Netherlands Red Cross, Amsterdam, NL

M.K. Brenner – The Royal Free Hospital, London, UK

B. Brozović – North London Blood Transfusion Centre, Edgware, UK

D.H. Buchholz – Travenol Laboratories, Round Lake, IL, USA

J.W. ten Cate – Academic Medical Centre of the University of Amsterdam, Amsterdam, NL

M.K. Elias – Red Cross Blood Bank Groningen-Drenthe, Groningen, NL

A.B. Glassman – Medical University of South Carolina, Charleston, SC, USA

S.F. Leitman – National Institutes of Health, Bethesda, MD, USA

B. Löwenberg – Dr. Daniel den Hoed Clinic, Rotterdam, NL

N.H. Mulder – Dept. of Internal Medicine, University of Groningen, Groningen, NL

R.T. Schooley – Harvard Medical School, Boston, MS, USA

J. Seidel – Blood Bank, University of Hannover, Hannover, FRG

S.J. Slichter – Puget Sound Blood Center, Seattle, WA, USA

J.W. Smit – Dept. of Internal Medicine, University of Groningen, NL

P. Terness – Ruprecht Karls University, Heidelberg, FRG

T.H. The – Dept. of Internal Medicine, University of Groningen, NL

J.Th.M. de Wolf – Dept. of Internal Medicine, University of Groningen, NL

Prepared discussants

C. Kaplan – National Blood Transfusion Service, Paris, F

K. Sintnicolaas – Dr. Daniel den Hoed Clinic, Rotterdam, NL

FOREWORD

As a clinical discipline blood transfusion encompasses enormous vista, varying from biotechnology to molecular biology, from plasma products, cell biology and growth factors to interleukines. Growth of knowledge in this field has been rapid, and expertise is now required to be mastered and renewed in translating these ideas for patient care. Various types of cells could be harvested – progenitor stem cells derived from bone marrow or from circulating blood as a source for transplants; in the hemostatic armoury platelets could be used prophylactically; granulocytes and mononuclear cells are available for treatment of infections or immune modulations. However, their therapeutic use carries potential complications including graft versus host disease and CMV-infection. Prevention of such complications by irradiation and by removal of immunocompetent leukocytes are important issues. Thus, production of such therapeutic materials ought to address the issues at the earliest, to eliminate those problems while adhering to the concept of high quality; the impact of storing platelets for longer periods by using improved plastic containers or storing almost indefinitely in frozen state should be explored. Rapid progress in cell culture techniques and biotechnology have enriched the transfusion medicine armoury with lymphokines, interferons and cell colony growth factors which have great potentials for enhancement of basic knowledge as well as considerable therapeutic applications in patients. The laboratory has crucial roles to play – it could preselect blood components and tissue by HLA-typing, it may also be in the forefront of innovations when specific cell-lines would produce suitable reagents, and cultured cells become available for therapy.

The purpose of this book is to inform physicians and laboratory workers of the developments in these areas with special emphasis on white cells and platelets, and their potential application in Transfusion Medicine.

Cees Th. Smit Sibinga, MD, PhD
Prakash C. Das, MD, PhD, FRCPath
C. Paul Engelfriet, MD, PhD

I. PRINCIPLES AND FUNCTIONAL ASPECTS

THE HUMAN MHC (HLA) AND ITS IMMEDIATE RELEVANCE IN TRANSFUSION PRACTICE

S.B. Moore

The human major histocompatibility complex (MHC) or HLA (human lymphocyte antigens) has a major role in the functioning of the immune system at several key points. The presence of these antigens was first recognized in mice by the pioneering work of Snell and his colleagues, who, in the mid-1930s, realized that the antigens were in some way related to the rejection of experimental skin allografts in these animals. In the early 1950s, the presence of a similar group of antigens in humans was independently discovered by Daussett in France and Payne in the United States. In The Netherlands, van Rood contributed to the elucidation of the actual genetic systems involved in the human MHC and in the characterization of sera from multiparous women so that tentative specificities could be assigned. A series of regular international workshops have continued this painstaking work and have paved the way for the detection of several genetic loci within the MHC. These workshops have also stimulated much of the work on the establishment of the clinical relevance of HLA in the fields of organ transplantation and the genetic predisposition to specific diseases.

While the general chromosomal alignment of the various loci has been well established for several years (Fig. 1), the development of monoclonal antibodies and DNA probes has led to a flurry of recent activity in the field of HLA. These new tools have permitted workers to look not only at the cell-surface antigens but also at the genes that underlie the expressions of these antigens. These new studies have begun to unravel the complexity of the

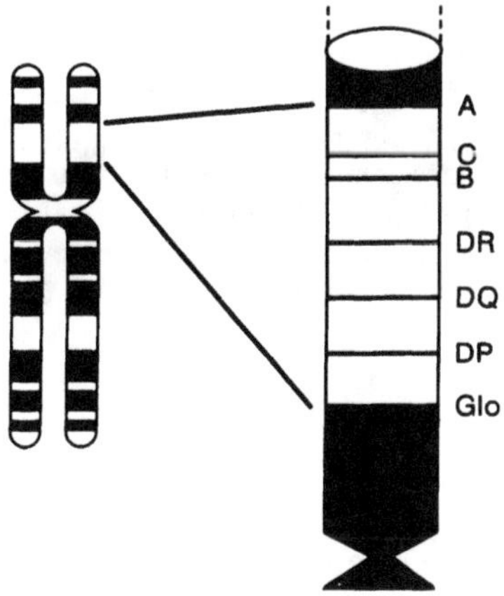

Figure 1. Major histocompatibility gene arrangement on chromosome 6.

genes of what are termed class II antigens and promise to supersede many of the older studies on both diseases and transplantation, which were based on the detection of cell-surface antigens alone.

Genetics

The human MHC is located on the short arm of chromosome 6 and is believed to consist of the following loci: A, C, B, D/DR, DQ, and DP, proceeding centromerically. A, C, and B locus antigens are termed class I, while D/DR, DQ, and DP antigens are class II. Serologic typing is performed for class I antigens and for the DR and DQ antigens of class II, while cellular typing culture methods are used to detect D and DP locus antigens. Interestingly, between the class I and class II regions on chromosome 6 resides an area containing loci that carry genes which code for various components of the complement system. Sometimes the products of these complement loci alleles are called MHC class III antigens. The gene for β_2-microglobulin (the β chain of class I) is located on chromosome 15. The genes that code for the various α and β chains in the class II subregions are outlined in Figure 2.

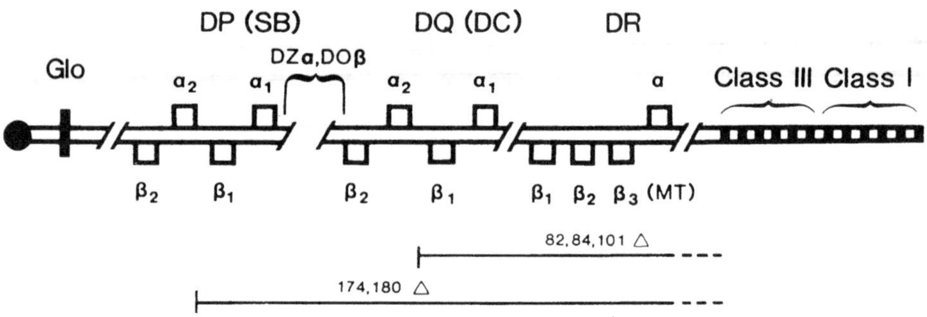

Figure 2. A provisional map of the HLA class II region. The map order shown here is provisional since the distal breakpoints of the two deletions have not been determined. (From Erlich H, Lee JS, Petersen JW, Bugawan T, DeMars R. Molecular analysis of HLA class I and class II antigen loss mutants reveals a homozygous deletion of the DR, DQ, and part of the DP region: implications for class II gene order. Hum Immunol 1986; 16;205-19. By permission of Elsevier Science Publishing Co. and the authors.)

Structure

Class I

HLA antigens can be divided into two major subgroups on the basis of structure, function, and distribution. Class I antigens are found on virtually all nucleated cells of the body as well as in plasma. They are also found in greatly reduced quantities on nonnucleated cells such as red blood cells and corneal epithelium. These antigens are present in abundance on platelets and lymphocytes and in lesser amounts on granulocytes. Class I antigens are composed of a variant 'heavy chain' α glycopeptide with a molecular weight of 44,000 and an invariant 'light chain' β polypeptide with a molecular weight of 12,000. This latter chain is a β_2-microglobulin, and it shows considerable amino acid homology at the molecular level not only within species but also between species. Clearly, the alloantigenic epitopes on class I molecules are not on this β chain. The class I antigens are remarkable in that the α chain, including its N-terminal, protrudes externally from the surface membrane and the carboxy terminal extends internally into the cytoplasm of the cell. The β_2-microglobulin is only found external to the lipid bilayer of the cytoplasmic membrane [1]. The β_2-microglobulin may function as a conformational stabilizer for the α chain. The α chain is divided into several 'domains': α_1, α_2, and α_3. Amino acid sequence studies of various class I antigens have revealed considerable heterogeneity between non-cross-reacting antigens, while there is much more amino acid homology between antigens that demonstrate serologic cross-reactivity. For example, of the several hundred amino acids in the α chain of A2 and A28 antigens, differences reflecting perhaps a single base change at the DNA level may explain the antigenic difference between these two highly cross-reactive antigens [2].

Class II

Class II antigens are found on a much more restricted spectrum of resting cells. A notable feature of these antigens is the fact that resting cells, which do not normally express or display these epitopes, will do so when they become activated in various ways. The structure of class II antigens displays superficial resemblances to that of class I antigens in that each antigen has two chains of peptides (α and β) and that both chains protrude externally from the cytoplasmic membrane surface. However, in class II antigens both chains extend through the membrane into the cytoplasm of the cell. The α chain has a molecular weight of 34,000, while the β chain has a molecular weight of 29,000. These chains are noncovalently linked to one another, and the alloantigenic epitopes are on the β chain. The β chain has two disulfide loops, similar to the configuration of the class I α chain [3].

Distribution

Studies of class I antigens and their distribution have demonstrated their presence on most nucleated cells but only weak expression on endocrine cells in the thyroid, parathyroid, and pituitary glands and the islets of Langerhans in the pancreas and on gastric mucosa, the myocardium, hepatocytes, and skeletal muscle. The antigens are not found on central-nervous-system neurons, endocrine (non-Langerhans) pancreatic cells, parotid acinar cells, and villous trophoblasts [4].

Class II antigen expression is much more limited than class I. Initially detected on B lymphocytes only, class II antigens have subsequently been seen on epidermal Langerhans cells, on endothelial cells and macrophages, and on activated T cells [5]. They have also been seen during different stages of the maturation of various myeloid and erythroid precursors [6]. They are seen on epithelial cells of the tongue, tonsil, epiglottis, trachea, small intestine, urethra, epididymis, and proximal renal tubules. Capillary endothelial cells express these antigens strongly, except in the testes and brain and in the placenta [5].

On myeolid progenitor cells, there seems to be a differential degree of expression of class II antigens as cells progressively mature. Pre-CFU-GM (colony forming units-granulocyte, macrophage) cells are the more immature, and they give rise to the day 14 CFU-GM cells, which in turn generate day 7 CFU-GM cells, which are more mature. DR antigens are expressed on all three of these cells, but their expression progressively increases with maturation. DQ antigens seem much more difficult to detect, and their detectability increases with progressive maturation. It has been postulated that the change in expression of these class II antigens reflects a role for HLA in the normal regulation of myeloid cell differentiation [6]. Class II antigens have not been found on platelets. It is also of interest that studies have shown that DQ antigens seem to be present on only certain subpopulations of monocytes [7], and class II antigens in general seem to be absent from mature granulocytic cells [8]. The role that class II antigens has in the innate immunogenicity of certain cells remains unresolved.

HLA typing the gene, not the gene product

Workers in the field of HLA testing have known that the classification of class II genes and their respective interrelationships have been both incomplete and inconsistent, because certain well-established serologic specificities at the DR locus could be shown to contain serologic subspecificities [9] and because of the demonstrated correlations between a single specificity such as DR4 with at least five different HLA-D clusters [10]. Subsequent studies by Bach and colleagues have extended this finding to several other specificities [11]. An exciting new tool in the elucidation of the actual genetic basis for class II molecules is the use of restrictive endonuclease enzymes to essentially dissect the DNA. The fragmented DNA can then be plated on membranes, and cDNA probes can be used to hybridize to the membrane-bound DNA and thus to detect specific segments of DNA. This method is already showing promise in the dissection of DR β gene polymorphisms and their correlation with the parent DR serologic typing and in the examination of MHC/disease correlations [12,13]. In fact, this method has even been used to HLA type patients who have immunodeficiency and lack HLA antigenic expression [14]. There is still controversy over the number of actual α and β genes for each of the class II loci, and this uncertainty may be a reflection of the role of pseudogenes that are detected at the DNA level but do not express products [15].

Immunogenicity

The question of the innate immunogenicity of HLA antigens is not as simple as one might suspect at first glance. Undoubtedly, HLA class I and class II antigens can elicit immune responses, both humoral and cellular. If they did not do so, there would be no tools with which to study them. The tools conventionally used are antibodies and lymphocytes. HLA alloimmunization in the form of antibodies is seen in patients who have been exposed to these antigens as a result of transfusions, pregnancies, or prior allografting. Each one of these immunizing events exposes the host to a plethora of different alloantigenic systems, only one of which is HLA. Therefore, the specificities of the induced antibodies have been difficult to clearly ascertain. Most studies have used panels of lymphocytes as targets to measure alloimmunization and have used the differential reactivity with subpopulations as an index of the general specificity. For example, an antibody that reacts with B cells but not T cells is considered likely to be directed to a class II antigen or antigens. Similarly, if platelets are used as targets, reactivity with lymphocytes and absorption by platelets are believed to indicate class I specificity.

Each of the aforementioned immunizing events has a different potential for inducing antibodies. We have studied this question in relation to patients awaiting renal allografts [16]. We examined the influence of pregnancy, allograft rejection, and transfusions on the levels of lymphocytotoxic antibodies in the sera of patients. Our results indicated that, with transfusion alone, 77% of men and 86% of women show less than 10% panel reactive antibodies as a result of the transfusions. Allograft rejection was by far the most likely of the three events to induce antibodies [16]. Similarly, we found that splenectomy prior to donor-specific transfusions seemed to minimize alloimmunization [17]. Allograft rejection induces both class I and class II antibodies, as does each of the other immunizing events. In a recent study of 50,000 post-pregnancy sera, Konoeda et al. [18] postulated that most of the antibodies found were directed against 'public' determinants or cross-reactive groups (CREG) of HLA (Table 1). This not a new idea, but Konoeda et al. provided

Table 1. Major HLA class I cross-reactive groups (CREG) groups defined by serologic reagents.*

Major CREG	Included specificities
1 CREG	1,3,11,9(23,24),10(25,26,34,66),29,30,31,32,33,36,43
2 CREG	2,28(68,69),9(23,24),17(57,58)
28 CREG	28(68,69),33,34,26
5 CREG	5(51,52),53,35,18,70(71,72),15(62,63),17(57,58),21(49,50)
12 CREG	12(44,45),21(49,50),40(60,61),13,41
7 CREG	7,22(54,55,56),27,40(60,61),13,42,47,48
22 CREG	22(54,55,56),16(38,39),67,42
8 CREG	8,14(64,65),18,59,16(38,39),51
Bw4	. . .
Bw6	. . .

* For brevity, the 'w' prefix is omitted from nomenclature.

compelling evidence with their data. Earlier data had indicated similar findings in a few cases [19]. Konoeda et al. also examined the relative immunogenicity of various HLA class I antigens and found that B locus antigens were highest while C locus antigens were lowest in this regard. There was considerable variation in immunogenicity within each locus. In addition, it was shown that the exposure to a narrow or restricted array of paternal antigens often led to broad sensitization as a result of the cross-reactions seen within the 'public' or cross-reactive groups. Similar to most antigen systems, there are 'naturally occurring' HLA antibodies in about 1% of normal blood donors. Interestingly, about half of these antibodies are directed to HLA-B8 [20]. Antigens that are cross-reactive with the hosts may occasionally immunize [21]. It would seem that on most occasions the host does not become alloimmunized against such cross-reactive antigens.

Thus, the immunogenicity of particular HLA antigens is much more complex than the mere expression on immunizing cell surfaces. Apart altogether from the myriad of host factors that determine whether a particular immune reaction will occur in response to the appearance of a particular immunogen within the system, there are factors in the immunizing event itself that have major roles.

With respect to alloimmunization induced by the transfusion of platelets, common experience is that patients subjected to many platelet concentrate transfusions tend to become refractory, with most of the refractory state apparently due to the development of antibodies to antigens of class I HLA. However, it has also been shown that the development of this refractory state can be delayed by minimizing the leukocyte content of the platelet concentrates [22]. These data suggest that leukocytes themselves actually present HLA antigens more efficiently than platelets do or that some of the 'contaminating' leukocytes provide some type of enhancement of the immunizing process. Viable mononuclear cells in the product may actually provide an added stimulus to the process. Such an event would be analogous to the concept of the 'second signal' for the elicitation of transplant immune response by so-called passenger leukocytes, a concept that is gathering considerable support as data accumulate [23-26]. Generally, the cells providing this 'second signal' are antigen-presenting cells; macrophages, lymphoid cells, or so-called dendritic cells [27].

It has now been shown that cloned T cells can be stimulated by interleukin-2 to express several class II antigen types but primarily to express DR. These cells have then been shown in vitro to present antigen and to stimulate in mixed leukocyte culture, autologous mixed leukocyte reaction, and primed lymphocyte test; and such stimulation can be blocked by monoclonal anti-DR antibodies [28]. The major factor is platelet alloimmunization may be the 'contaminating' mononuclear cells in the product. Interestingly, noninvasive methods of abrogating the immune reactivity of contaminating leukocytes in plate concentrates are being actively examined. The use of ultraviolet light irradiation seems to hold promise in this regard [29]. Such irradiation abolishes the ability of lymphocytes to stimulate or react in a mixed lymphocyte reaction [30]. The effect apparently is not mediated by alteration in the phenotypic expression of class II antigens [31]. Ultraviolet light irradiation has been claimed to interfere with the synthesis or elaboration of interleukin-1 [32] and has also been reported to lead to the activation of suppressor cells [33]. From a practical standpoint, about 20% of the alloimmune antibodies seen in multitransfused patients are apparently directed to non-HLA antigens. This is probably why HLA-matched donors provide an excellent increment in only about 70% to 80% of such patients. It also lends emphasis to the point that noninvasive methods to actually prevent the development of alloimmunization (not just to HLA) are much more promising than further refinements of the HLA-typed donor pool for the support of patients who are already compromised by the alloimmune state. Slichter [34], who has contributed so much to our understanding of platelet alloimmunization, has lucidly reviewed this topic. The possession of certain class II antigens may confer the capacity for forming an immune response that is more heavily weighted toward the suppressive side of the balance. This immune response is somewhat analogous to the concept of immune response genes, and in man the response seems to be associated more particularly with DRw6 than with other class II antigens [35]. There is some evidence that under certain conditions, class I antigens *in the absence of class II antigens* may be immunosuppressive and could conceivably lead to active allograft enhancement [36].

The HLA system and adverse transfusion reactions

Febrile nonhemolytic reaction

While there are small quantities of HLA class I antigens on red blood cells, antibodies to HLA have not been implicated in clinical hemolytic reactions. However, febrile nonhemolytic reactions have been clearly associated with antibodies to blood cells other than erythrocytes. In our experience febrile nonhemolytic reactions cause between 55% and 75% of all immediate adverse reactions to blood and blood products. Other centers have published data indicating that between 65% and 70% of reactions are febrile [37], and the incidence of such reactions is approximately 0.5% of units of blood transfused. The rate is higher in patients who are transfused frequently and at regular intervals [32]. Recent studies have indicated that many different antibodies may be associated with these reactions and that no one test is highly sensitive (or specific). One of the most obvious problems with any study of febrile nonhemolytic reaction is the lack of established and uniformly accepted definition of the clinical criteria. For example, if one demands that in all cases one of the serologic tests be positive, then by definition, all cases will be associated with a positive test. However, if one uses rather broad clinical limits, one inevitably will include patients whose reactions cannot be proved to be due to transfusions at all. Everyone is aware of the dilemma of 'reactions' in patients who are septic or have an underlying febrile course that confuses the issue. Most clinicians tend to use rather broad clinical criteria, and perhaps because of this, serologic studies in these cases frequently show positivity in only about 50% of cases using various techniques, including leukocyte agglutination, lymphocytotoxicity, granulocyte cytotoxicity, indirect granulocyte immunofluorescence, and indirect platelet immunofluorescence.

One recent study [38] showed lymphocytotoxicity with B cells as the most sensitive test (that is: 64%). This test seemed to be about twice as sensitive as that using unseparated peripheral blood mononuclear cells. It has been considered that class I HLA antigens are more prominent on B cells than on T cells, so perhaps this study was indicating that HLA class I was the major culprit. Unfortunately, more extensive serologic absorption/elution studies are needed to provide more substantial evidence for this surmise. De Rie et al. [39], using an extensive array of tests, concluded that most of the alloantibodies were to HLA but that platelet-specific antibodies were also seen frequently. Interestingly, granulocyte-specific antibodies seemed to be least frequent. This last-mentioned study also pointed out that patients whose clinical reactions include rigors, do not differ serologically from those in whom fever is unaccompanied by rigors.

Using ^{111}indium-labeled granulocytes to examine the in vivo kinetics of granulocyte recovery and tissue localization, McCullough et al. [40] recently demonstrated that the granulocyte agglutination test is the most reliable predictor of altered granulocyte activity. Although the study utilizes six different serologic test systems, the mixed nature of the patients' antibodies makes it extremely difficult to dissect out the role of HLA alone. However, the data suggested that both HLA class I antigens and lymphocytotoxic antibodies were involved in the in vivo destruction of transfused granulocytes [40]. It has also been shown that granulocyte transfusions are the most frequent component associated with febrile nonhemolytic reactions [38].

Transfusion-related acute lung injury

Posttransfusion pulmonary edema is seen infrequently, but the diagnosis is often not reported to the blood bank, so it is difficult to ascertain the true incidence. This transfusion reaction is most frequently encountered after massive transfusion therapy for trauma or catastrophic hemorrhage. It is also a complication of the transfusion of infants or the elderly with compromised cardiovascular compliance. In all of these situations, the cardiovascular system is compromised, and the patients have the clinical hallmarks of congestive cardiac failure such as elevated jugular venous presure, third heart sound, cardiomegaly, and audible pulmonary edema. Occasionally, massive trauma/transfusion is followed by noncardiogenic pulmonary edema, giving rise to the adult respiratory distress syndrome (ARDS). This is often termed 'shock lung'.

In addition to the previously mentioned clinical entities, a form of noncardiogenic pulmonary edema can arise when massive transfusion has not been given. This particular form of ARDS seems to be mediated by antibodies to white cells or at least is strongly associated with their presence. Interestingly, in this setting, which is termed 'transfusion-related acute lung injury' [41], the antibody in question is in the plasma of the donor, not the patient. We have noted 36 cases in a period during which 194,715 units of blood products were transfused to approximately 22,300 patients [41]. This reaction was characterized by the onset of profound hypotension and hypoxemia, with a mean initial Pa_{O_2} of 40 mm Hg. All patients required mechanical ventilation, and the reaction generally occurred within 1 or 2 hours of infusion. The patients had extensive pulmonary infiltrates that tended to predominate in dependent areas. The reaction was characterized by complete resolution within 96 hours (most cases resolved within 48 hours). Laboratory data are summarized in Table 2. While the association of HLA class I antibodies (corresponding to

Table 2. Antibodies in 36 cases of transfusion-related acute lung injury.

Test	Number of cases
Granulocyte antibody (immunofluorescence)	
Patient (pretransfusion)	2
Donor	32
Lymphocytotoxic antibodies	
Donor	26
HLA class I specific antibody	11*
HLA antibody corresponding to patient HLA	10*

* Seventeen patients were tested. (Modified from Popovsky MA, Moore SB [41].

patient HLA phenotype) is striking, our data are by no means conclusive because several key questions remain to be answered satisfactorily. First, only some HLA antibodies in donor plasma seem to cause this reaction. We have not been able to ascertain the reason for this [41]. Second, while it is very tempting to postulate a role for the liberation of complement components C5a or C3a in the pathogenesis of this entity, thus far no firm clinical data have been gathered. The role of complement in similar clinical syndromes has been elucidated [42]. Third, some reactions occur without demonstrable HLA antibodies involved.

In summary, the evidence is strong that HLA antigens and antibodies are involved in this transfusion reaction but perhaps only as one of several possible systems that may trigger the final common clinical pathway.

The HLA system is clearly relevant to blood bankers and to transfusion therapy; however, its role should not be overemphasized, but rather the system should be used as a model with which to study some basic immunlogic phenomena that need clarification.

References

1. Fuller TC, Rodey GE. Specificity of alloantibodies against antigens of the HLA complex. In: Hackel E, Mallory D, eds. Theoretical aspects of HLA: A technical workshop. Arlington, Virginia: The American Association of Blood Banks 1982:51-80.

2. Ploegh HL, Orr HT, Strominger JL. Major histocompatibility antigens: the Human (HLA-A, -B, -C) and murine (H-2K, H-2D) class I molecules. Cell 1981; 24:287-99.
3. Larhammar D, Wiman K, Schenning L, et al. Evolutionary relationship between HLA-DR antigen β-chains, HLA-A, B, C antigen subunits and immunoglobulin chains. Scand J Immunol 1981;14:617-22.
4. Daar AS, Fuggle SV, Fabre JW, Ting A, Morris PJ. The detailed distribution of HLA-A, B, C antigens in normal human organs. Transplantation 1984;38: 287-92.
5. Daar As, Fuggle SV, Fabre JW, Ting A, Morris PJ. The detailed distribution of MHC class II antigens in normal human organs. Transplantation 1984;38:293-8.
6. Sparrow RL, Williams N. The pattern of HLA-DR and HLA-DQ antigen expression on clonable subpopulations of human myeloid progenitor cells. Blood 1986;67:379-84.
7. Alonso MC, Navarrete C, Solana R, Torres A, Pena J, Festenstein H. Differential expression of HLA-DR and HLA-DQ antigens on normal cells of the myelomonocytic lineage. Tissue Antigens 1985;26:310-17.
8. Winchester RJ, Ross GD, Jarowski CI, Wang CY, Halper J, Broxmeyer HE. Expression of Ia-like antigen molecules on human granulocytes during early phases of differentiation. Proc Natl Acad Sci USA 1977;74:4012-6.
9. Bontrop RE, Schreuder GMT, Mikulski EMA, van Miltenburg RT, Giphart MJ. Polymorphisms within the HLA-DR4 haplotypes: Various DQ subtypes detected with monoclonal antibodies. Tissue Antigens 1986;27:22-31.
10. Reinsmoen NL, Bach FG. Five HLA-D clusters associated with HLA-DR4. Hum Immunol 1982;4:249-58.
11. Segall M, Noreen H, Schluender L, Bach FH. DNA restriction fragment length polymorphisms characteristic for DW subtypes of DR2. Hum Immunol 1986;15: 336-46.
12. Kohonen-Corish MRJ, Serjeantson SW. HLA-DR-beta gene DNA polymorphisms revealed by taq I correlate with HLA-DR specificities. Hum Immunol 1986; 15:263-71.
13. Owerbach D, Hägglöf B, Lernmark A, Holmgren G. Susceptibility to insulin-dependent diabetes defined by restriction enzyme polymorphism of HLA-D region genomic DNA. Diabetes 1984;33:958-65.
14. Marcadet A, Cohen D, Dausset J, Fischer A, Durandy A, Griscelli C. Genotyping with DNA probes in combined immunodeficiency syndrome with defective expression of HLA. N Engl J Med 1985;312:1287-92.
15. Möller E, Carlsson B, Wallin J. An unorthodox interpretation of the genetic basis for DR antigens. Transplant Proc 1986;18:5-8.
16. Moore SB, Sterioff S, Pierides AM, Watts SK, Ruud CM. Transfusion-induced alloimmunization in patients awaiting renal allografts. Vox Sang 1984;47:354-61.
17. Sterioff S, Marsh JW, Moore SB, Engen DE, Zincke H, Frohnert PP. Splenectomy prior to donor-specific transfusions with azathioprine is associated with low incidence of sensitization. Transplant Proc 1985;17:2349-53.
18. Konoeda Y, Terasaki PI, Wakisaka A, Park MS, Mickey MR. Public determinants of HLA indicated by pregnancy antibodies. Transplantation 1986;41: 253-9.
19. Oldfather J, Mora A, Phelan D, et al. The occurrence of cross-reactive 'public' antibodies in the sera of highly sensitized dialysis patients. Transplant Proc 1983; 15:1212-5.
20. Tongio MM, Falkenrodt A, Mitsuishi Y, et al. Natural HLA antibodies. Tissue Antigens 1985;26:271-85.

21. Darke C. The first example of an HLA-Bw45 antiserum produced in a HLA-Bw44 positive woman. Tissue Antigens 1980;15:75-80.
22. Eernisse JG, Brand A. Prevention of platelet refractoriness due to HLA antibodies by administration of leukocyte-poor blood components. Exp Hematol 1981;9:77-83.
23. Lafferty KJ, Simeonovic CJ. Immunology of graft rejection. Transplant Proc 1984;16:927-30.
24. Dausset J, Contu L. MHC in general biologic recognition: Its theoretical implications in transplantation. Transplant Proc 1981;13:895-9.
25. Bach FH, Gose JE. Cellular basis of allograft rejection. Transplant Proc 1981;13: 1063-7.
26. Fisher M, Chapman JR, Ting A, Morris PJ. Alloimmunisation to HLA antigens following transfusion with leukocyte-poor and purified platelet suspensions. Vox Sang 1985;49:331-5.
27. Deeg JH. Modification of immunogenicity of transfusion products. In: Murawski K, Peetoom F, eds. Transfusion medicine: Recent technological advances. New York: Alan R Liss 1986:117-27.
28. Triebel F, De Roquefevil S, Blanc C, Charron DJ, Debre P. Expression of MHC class-II and tac antigens on IL-2 activated human T-cell clones that can stimulate in MLR, AMLR, PLT and can present antigen. Hum Immunol 1986;15:302-15.
29. Kahn RA, Duffy BF, Rodey GG. Ultraviolet irradiation of platelet concentrate abrogates lymphocyte activation without affecting platelet function in vitro. Transfusion 1985;25:547-50.
30. Lindahl-Kiessling K, Säfwenberg J. Inability of UV-irradiation lymphocytes to stimulate allogeneic cells in mixed lymphocyte culture. Int Arch Allergy 1971;41: 670-8.
31. Slater LM, Murray S, Liu J, Hudelson B. Dissimilar effects of ultraviolet light on HLA-D and HLA-DR antigens. Tissue Antigens 1980;15:431-5.
32. Ullrich SE, Kripke ML. Mechanisms in the suppression of tumor rejection produced in mice by repeated UV irradiation. J Immunol 1984;133:2786-90.
33. Lafferty KJ, Andrus L, Prowse SJ. Role of lymphokine and antigen in the control of specific T cell responses. Immunol Rev 1980;51:279-314.
34. Slichter S. Prevention of platelet alloimmunization. In: Murawski K, Peetoom F, eds. Transfusion medicine: Recent technological advances. New York: Alan R Liss 1986:83-116.
35. Hendriks GFJ, D'Amaro J, Persijn GG, et al. Excellent outcome after transplantation of renal allografts from HLA-DRw6-positive donors even in HLA-DR mismatches. Lancet 1983;ii:187-9.
36. Baird MA, Bradley MP, Heslop BF. Prolonged survival of cardiac allografts in rats following the administration of heat treated donor lymphocytes. Transplantation 1986;42:1-7.
37. Brubaker DB. Immunologically mediated immediate adverse effects of blood transfusions (allergic, febrile nonhemolytic and noncardiogenic pulmonary edema). Plasma Ther Transfusion Technol 1985;6:19-30.
38. Decary F, Ferner P, Giavedoni L, et al. An investigation of nonhemolytic transfusion reactions. Vox Sang 1984;46:277-85.
39. De Rie MA, van der Plas-van Dalen CM, Engelfriet CP, von dem Borne AEG Kr. The serology of febrile transfusion reactions. Vox Sang 1985;49:126-34.
40. McCullough J, Clay M, Hurd D, Richards K, Ludvigsen C, Forstrom L. Effect of leukocyte antibodies and HLA matching on the intravascular recovery, survival, and tissue localization of ^{111}indium granulocytes. Blood 1986;67:522-8.

41. Popovsky MA, Moore SB. Diagnostic and pathogenetic considerations in transfusion-related acute lung injury. Transfusion 1985;25:573-7.
42. Boogaerts MA, Roelant C, Goossens W, Verwilghen RL. Complement activation and adult respiratory distress syndrome during intermittent flow apheresis procedures. Transfusion 1986;26:82-7.

ALLOIMMUNIZATION AGAINST PLATELETS AND GRANULOCYTES

C.P. Engelfriet

Before discussing the mechanisms involved in alloimmunization against platelets and granulocytes, it is important to realize which categories of alloantigens are present on these cells. The presence on platelets of antigens, shared with red cells, has been clearly established i.e. the ABH, Lewis, Ii and P antigens. There is no evidence that alloimmunization against these antigens may follow transfusion of incompatible platelets. However, once a patient has antibodies against these antigens part of a population of transfused incompatible platelets will have a shortened survival time. That only part of the platelets are destroyed is due to a heterogeneous distribution of these antigens over the platelet population [1]. These antigens are also heterogeneously distributed over the megakaryocytes in the bone marrow [2]. However the progeny of an individual megakaryocyte carry an equal number of these antigens. Important for alloimmunization against platelets are the HLA-A, B and C antigens (class I) and platelet-specific antigens. Although it has been thought that granulocytes also carry alloantigens shared with red cells, this has not been confirmed in recent studies with more reliable techniques [1,3]. Alloantigens present on granulocytes are either shared with monocytes and lymphocytes or monocytes alone. In addition the HLA-A, B and C antigen and antigens specific for granulocytes are present on granulocytes.

The question is whether immunization against the above alloantigens follows the same rules as immunization against antigens, foreign to the host in general. In that case the antigens must be presented to T helper cells by antigen presenting cells (APC) in conjunction with HLA class II antigens identical to those of the host. Thus foreign antigens are normally presented by APC of the host. This is probably also true for alloantigens with one very important exception (see below).

If indeed alloantigen presentation in general follows the same rules as presentation of other foreign antigens, there should be evidence for the involvement of immune response genes located in the HLA-D region in alloimmunization. The following evidence has been found: the frequency of HLA-B8 was strongly increased in a group of $Zw^{(a-)}$ women, who were immunized against Zw^a in pregnancy [4]. This was confirmed in a larger group of patients [5]. It was then established that the frequency of HLA-DR3 was even more strongly increased [6] and this was confirmed by others [7,8].

It was also shown that the frequency of DR3 in $Zw^{(a-)}$ women who were not immunized in pregnancy was not different from that in the general population [7]. All of 24 women immunized in pregnancy were found to be DRw52 positive and the frequency of DRw3 and DR52 was as high in a group of 12 patients who had developed posttransfusion purpura due to anti-Zw[a][8].

It has also been shown that the formation of antibodies against alloantigens expressed on both monocytes and some epithelial cells (ME antigens) occurs almost exclusively in DRw6 positive individuals [9]. Also alloantigens against B cell and monocyte antigens were found to be formed much more frequently in DRw6 positive than in DRw6 negative individuals [10].

Thus although still scanty, there is clear evidence that genes in the HLA-D region are involved in alloimmunization against some alloantigens.

The important exception to the rule that alloantigens are presented by APC of the host is as follows: clear evidence was obtained that in contrast to other alloantigens, the antigens of the Major Histocompatibility System are presented to T-helper cells of the host by APC of the donor [11]. Removal of donor APC (dendritic cells) from a kidney graft prevented alloimmunization. Moreover the donor APC had to be metabolically active cells. This important exception was confirmed [12], but it was shown that to a much lesser extent APC of the host are also capable of presenting antigens of the Major Histocompatibility System. Following alloimmunization of mice it was shown that the APC of the immunized mice were capable of inducing alloimmunity in non-immunized syngeneic (to the host) mice. Moreover it was shown that both donor and host alloantigens were detectable on some of the APC and that immunization of the non-immunized syngeneic mice could be prevented by incubating the APC with antibodies against host class II antigens [12].

What is the significance of these findings with regard to alloimmunization against HLA-A, B and C antigens depends largely on the presence of class II positive APC from the donor in the platelet concentrate, would explain why the removal of leukocytes and therefore also class II positive APC from platelet concentrates has been found to be effective in preventing alloimmunization against HLA-A, B and C antigens. Since, though much less effectively, these antigens can also be presented by APC from the host, this could explain why sometimes anti-HLA are formed, even when leukocyte-free concentrates are transfused. Moreover alloimmunization against platelet-specific antigens cannot be prevented, because these are presented by APC from the host.

Alloimmunization against granulocytes probably follows the same rules. However, removal of class II positive APC from granulocyte concentrates, is obviously much more difficult than the removal of leukocytes from platelet concentrates.

Another important question is whether recipients of platelet concentrates may be non-responders to platelet alloantigens. It is a well-known fact that whereas some Rh-negative subjects produce anti-D antibodies after a single injection of Rh-D positive red cells, other Rh-D negative subjects do not become immunized even after a series of many such injections. Is this also true for immunization against platelet alloantigens? That unresponsiveness against platelet alloantigens exists was shown in a patient described in 1979 [13]. This patient had received platelet concentrates from 700 random donors without becoming refractory. No platelet-reactive antibodies were detectable in his serum, although antibodies against granulocyte-specific and lymphocyte-specific antigens were detectable. It would be important to be able to recognize non-responders, but alloimmunization against platelets was found to be dose-dependent [14 and Slichter at al. (personal communication)].

The consequences of alloimmunization against platelets are as follows: the survival time of incompatible platelets is severely shortened by both anti-HLA-A, B and C antibodies and antibodies against platelet-specific antigens. Moreover the reaction between antibodies and donor platelets may lead to transfusion reactions. These may be mild febrile reactions, but a much more serious event is posttransfusion purpura which so far has been found to be due to alloantibodies against antigens on glycoprotein IIb (anti Bak^a/Lek^a) or IIIa (anti-Zw^a, anti-Zw^b).

Alloimmunity against granulocytes has the following consequences: the increment of incompatible granulocytes in patients with HLA-A, B or C antibodies is decreased. Granulocyte-reactive antibodies are responsible for the well-known, typical febrile transfusion reaction in which the temperature begins to rise a few hours after the start of the transfusion, while it usually drops to normal values within 8 hours. The fever may be severe and may be accompanied by the presence of leukoagglutinins in donor blood, is characterized by dry cough, cyanosis, shock and pulmonary infiltrates.

The final question to be answered is in which frequency alloantibodies against the various alloantigens present on platelets are formed. In Table 1 the results are shown of serological investigations with the serum of 40 patients, who developed a typical febrile transfusion reaction, using the leukoagglutination test, the lymphocytotoxicity test and the immunofluorescence test on granulocytes, platelets and lymphocytes, using cells from 9-12 donors [15]. Alloantibodies were detectable in the serum of all patients. It can be seen that HLA antibodies were detected in 34 of the 40 patients, platelet specific antibodies in 7 patients and granulocyte specific antibodies in only 1 patient. Thus, HLA-A, B, C antibodies are formed the most frequent. It is interesting that the incidence of platelet specific antibodies (about 20% of the patients) corresponds very well with the finding by many investigators, that in alloimmunized patients the increment of HLA compatible platelets is unsatisfactory in about 20% of the cases.

Table 1. Serological investigation in 40 cases of a typical febrile transfusion reaction.

Techniques:	LAT, LCT, IF on granulocytes, lymphocytes, platelets. Cells from 9-12 donors.
Results:	Alloantibodies detectable in all 40 cases.

– HLA antibodies in	28
– HLA-, + granulocyte specific antibodies in	3
– HLA-, + platelet specific antibodies in	3
– Platelet specific antibodies in	4
– Granulocyte specific antibodies in	1
– Lymphocyte specific antibodies in	1

(From [15] de Rie et al. 1985.)

References

1. Dunstan RA, Simpson MB, Knowles RW, Rosse WF. The origin of ABH antigens on human platelets. Blood 1985;3:615-9.
2. Dunstan RA. The expression of ABH antigens during in vitro megakaryocyte maturation: origin of heterogeneity of antigen density. Brit J Haemat 1986;62: 587-93.
3. Gaidulis L, Branch DR, Lazar GS, Petz LD, Blume KG. Failure to detect the red cell antigens A, B, D, V, Ge, Jk3 and Jta on granulocytes by direct measurement using J-125 staphylococcal protein or avidin-biotin-complex assay. (Abstract) Blood 1984;64:85a.
4. Reznikoff-Etievant MF, Dangu C, Labet R. HLA-B8 antigen and anti-PL^{al} allo-immunization. Tissue Antigens 1981;18:66.
5. Taaning E, Antonsen H, Peterson S, Svejgaard A, Thomsen M. HLA antigens and maternal antibodies in allo-immune neonatal thrombocytopenia. Tissue Antigens 1983;21:351.
6. Reznikoff-Etievant MF, Muller JY, Julien F, Patereau C. An immune response gene linked to MHC in man. Tissue Antigens 1983;22:312.
7. Mueller-Eckhardt C, Mueller-Eckhardt G, Willen-Ohff H, et al. Immunogenicity of an immune response to the human platelet antigen Zw^a is strongly associated with HLA-B8 and -DR3. Tissue Antigens 1985;26:71.
8. De Waal LP, van Dalen CM, Engelfriet CP, Von dem Borne AEG Kr. Allo-immunization against the platelet-specific Zw^a antigen, resulting in neonatal alloimmune thrombocytopenia or posttransfusion purpura, is associated with the supratypic DRw52 antigen including DR3 and DRw6. Human Immunology 1986;17:45-54.
9. Baldwin WU, Claas FHJ, van Es LA, van Rood JJ, Paul LC, Persijn GG. Renal graft rejection and the antigenic anatomy of human kidneys. Thirteenth Congress on Transplantation and Clinical Immunology, Lyon. Amsterdam: Excerpta Medica 1981:140-6.
10. Hendriks GFJ, D'Amors J, Persijn GG, et al. Excellent outcome after transplantation of renal allografts from HLA-DRw6 positive donors even in HLA-DR mismatches. Lancet 1983;ii:187-9.
11. Lechler RJ, Batchelor JR. Restoration of immunogenecity to passenger cell-depleted kidney allografts by the addition of donor strain dendritic cells. J Exp Med 1982;155:31-41.
12. Sherwood RA, Brent L, Rayfield LS. Presentation of alloantigens by host cells. Europ J Immunol 1986;16:569-74.
13. Decary F, Verheugt FWA, van Helden-Heuningheim L, et al. Recognition of a non-HLA-ABC antigen present on B and T lymphocytes and monocytes only detectable with the immunofluorescence test. Vox Sang 1979;36:150-8.
14. Pegels JF, Bruynes ECE, Engelfriet CP, von dem Borne AEG Kr. Serological studies in patients on platelet and granulocyte substitution therapy. Brit J Haemat 1982;52:59-68.
15. De Rie MA, van der Plas-van Dalen CM, Engelfriet CP, von dem Borne AEG Kr. The serology of febrile transfusion reactions. Vox Sang 1985;49:126-35.

LEUKOCYTES IN TRANSFUSION MEDICINE – AN OVERVIEW OF FUNCTIONS AND CLINICAL IMPLICATIONS

J. Seidel, W. Stangel

Introduction

The ways to approach the role of leukocytes in the wide range of blood transfusion has many ramifications. The first thing that has to be considered is the class of leukocytes to be discussed: are they polymorphonuclear leukocytes (PMNL), T-lymphocytes, B-lymphocytes, NK-cells or monocytes which are to be dealt with? Is it the behaviour of these cellular elements in the saved blood unit or the fate in the recipient and his reactions after transfusion that is to be reviewed? Or, does the blood donor show any reactions as a consequence to the donation procedure?

In this contribution we would like to focus on transfusion medicine in a stricter sense, that is the production, storage and transfusion in clinical settings leaving aside for instance cytapheresis procedures.

As has been said above the first thing to be defined is the class of leukocytes under consideration. Secondly, dealing with the role of these cells in the context of transfusion medicine, one has to define the compartment in which these cells are to be reviewed: the donor and his possible reactions to the donation procedure, the blood unit and the changes during storage or processing and, of course, the recipient; the functions of those cells within the recipient and his possible serological reactions as well as his alterations of immunofunctions following transfusion.

As a matter of convenience we have set up a scaffolding – a table where the lines give the different classes of leukocytes and the columns the compartment in which the behaviour of these cells is to be described. This way has been chosen only in order not to get lost in the variety of different matters to be addressed in the course of this overview and is not meant to document any interrelationships. Some items will be discussed in more detail and some others will only be mentioned for the lack of space.

The role of polymorphonuclear leukocytes in transfusion medicine

A. Donor

Donor reactions to donation procedures of PMNL are well known and documented in the literature. We shall not comment on the influences of the various anticoagulants, sedimentation agents or eluation media reported in

Table 1. Behaviour of leukocytes in different 'compartments' (see text).

	Donor	Blood unit	Recipient
PMNL	Pulmon. leukostasis by complement activ. in filtration proc.	Rapid deterioration of functional capacities	In general good functional activity danger of NCPE
T-lymphocytes	No untoward effects known	Disappearance of HLA-bearing cells	Normal or slightly depressed T4/T8-ratio, increased SCA
B-lymphocytes	No untoward effects known	Persistance	Increase in CIgG+ and SIgG+ cells
NK-cells	No untoward effects known	(?)	Marked reduction of NK-activity
Monocytes	No untoward effects known	Persistance	Help depress MLC-reactivity

the literature. Continuous and discontinuous (intermittent flow) centrifugation procedures as a rule produce only mild side effects like trembling, dysesthesia or muscular cramps which are more or less related to the serum calcium depletion effected by the citrate anticoagulant employed and subside within 20 minutes after terminiation of the separation process [1-3]. One case of cardiac arrest has been reported in the literature using an intermittend flow blood cell processor [4].

The situation is somewhat different for the method of filtration leukapheresis which not only produces a profound transient neutropenia early in the procedure followed by a rebound neutrophilia but may also precipitate a pulmonary leukostasis with respiratory distress in the donor with a reported incidence of about 2% [5-7]. Plasma into contact with plastic surface or nylon fibers like the one used in filtration leukapheresis is stimulated to produce C5a [8], the activated part of the fifth component of complement. This is probably done by the activation of the alternative pathway. C5a produces an irreversible aggregation of PMNL in vitro and a sharp drop of PMNL numbers in the peripheral blood of the donors as well as a pulmonary leukostasis accompanied by a respiratory distress syndrome [8]. Comparable situations are known in hemodialysis procedures [9] as well as by use of artificial oxygenators [10,11] in open-heart surgery.

B. Blood unit

In this section we will deal with the behaviour and changes of functional capacities of PMNL in blood units. Evaluating the functional capacities of PMNL one has to take into account, of course, the procedure by which the PMNL have been collected as well as the storage conditions. A marked functional impairment of degranulation, phagocytosis and killing of test-bacteria has been noted in PMNL-preparations collected by filtration leukapheresis [12,13].

Furthermore, the in vivo recovery of PMNL prepared by filtration leukapheresis seems to be impaired as compared to the recovery of PMNL procured by continuous flow centrifugation [14].

PMNL prepared by continuous or discontinuous flow procedures seem to be more or less unimpaired as compared to freshly drawn PMNL [15] although storage of such PMNL-preparations should probably not be extended more than 8 hours at longest [16]. The same holds true for PMNL which have been submitted to irradiation [17]. Strongly reduced functional capacities have been found after freezing and thawing of purified PMNL-preparations [18,19]. Functional integrity of PMNL harvested after steroid premedication of the donor, which may be done in order to increase the PMNL-count in the donor and subsequently to enhance the yield of PMNL harvested seems to be unimpaired [20].

PMNL-functions in whole blood (own studies)

In our laboratory we have investigated a) the changes of PMNL-functions during storage in whole blood and b) in autologous blood in the course of intraoperative cell saving with a Haemonetics Cell Saver. The following tests for assessing PMNL-functions were performed: adherence to nylon wool, random migration, chemotaxis under agarose against gradients of FMLP (formyl-methionyl-leucyl-phenylalanine) and YAS (yeast activated serum), phagocytosis and killing of *Staphylococcus areus*, killing of *Candida tropicalis*, generation of superoxide anion (O^{-}_2) and peroxide (H_2O_2) after stimulation with opsonized zymosan. We further determined the cellular contents of the lysosomal constituents myeloperoxidase (MPO) in primary granula and lysozyme in primary plus secondary granula.

Materials and methods

a. Changes of PMNL-functions in stored whole blood

We investigated the changes of PMNL-functions in whole blood units during 48 hours of storage under routine conditions at 4°C. 23 units of blood (450 ml) were collected in polyvinylchloride bags (Fenwal Laboratories) containing CPDA-1 as an anticoagulant. Testing was done immediately after collection as well as after 6, 24 and 48 hours of storage.

b. Changes in PMNL-functions during intraoperative cell saving

In seven patients undergoing major cardio-thoracic surgery the Haemonetics Cell Saver model III was employed to reduce the amount of blood units otherwise necessary to compensate for the massive blood loss. We were interested in the functions of PMNL after processing, that is in the preparation that has been made ready for autologous retransfusion to the patient after suction from the operation site, filtration to remove debris, centrifugation and washing with saline. In three patients the salvaged blood was investigated once; in the other patients we were able to study the salvaged blood in several consecutive runs.

In each study undertaken normal healthy blood donors served as day controls.

In short, purification of PMNL was accomplished using a modification of the method of Boyum [21] with hydroxyethyl-starch (Plasmasteril®) used as a sedimentation agent. Contaminating erythrocytes were removed by hypotonic shock.

Adherence

Adherence to nylon wool was assessed employing the method as detailed by McGregor [22]. The number of PMNL before and after passage through a premoistened and prewarmed (37°C) nylon wool column with defined density (50 mg in an insulin syringe compressed to 1 ml) was determined and the percentage of adherent PMNL calculated.

Spontaneous migration and chemotaxis

We performed the 'chemotaxis under agarose' method as lined out by Chenoweth et al. [23]. There were two substances with chemotactic activity employed: yeast activated serum (YAS) containing the complement activation product C5a and formyl-methionyl-leucyl-phenylalanine (FMLP), a tripeptide with exquisite chemotactic properties.

Phagocytosis and killing of Staphylococcus aureus

The method employed was a modification of the procedure proposed by Van Furth et al. [24]. After phagocytosis the number of surviving bacteria (a coagulase positive strain of *Staphylococcus aureus*) was determined in the supernatant and after osmotic disrupture of the PMNL by plating out and counting the number of colony forming units. In preliminary experiments it was shown that the strain in use was resistant against serum factors by incubating the bacteria in 10% pooled AB-serum. There was a relation of 1:1 of bacteria:PMNL in the assays. A Phagocytosis Index and a Killing Index were calculated after 90 minutes of incubation.

Fungicidal activity

The test-germ used was *Candida tropicalis* which had previously shown to be resistant against 10% human AB-serum. The assessment of fungicidal activity was analogous to the procedure lined out for the determination of bactericidal capacity with the exception that the incubation time had been extended to 120 minutes and the relation germs:PMNL was 10:1.

Generation of superoxideanion (O^-_2)

Following the procedure proposed by Weening et al. [25] the PMNL were stimulated by preopsonized zymosan and the amount of superoxideanion generated determined by the reduction of cytochrome c by measuring at 546 nm against a blank prepared without zymosan.

Generation of hydrogen peroxide (H_2O_2)

The assessment of hydrogen peroxide generation was carried out according to the method described by Pick and Keisari [26]. Horse-radish peroxidase

(HRPO) catalyses the oxidation of phenol red utilizing H_2O_2 set free by zymosan stimulated PMNL. The supernatant was supplemented with 25 μl NaOH and then photometrically measured at 623 nm.

Cellular content of myeloperoxidase (MPO)
The oxidative capacity of the freed myeloperoxidase after lysis of PMNL was determined by photometry following the oxidation of diansidine (3.2 mM in 0.1 M citrate buffer, pH 5.5). The reaction mixture consisted of 890 μl dianisidine solution, 50 μl 0.2% Triton-X-100, 10 μl 10 mM μl H_2O_2 in aqua dest. and 50 μl of PMNL-suspension (2×10^6/ml PBS). The reaction was kept at 25°C in a thermostatically controlled vial and read after 30, 60 and 90 sec at 436 nm.

Cellular content of lysozyme
After lysis of PMNL the cellular content of lysozyme was determined using a commercially available test kit (Behringwerke, Marburg/Lahn FRG). PMNL (1×10^7) were suspended in 1 ml 1% Triton-X-100 and left standing for 1 hour at room temperature. An aliquot of 25 μl was dissolved in 1.5 ml of lysozyme reactant and immediately read at 546 nm.

Results

a. Changes of PMNL-functions in stored whole blood

Results are summarized in Figure 1. Adherence to nylon wool, random migration, phagocytosis of *Staph. aureus* and killing of *Candida tropicalis* were significantly reduced after 24 hours ($p < 0.05$). Chemotaxis against a gradient of FMLP was depressed after 6 hours of storage whereas chemotaxis against a grandient of YAS remained stable within this period before falling. The ability to generate H_2O_2 was already significantly impaired after 6 hours ($p<0.01$), whereas the depression in O^-_2-generation became evident only after 48 hours of storage ($p<0.01$). At this time all the other functional parameters were deeply depressed as compared to the initial values ($p<0.01$). The lysosomal contents of MPO and lysozyme remained largely unchanged.

Summarizing these results there seems to be a rapid deterioration of PMNL-functions in stored whole blood taking effect after about 6 to 24 hours of storage. The functional impairment is severe enough so that those cells seem not to be capable to play a decisive role in fighting infections or sepsis once transfused after a period of storage longer than a few hours after collection.

b. Changes of PMNL-functions during intraoperative cell saving

Patients 1, 2 and 3 were tested once, patient 4 was tested 5 times, patients 5 and 6 were tested 3 times each and patient 7 was tested 4 times so that a total of 18 testruns were available for evaluation. Results are summarized in

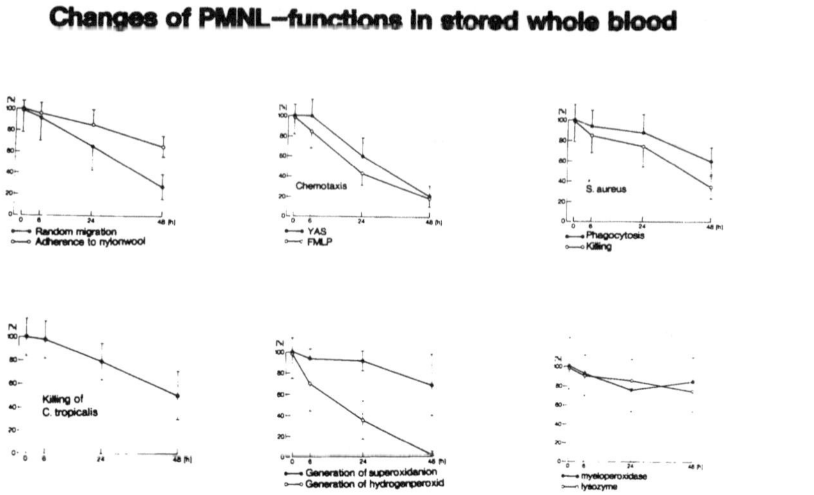

Figure 1. Changes of PMNL-functions in whole blood monitored over a period of 48 hours.

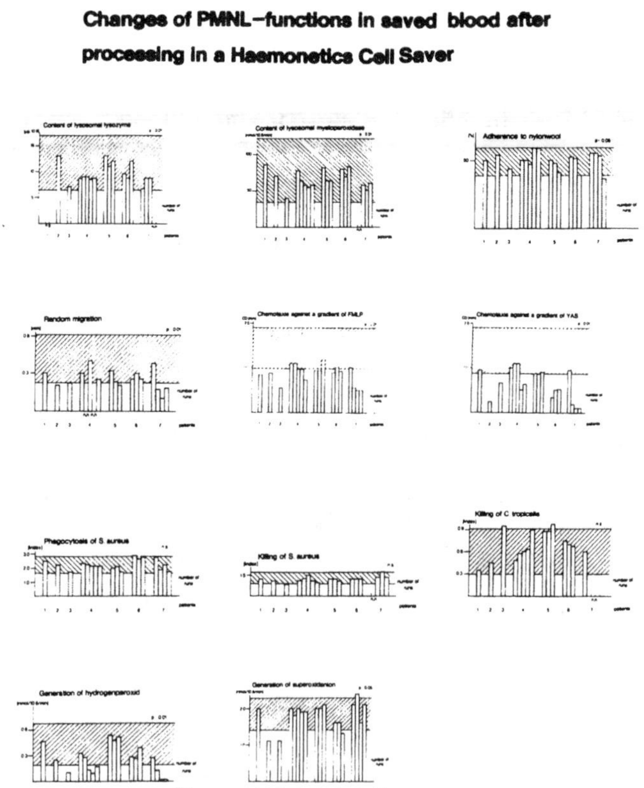

Figure 2. Changes of PMNL-functions in saved blood after processing in a Haemonetics Cell Saver.

Figure 2: As compared to the group of healthy blood donors the PMNL showed marked impairment in adherence to nylon wool ($p<0.05$), random motility ($p<0.01$), chemotaxis against gradients of YAS and FMLP ($p<0.01$), generation of H_2O_2 and O^-_2 ($p<0.01$). Unaffected remained the ability to phagocytize and kill *Staph. aureus* and *Candida tropicalis* as well as cellular contents of MPO and lysozyme.

The reported results show that after cell saving the retransfused PMNL are more or less unable to respond to membrane activating stimuli like chemotaxins and to generate a respiratory burst. It seems questionable that those cells might produce a respiratory distress syndrome after retransfusion.

Preparation of leukocyte free blood units

In order to avoid sensitation of recipients which might lead to non-hemolytic transfusion reactions and/or impaired graft survival after renal transplantation [27] several procedures have been designed to remove leukocytes (PMNL and others) from blood units. Among the methods employed are: washing of red cells [28], centrifugation in upright [29] or inverted positions [30], freezing and thawing [31], dextran sedimentation [30,32] and filtration through cotton wool [33] or polyester wool columns [34,35]. By filtration through a cotton wool column 98% of leukocytes and 89% of platelets could be removed from the blood unit [36]. Applying a filtration technique it should be assured that no PMNL-aggregating activity is produced in the plasma after passage through the filter (see above).

We in our laboratory tested the aggregating activity in plasma before and after filtration of whole blood units through a filter consisting of polyester mesh (Sepacell R 500; Asahi Medical Comp. Ltd). A total of 10 blood units were investigated. Aggregometry was done according to the method described by Hammerschmidt [9,37]. Concomitantly the release of lysozyme into supernatants was investigated. There is no difference in the aggregation response elicited by adding sample plasma before and after passage through the filters. There is also no difference in the amount of lysozyme released into supernatants, which might be indicative of membrane perturbation of PMNL.

As a conclusion there seems to be no risk of generating an aggregating activity in the plasma that might lead to a respiratory distress syndrome or leukopenia [38] in the recipient like the one occasionally happening to donors undergoing filtration leukapheresis (see above).

C. Recipient

As clinical indications for PMNL-substitution the following have been widely accepted [39-41]:

- profound neutropenia of expectedly more than three days;
- septic fever with suspected bacterial or fungal infection or ulcerations in stomach/intestine.

Substitution of PMNL was especially successful in treatment of neonate septicemia where no severe side effects have been reported [42,43]. Incidence of PMNL-substitution as a form of supportive therapy in chemotherapy of malignancies has decreased notably in recent years. In our facility, for instance, in the year 1983 191 PMNL-concentrates were prepared; in the year 1985 only 42 (results not published).

Clinical effectiveness of PMNL-substitution may be gauged by [33,44-50]:

- recovery of PMNL in peripheral blood;
- resolve of fever;
- resolve of infections (blood and urine cultures become negative);
- appearance of orogranulocytes/PMNL in skin windows;
- improvement of patient survival.

Assessment is generally hampered by the occurrence of febrile transfusion reactions [51] which are likely to reverse resolve of fever as well as by the appearance of infections and/or purulent effusions precipitated by the provision of PMNL. Especially deleterious is the appearance of diffuse pulmonary infiltrates with ensuing respiratory failure after PMNL-substitution [51]. The recommended dose for substitution of functionally intact PMNL is 0.5–2.0$\times 10^{10}$ PMNL/m^2/day for PMNL collected by continuous or intermittent flow centrifugation procedures and a number 2-4 times as much for filtration leukapheresis [52]. The transfusion of PMNL should be divided in 2 to 3 doses a day. Simultaneous antibiotic treatment is generally advised [52].

In a study involving 26 patients suffering from AML Ford et al. [44] found a mean 1-hour-recovery of 11.1% of ^{111}In-labeled PMNL calculated from a total number of 191 transfusions (mean of 1.4×10^{10} PMNL collected by Haemonetics Model 30 intermittent flow centrifugation). In patients with transfusion reactions the recovery dropped to 4.7% and in patients under prednisone treatment recovery was an astonishing 27.6%.

Sensitization against PMNL-specific antigens and transfusion reactions are not rare and may interfere with the effectiveness of PMNL-substitution as has been stated above. Kretschmer [52] compared outcome and incidence of cross-match results with the incidence of clinically observed transfusion reactions warranting symptomatic therapy:

Cross-match	**n**	**Transfusion-R**
LCTT* positive	5	5
IGIFT**/GAT*** positive, LCTT negative	10	4
LCTT/IGIFT/GAT negative	51	6
Total	66	16

* LCTT = lymphocytotoxicity
** IGIFT = indirect granulocyte fluorescence test
*** GAT = granulocyte agglutination test

A total of 66 cross-matches were performed and evaluated. PMNL-specific (IGIFT/GAT) reactions were found in 15% of the cross-matches; in 40% of the serologically positive cases there was also a transfusion reaction seen. The overall rate of transfusion reactions in this study was 24.2%.

A list of known PMNL-specific antigens possibly involved is given below [53]:

System	Antigen	Frequence (%)
9	9a	0.39
NA	NA_1	0.31
	NA_2	0.69
NB	NB_1	0.72
NC	NC_1	0.80
ND	ND_1	0.88
NE	NE_1	0.12
G-A, G-B, G-C		

Next to these there is quite a row of other antigens on PMNL shared with other blood cells like ABO, I, i and especially HLA, to mention only some [54].

Non-cardiac pulmonary edema (NCPE)

In recent years attention has been called to the transfusion related occurrence of pulmonary edema – the non-cardiac pulmonary edema (NCPE). The NCPE is an acute complication with an estimated incidence of 1:5,000 transfusions with the following signs as its hallmarks [52,55-59]:

- symptoms developed within hours after transfusion;
- hypoxia and process to respiratory failure necessitating mandatory ventilation;
- hypotension;
- bilateral pulmonary edema and fluffy infiltrates in röntgenograms;
- no signs of left heart failure;
- fever, cough, urticarial rash;
- resolve within a few days;
- in the course no progress toward ARDS*

As a possible cause *passive* transfer of antileukocytic cytotoxic antibodies or leukoagglutinins [57,58] as well as the existence of *preformed antileukocytic antibodies* in the recipient have been identified [55,56]. In order to prevent passive transfer of antileukocytic antibodies it has been advocated by some [57,60] to use only packed RBC-preparations when salvaging blood from multiparous female donors.

Summarizing what has been said in this section one might enter in the table under the column 'recipient': in general good functional activity and danger of NCPE.

* ARDS = adult respiratory distress syndrome with a mortality of 40%.

The role of mononucleated cells in transfusion medicine

A. Donors

In this part of the overview we shall try to gain some insight into the behaviour of T- and B-lymphocytes, NK-cells and monocytes within the context of transfusion medicine.

Untoward side effects concerning the donor due to the donation and loss of mononucleated cells have hitherto not come to attention. This is also true considering the different collection methods employed. Increased incidence of infections or occurrence of malignancies that might be attributed to loss of specific immunity after blood donation have not yet been reported.

B. Behaviour of mononucleated cells in blood units

After 24 hours of storage there is a considerable loss of E-rosette forming cells, while cells displaying dot-like non-specific esterase activity which is also a marker for T-lymphocytes persist longer than 7 days [61]. The number of viable lymphocytes remains largely unchanged. From these findings it cannot be excluded that there is a loss of E-receptors on T-cells taking place under storage conditions leaving the T-cells without E-receptor but possibly otherwise intact [61]. Cells forming EA-rosettes responsible for cytotoxicity and T-suppressor cells also remain unchanged for at least one week which is also true for SIgG-bearing cells [61]. In a more recent study it was shown that T-helper and T-suppressor cells as well as cells bearing HLA-A, -B, -C, and -DR remain stable for two weeks of storage [62,63]. No information is available so far about the behaviour of NK-cells in stored blood.

C. Recipient

The behaviour of transfused mononucleated cells in the recipient after transfusion is not well understood except for the case of graft-versus-host-disease (GVHD). GVHD results when immunologically competent cells are introduced into an immunodeficient host [64] as is the case for instance in bone marrow transplantation. There are a number of monographs and reviews available discussing this matter in detail [64-68]. Most likely the transfused cells are cleared via immunologically mediated destruction in the immunocompetent host [68].

There are a number of immunologic reactions elicited in the host following blood transfusion. The generation of specific antibodies to membrane antigens (cytotoxic or agglutinating antibodies) is only one of the possible mechanisms by which the recipient tries to cope with the massive transfer of antigenic material [69]. Changes in immunoreactivity are also involved and some aspects will be reviewed in the following section.

After transfusion of RBC to patients awaiting renal transplant a rise of suppressor-T-cell activity assessed by the concanavalin A enhancement method has been noted: In 15 male patients on hemodialysis who had previously not yet been transfused suppressor-cell activity was studied after receiving two units of RBC [70]. Following an initial decline of suppressor-cell activity after one week there was an 5 to 10-fold increase in suppressor-cell activity at three weeks. At 20 weeks following transfusion this situation had turned back to normal. Attempts to further characterize nature and specifity of the suppression observed are not yet conclusive [71,72]. A suppression of plant mitogen mediated lymphocyte transformation as a consequence of blood transfusion with return to normal within four weeks have also been observed by others [73].

Studying changes of suppressor cell status and NK-activity after repeated blood transfusions in patients with sickle cell disease a depression of NK-cell activity has been described while healthy controls and non-transfused patients with sickle cell disease retained normal NK-cell activity [74]. In the same study an increase of OKT-8-positive T-lymphocytes after transfusion was noted thus significantly lowering the T4/T8-ratio as compared to healthy controls [74]. These findings gain some weight by the fact that in the same study non-transfused patients also suffering from sickle cell disease do not show those alterations. These changes thus seem to be truely transfusion-related and not an inherent defect of the underlying disease. The findings mentioned before were corroborated in a study investigating changes of NK-cell activity, HLA-DR expression on T-cells and T4/T8-ratios in multitransfused patients suffering from sickle cell anemia, thalassemia and other forms of chronic anemia. Next to the suppression of NK-cell activity in the transfused pateints there was also seen a marked increase in HLA-DR expression on patient T-lymphocytes which signals a state of chronic antigenic stimulation [75]. A linear increase of the percentage of T8-positive cells with the number of units of blood transfused to patients with thalassemia could be demonstrated [76]. A reversal of T4/T8-ratio in a small subgroup (n=10) of 65 multitransfused patients suffering from thalassemia was observed although an explanation could not be given [77].

Furthermore following multiple transfusion an increase in B-cell-immunoglobulin production in vitro may be seen which goes along with an elevation of serum immunoglobulin levels [78,79]. In thalassemia patients a transfusion-related increase in CIg-positive cells was demonstrated [80].

MLC-reactivity of lymphocytes of uremic patients was significantly lowered after transfusions [71]. In an investigation involving uremic patients again a low MLC-reactivity of patient lymphocytes challenged with pooled lymphocytes from 30 healthy donors as stimulator cells could be correlated to a high number of transfusions (more than 20) as compared to a state where less than 20 blood units had been given [81]. Using a third-party donor MLC-assay system it was shown that mononuclear cells from uremic patients having received more than five blood units mediated a significantly higher suppression of responder cells than mononuclear cells collected from patients who had received no or less than five units of blood [82]. It is worth noting that in this study patients with normal percentage of OKT-8-positive cells and more than 5 units blood transfused caused a 60% suppression of third-party-donor MLC while patients receiving less than 5 blood units caused a 31% suppression. Next to the quality of the HLA- and DR-match the number of transfusions and the degree of immunosuppression thus achieved is regarded to be decisive for graft survival after renal transplantation [82].

In order to rule out that renal failure and chronic hemodialysis alone are responsible for the depression in MLC-reactivity a group of uremic patients was compared to healthy controls as well as to a group of multitransfused patients with chronic anemia [83]. Although compared to multitransfused non-uremic patients polytransfused uremic patients displayed a more pronounced suppression of immuneresponsiveness. As far as MLC- and PHA-responses were concerned both groups showed signs of lower immunoresponsiveness than healthy controls in the assay systems chosen. Interestingly cytotoxic antibody formation in the group of polytransfused non-uremic patients was associated with relative high MLC-responses – as would be expected reflecting a state of sensitization. In contrast, in patients with chronic renal failure lowest MLC-responses were seen in conjunction with multispecific antibodies [83].

Impairement of T-cell activation on an earlier stage was suspected when monocytes/macrophages challenged with lysates of RBC produced a nearly complete suppression of MLC on cocultivation [84]. In a similar way depressed MLC-reactivity in uremic patients could be restored after removal of adherent cells [81]. A serum factor mediating lymphocyte suppression occurring after polytransfusion [85] or major surgical procedures [86,87] could be removed after plasmapheresis [88]. The ability of plasma samples to inhibit autologous lymphocyte responses to PPD could be attributed to a factor of low molecular weight associated with alpha-2-macroglobulin in polytransfused uremic patients [89]. A suppression of donor-specific MLC after transfusion of donor-specific stored blood units to patients awaiting kidney grafts from related donors was explained by the action of both humoral and cellular adaptive changes of immunoregulatory circuits in the patient [90]. These findings correlated with a high graft survival in the study referred to.

The findings just cited without paying attention to methodological considerations, as has to be admitted, all do suggest a more or less depressive effect of blood transfusions on the adaptive immunesystem. As has been stated above, these alterations may even be dependent on the number of blood units given [81,82]. It has to be stated, however, that the changes on the immunoregulartory circuits that are due to the underlying disease per se are not yet well understood. Of clinical relevance seem to be the beneficial effects of blood transfusions on graft survival in renal transplant patients. Depression of MLC-reactivity [71,82,83], induction of suppressor-T-cell activity [70], lowering of plant mitogen transformation of lymphocytes [73], presence of non-cytotoxic Fc-receptor blocking antibodies [91], immunodepressive action of serum factors [88-90] and monocytes/macrophages [81,84], appearance of anti-idiotypic antibodies against T-lymphocytes [92], and anti-immunoglobulins [93], avoiding of sensitization with cytotoxic antibodies against B- [94,95] and T-lymphocytes [27,96-98] are some examples of changes induced by blood transfusions to uremic patients that are said to contribute to the transfusion-related improvement of graft survival after renal transplantation.

Use of leukocyte-free blood units in a donor-specific transfusion protocol did not altogether prevent development of sensitization and generation of antibodies against granulocytes and monocytes [100]. Generation of lymphocytotoxic antibodies as a result of regular leukocyte-free blood transfusions leading to broad sensitization was documented studying 26 patients with graft failure. Only 2 of 27 patients had lymphocytotoxic antibodies detectable at time of graft rejection; after blood transfusions 76% eventually became broadly sensitized [27].

Skin allograft survival in healthy volunteers after administration of donor-specific cell-free leukocyte extracts was greatly enhanced when mixtures of these extracts kept at −20°C followed by 1-2 hours thawing at 37°C were injected subcutaneously [101]. This finding contrasted with an observation made by the same authors that administration of isolated particulate components of cytoplasm produced a state of sensitization in the recipient with subsequent rapid graft rejection within 10 days. It is speculated that action of intraleukocytic RNA-ase may be responsible for the abrogation of allogenicity. Increased sensitization of possible recipients of kidney transplants after donor-specific haploidentical transfusion of fresh blood compared to negative donor cross-match outcomes after regular transfusion of stored (for 1, 3 and 5 weeks) donor-specific blood was observed thus suggesting a protective effect of storing blood on sensitization to HLA antigens [63,101]. In the study just cited no transplant rejection has been observed in the group transfused with stored blood. For the improvement of graft survival there seems to be also of importance a time space between transfusion and kidney transplantation as well as a certain dosage effect – that is the need for more than one transfusion [101,75,76].

Looking at the incidence of antileukocytic antibodies after polytransfusion lymphocytotoxins were found in 9.14% of the 383 sera tested [100]. Granulocytotoxins and granulocytoagglutinins were found in 8.35% and 2.87% respectively. Various combinations of the just mentioned classes of antileukocyte antibodies were found in 9.65%. More or less similar percentages were detected investigating 521 sera obtained from multiparous women [102].

Allogenic lymphocytic transfusion for correction of disorders that go along with impaired helper or suppressor T-cell functions have been opposed [103]. A long lasting beneficial clinical effect and normalization of rheumatoid factor after transfusion of allogenic lymphocytes has been described in a small number of patients suffering from rheumatoid arthritis [103]. Transfer of immunity to leprosy patients by transfusion of lymphocytes harvested from lepromin positive healthy donors has been suggested [104].

The results reported in this section are again summarized in Table 1 in a compressed form.

Conclusion

Many questions remain to be answered before the role of mononucleated leukocytes in transfusion medicine is fully elucidated. Because of the many interdigitations between cells and modifying serological factors on one side and the different states of immunocompetence of the patient and his reactions after transfusion on the other side the picture remains blurred and the relative importance of the different mechanisms obscure. Thanks to the advent and application of cyclosporin as an immunomodulator focus has somewhat shifted to the beneficial properties of this agent in transplantation immunology. But to expand our knowledge and understanding of functions and associated reactions of immunocompetent leukocytes in transfusion medicine is still desirable because given the enormous number of blood transfusions applied in many different clinical situations this challenge with more or less defined antigens serves as an excellent model for the study of immune function in man.

References

1. Mishler JM, Highby DJ, Rhomberg W, Nicora RW, Holland JF. Leukapheresis: increased efficiency of collection by the use of hydroxyethyl starch and dexamethasone. In: Goldman JM, Lowenthal RM(eds). Leukocytes: separation, collection and transfusion. New York: Academic Press 1975:61-74.
2. Mishler JM. Hydroxyethyl starch as an experimental adjunct to leukocyte separation by centrifugal means. Transfusion 1975;15:449-53.
3. Huestis DW, White RF, Price MJ, Inman M. Use of hydroxyethyl starch to improve granulocyte collection in the Latham blood processor. Transfusion 1975;15: 559-64.
4. Sirchia G. Erfahrungen mit dem Zellseparator Haemonetics 30 (H-30). Advanced component therapy, Seminar 1975, London.
5. Higby DJ, Burnett D, Ruppert K, Hendersen ES. Filtration leukapheresis: studies on donors. In: Goldman JM, Lowenthal RM (eds). Leukocytes: separation, collection and transfusion. New York: Academic Press 1975:153-62.
6. Buchholz DH, Schiffer CA, Wiernik PH, Reilly JA. Granulocyte harvest for transfusion: donor response to repeated leukapheresis. Transfusion 1975;15: 96-103.
7. Fehr J, Craddock PR, Jacob HS. Complement (C) mediated granulocyte (PMN) and pulmonary dysfunction during nylon fiber leukapheresis. Blood 1975;46: 1045-61.
8. Fehr J. Complement as a mediator of granulocyte adherence and margination. Studies based on the acute neutropenia of filtration leukapheresis. In: Greenwalt TJ, Jamieson GA (eds). The granulocyte: function and clinical utilization. New York: Alan R. Liss, Inc. 1977:243-61.
9. Hammerschmidt D, Weaver L, Hudson L, Craddock P, Jacob H. Association of complement activation and elevated plasma-C5a with adult respiratory distress syndrome. Lancet 1980;i:947-9.
10. Ivanovich P, Chenoweth D, Schmidt R, Klinkmann H et al. Symptoms and activation of granulocytes and complement with two dialysis membranes. Kidney Int 1983;24:758-63.

11. Hammerschmidt D, Stroncek D, Bowers T et al. Complement activation and neutropenia occurring during cardiopulmonary bypass. J Thorac Cardiovasc Surg 1981;81:370-7.
12. Wade PH, Skrabut EM, Vinciguerra L, Valeri CR. In vitro function of granulocytes isolated from blood of normal volunteers using continuous-flow centrifugation in the IBM-Aminco Celltrifuge and adhesion-filtration leukapheresis using nylon fiber. Transfusion 1977;17:136-40.
13. Klock JC, Bainton DF. Degranulation and abnormal bactericidal function of granulocytes procured by reversible adhesion to nylon wool. Blood 1976;48: 149-61.
14. McCullough J, Weiblein BJ, Deinard AR, Boen J, Fortuny IE, Quie PG. In vitro function and post-transfusion survival of granulocytes collected by continuous-flow centrifugation and by filtration leukapheresis. Blood 1976;48:315-26.
15. Price TH. Neutrophil transfusion: In vivo function of neutrophils collected using cell separators. Transfusion 1983;23:504-7.
16. McCullough J, Weiblein BJ, Fine D. Effects of storage of granulocytes on their fate in vivo. Transfusion 1983;23:20-4.
17. Wheeler JG, Abramson JS, Ekstrand K: Function of irradiated polymorphonuclear leukocytes obtained by buffy-coat centrifugation. Transfusion 1984;24: 238-9.
18. McCarthy DM, Skacel P, Raja K, Martin F, Peters T, Goldman JM. Granulocyte cryopreservation: further studies on the pathogenesis of impaired cellular function. Br J Haematol 1984;56:45-54.
19. Frim J, Mazur P. Interactions of cooling rate, warming rate, glycerol concentration and dilution procedure on the viabiity of frozen-thawed human granulocytes. Cryobiology 1983;20:657-76.
20. Glasser L, Huestis DW, Jones JF. Functional capabilities of steroid-recruited neutrophils harvested for clinical transfusion. N Engl J Med 1977;297:1033-6.
21. Boyum A. Separation of leukocytes from blood and bone marrow. Scand J Clin Lab Invest 1968;21(suppl 97):1-6.
22. MacGregor RR, Spagnuolo PJ, Lentek AL. Inhibition of granulocyte adherence by ethanol, prednisone, and aspirin measured with an assay system. N Engl J Med 1974;291:642-6.
23. Chenoweth DE, Rowe JG, Hugli T. A modified method for chemotaxis under agarose. J Immunol Meth 1979;25:337-53.
24. Van Furth R, van Zweet TL. In vitro determination of phagocytosis and intracellular killing by polymorphonuclear and mononuclear leukocytes. In: Weir DM. Handbook of experimental Immunology. Oxford: Blackwell Scientific Publications 1973;vol 2:36.1-36.24.
25. Weening RS, Wever R, Roos D. Quantitative aspects of the production of superoxide radicals by phagocytizing human granulocytes. J Lab Clin Med 1975;85: 245-52.
26. Pick E, Keisari Y. A simple colorimetric method for the measurement of hydrogen peroxide produced by cells in culture. J Immunol Meth 1980;38:161-70.
27. Scornik JC, Ireland JE, Howard RJ, Fennell RS, Pfaff WW. Role of regular and leukocyte-free blood transfusions in the generation of broad sensitization. Transplantation 1984;38:594-8.
28. Buchholz DM, Charette RJ, Bove JR. Preparation of leukocyte-poor red blood cells using the IBM 2991 blood cell processor. Transfusion 1978;18:653-61.
29. Miller WV, Vilson MJ, Kalb HJ. Simple methods for production of HLA antigen-poor red blood cells. Transfusion 1973;13:189-93.

30. Tenczar JJ. Comparison of inverted centrifugation, saline washing, and dextran sedimentation in the preparation of leukocyte-poor red cells. Transfusion 1973;13:183-8.
31. Crowley JP, Wade PH, Wish C, Valeri CR. The purification of red cells for transfusion by freeze-preservation and washing: V. Red cell recovery and residual leukocytes after freeze-preservation with high concentrations of glycerol and washing in various systems. Transfusion 1977;17:1-7.
32. Cassel M, Phillips DR, Chaplin H. Transfusion of buffy-coat-poor red cell suspension prepared by dextran sedimentation: Description of newly designed equipment and evaluation of its use. Transfusion 1962;4:216-20.
33. Diepenhorst P, Engelfriet CP. Removal of leukocytes from whole blood and erythrocyte suspensions by filtration through cotton wool. V. Results after transfusion of 1820 units of filtered erythrocytes. Vox Sang 1975;29:15-22.
34. Wenz B. Microaggregate blood filtration and febrile transfusion reaction: A comparative study. Transfusion 1983;23:95-8.
35. Myovic V, Brozovic B, Hughes ASB, Davies TD. Leukocyte depleted blood: A comparison of filtration techniques. Transfusion 1983;23:30-2.
36. Major KE, Child JA, Roberts BE. Transfusion of patients with leukocyte antibodies using cotton wool filtered blood. J Clin Pathol 1981;34:225.
37. Hammerschmidt D, Bowers T, Lammi-Kaefe C, Jacob H, Craddock P. Granulocyte aggregometry: a sensitive technique for the detection of C5a and complement activation. Blood 1980;55:898-902.
38. Craddock P, Hammerschmidt D, White J, Dalmasso A, Jacob H. Complement (C5a)-induced granulocyte aggregation in vitro: a possible mechanism of complement-mediated leukostasis and leukopenia. J Clin Invest 1977;60:261-4.
39. Graw RG, Herzig G, Perry S et al. Normal granulocyte transfusion therapy: treatment for septicemia due to Gram-negative bacteria. N Engl J Med 1972;287: 367-71.
40. Vallejos C, McCredie KB, Bodey GP et al. White blood cell transfusions for control of infections in neutropenic patients. Transfusion 1975;15:28-33.
41. Higby DJ, Burnett D, Ruppert K, Henderson ES, Cohen E. Granulocyte transfusions: experience at Roswell Park Memorial Instute. In: Greenwalt TJ, Jamieson GA (eds). The granulocyte: function and clinical utilization. New York: Alan R. Liss, Inc. 1977:293-304.
42. Christensen RD, Rothsein G, Anstall HB, Bybee B. Granulocyte transfusion in neonates with bacterial infection, neutropenia and depletion of mature bone marrow neutrophils. Pediatrics 1982;70:1-6.
43. Stegagno M, Pascone R, Colarizi P, Laurenti F, Isacci G, Bucci G, DeLuca EC. Immunologic follow-up of infants treated with granulocyte transfusions for neonatal sepsis. Pediatrics 1985;76:508-11.
44. Ford JM, Cullen MH, Brown LM, Roberts MM, Fulford AJC, Lister TA. Combined granulocyte and platelet transfusions: interrelationship between granulocyte and platelet recoveries in the presence and absence of complicating factors. Scand J Haematol 1984;32:65-75.
45. Dutcher JP, Schiffer CA, Johnston GS. Rapid migration of ^{111}Indium-labeled granulocytes to sites of infection. N Engl J Med 1981;304:586-9.
46. Arnold R, Pflieger H, Wiesneth M, Bhaduri S, Bültmann B, Heimpel H. In vitro and in vivo studies on filter collected granulocytes. Scand J Haematol 1981;26: 31-6.
47. Arnold R, Pflieger H, Dietrich M, Heimpel H. The clinical efficacy of granulocyte transfusion: studies on the oral cavity. Blut 1977;35:405-14.
48. Rebuck JW, Crowley JH. A method of studying leukocyte function in vivo. Ann NY Acad Sci 1955;59:757.

49. Schiffer CA, Buchholz DA, Aisner J, Betts SW, Wiernik PH. Clinical experience with transfusion of granulocytes obtained by continuous flow filtration leukapheresis. Am J Med 1975;58:373-81.
50. Pflieger H, Arnold R, Bhaduri S, Haghou F, Heimpel H. Parameters for determining the clinical efficacy of granulocyte transfusion therapy. In: Mandelli F (ed). Therapy of acute leukemias. Proc. 2nd Int Symposium. Rome: Lombardo Editore 1979:631-5.
51. Brubaker DB. Immunologically mediated immediate adverse effects of blood transfusions (allergic, febrile, nonhemolytic, and noncardiogenic pulmonary edema). Plasma Ther Transfus Technol 1985;6:19-30.
52. Kretschmer V. Leukozytenseparation und -transfusion. In: Reissigl H, Bässler KH, Henneberg U (eds). Beiträge zu Infusionstherapie und klinische Ernährung. Basel: S. Karger, 1981:133-57.
53. Lalezari P. Neutrophil antigens: Immunology and clinical implications. Prog Clin Biol Res 1977;13:209-25.
54. Engelfriet CP, Tetteroo PAT, van der Veen JPW, Weiner WF, van der Plas-van Dalen C, von dem Borne AEG KR. Granulocyte-specific antigens and methods for their detection. In: Advance in Immunobiology: Blood cell antigens and Bone Marrow Transplantation. New York: Alan R. Liss 1984:121-54.
55. Ward HN, Lipscomb TS, Cawley LP. Pulmonary hypersensitivity reaction after blood transfusion. Arch Intern Med 1968;122:362-6.
56. Ward HN. Pulmonary infiltrates associated with leukoagglutinin transfusion reactions. Ann Intern Med 1970;73:689-94.
57. Dubois M, Lotze MT, Diamond WJ, Kim YD, Flye MW, Macnamara TE. Pulmonary shunting during leukoagglutinin-induced noncardiac pulmonary edema. JAMA 1980;244:2186-9.
58. Popovsky MA, Abel MD, Moore SB. Transfusion-related acute lung injury associated with passive transfer of antileukocyte antibodies. Am Rev Respir Dis 1983;128:185-9.
59. Levy GJ, Shabot MM, Hart ME, Mya WW, Goldfinger D. Transfusion-associated noncardiogenic pulmonary edema. Transfusion 1986;26:278-81.
60. Andrews AT, Zmijewski CM, Bowman HS, Reihart JK. Transfusion reaction with pulmonary infiltration associated with HLA-specific leukocyte antibodies. Am J Clin Pathol 1976;66:483-7.
61. Fosse E, Svennevig JL, Harboe M. Cell markers in stored blood. Injury 1985;16: 393-7.
62. Prince HE, Arens L. Effect of storage on lymphocyte surface markers in whole blood units. Transplant 1986;41:235-8.
63. Light JA, Metz S, Oddendino K et al. Fresh versus stored blood in donor specific transfusion. Transplant Proc 1982;14:296-9.
64. Graze PR, Gale RP. Chronic graft versus host disease: a syndrome of disordered immunity. Am J Med 1979;66:611-20.
65. Shulman HM, Sullivan KM, Weiden PL et al. Chronic graft-versus-host-syndrome in man. A long-term clinicopathologic study of 20 Seattle patients. Am J Med 1980;69:204-17.
66. Sullivan KM. Graft-versus-host disease. In: Blume KG, Petz LD. Clinical bone marrow transplantation. New York: Churchill Livingstone 1983:91-129.
67. Möller G (ed). Graft versus host reaction. Immunological Reviews 1985. Copenhagen: Munksgaard.
68. Roitt I, Brostoff J, Male D. Immunology. London Gower Medical Publishing 1985:24.1-24.9.

69. Gleichmann H, Breininger J. Over 95% sensitization against allogenic leukocytes following single massive blood transfusion. Vox Sang 1975;28:66-73.
70. Smith MD, Williams JD, Coles GA, Salaman JR. Blood transfusions, suppressor T cells, and renal transplant survival. Transplantation 1983;36:647-50.
71. Lenhard V, Massen G, Seifert P, Johannsen R, Grosse-Wilde H. Characterization of transfusion-induced suppressor cells in prospective kidney allograft recipients. Transplant Proc 1982;14:329-32.
72. Jeannet M, Neri-Legendre C, Descoeudres C, Leski M. Does blood transfusion induce a nonspecific suppression of cell-mediated immunity. Transplant Proc 1982;14:325-8.
73. Fischer E, Lenhard V, Seifert P, Kluge A, Johannsen R. Blood transfusion induced suppression of cellular immunity in man. Hum Immunol 1980;3:187-92.
74. Kaplan J, Sarnaik S, Gitlin J, Lusher J. Diminished helper/suppressor lymphocyte ratios and natural killer activity in recipients of repeated blood transfusions. Blood 1984;64:308-10.
75. Gascon P, Zoumbros NC, Young NS. Immunologic abnormalities in patients receiving multiple blood transfusions. An Intern Med 1984;100:173-7.
76. Grady RW, Akbar AN, Giardina PJ, Hilgartner MW, DeSousa M. Disproportionate lymphoid cell subsets in thalassemia major: the relative contribution of transfusion and splenectomy. Br J Haematol 1985;59:713-21.
77. DeMartino M, Rossi ME, Muccioli AT, Vullo C, Vierucci A. Altered T cell subsets and function in polytransfused beta-thalassemia patients: correlation with sex and age at first transfusion. Vox Sang 1985;48:296-304.
78. Wang W, Herrod H, Presbury G, Wilimas J. Lymphocyte phenotype and function in chronically transfused children with sickle cell disease. Am J Haematol 1985; 20:31-40.
79. Shimizu K, Kitoh S. Increase in the number of lymphocytes secreting IgG following blood transfusion. Blood 1982;59:312-6.
80. Akbar AN, Giardina PJ, Hilgartner MW, Grady RW. Immunological abnormalities in thalassaemia major. I. A transfusion-related increase in circulating cytoplasmatic immunoglobulin-positive cells. Clin Exp Immunol 1985;62:397-404.
81. Fehrman I, Ringden O. Lymphocytes from multitransfused uremic patients have poor MLC reactivity. Tissue Antigens 1981;17:386-95.
82. Kerman RH, van Buren CT, Payne W et al. Influence of blood transfusion on immune responsiveness. Transplant Proc 1982;14:335-7.
83. Fehrman I, Ringden O. Reduced immunologic responsiveness in multitransfused anemic nonuremic patients. Transplant Proc 1982;14:341-3.
84. Keown P, Descamps B. Suppression de la reaction lymphocytaire mixte par les globules rouges autologues et leurs constituents: une hypothese nouvelle sur l'effet apparement tolerogene des transfusions sanguines en transplantation. C R Acad Sci 1978;287:749-52.
85. Maerker-Alzer G, Kugland K, Dienst C, Schumacher K, Dalichau H, Hügel W. In-vivo-Reaktiviering reduzierter T-zellaktivität nach Polytransfusion durch Immunaggregate in Immunglobulinpräparaten. Immun Infekt 1985;13:85-6.
86. Warden GD, Ninnemann J, Stratta RJ, Saffle JR. The effect of exchange therapy on postburn lymphocyte suppression. Surgery 1984;96:321-9.
87. Constantian MB. Association of sepsis with an immunosuppressive polypeptide in the serum of burn patients. Ann Surg 1978;188:209-15.
88. Ninnemann JL, Stratta RJ, Warden GD, Saffle JR, Weber ME. The effect of plasma exchange on lymphocyte suppression after burn. Arch Surg 1984;119:33-8.

89. Proud G. Blood transfusion and organ transplantation. Ann R Coll Surg Eng 1980;62:271-9.
90. Cheigh JS, Suthanthiran M, Kaplan M et al. Induction of immune alterations and successful renal transplantation with a simplified method of donor-specific blood transfusion. Transplantation 1984;38:501-6.
91. MacLeod AM, Mason RJ, Shewan WG, Power DA, Stewart KN, Edward N, Catto GRD. Possible mechanism of action of transfusion effect in renal transplantation. Lancet 1982;ii:468-70.
92. Fagnilli L, Singal DP. Blood transfusion may induce anti-T cell receptor antibodies in renal patients. Transplant Proc 1982;14:319-21.
93. Chia D, Horimi T, Terasaki PI, Hermes M. Association of anti-Fab and anti-IgG antibodies with high kidney transplant survival. Transplant Proc 1982;14: 322-4.
94. Bow LM, Schweizer RT, Cho S. Successful renal transplantation after transient warm B cell antibody to donor-specific transfusions. Transplantation 1984;37: 618-9.
95. Blank JL, Leo GM, Sollinger HW, Glass NR, Belzer FO. B-warm-positive crossmatch: a contraindication for transplantation in living related transplants undergoing donor-specific transfusion. Transplantation 1982;33:212-3.
96. Fehrman I, Ringden O. Increased incidence of sensitization among patients with polycystic kidney disease following pretransplant blood transfusions. Nephron 1985;40:41-7.
97. Ettenger RB, Jordan SC, Arnett J, Robinson BJ, Fine RN. Specific anti-donor lymphocytotoxic antibodies following blood transfusions from nonrelated donors. Transplant Proc 1982;14:347-8.
98. Soulillou JP, Bignon JD, Peyrat MA, Guimbretiere J, Guensel J. Systematic transfusion in hemodialyzed patients awaiting grafts. Kinetics of anti-T and -B lymphocyte immunization and its incidence on graft function. Transplantation 1980;30:285-9.
99. Gluckman JC, Bacri JL, Debas P, Foucault C, Harispe S, Cartron J. Alloimmunisation to monocytes and granulocytes after leukocyte-poor platelet transfusion. Lancet 1982;i:1471.
100. Rapaport FT, Dausset J. Facilitation of skin allograft survival by blood leukocyte extracts. A possible mechanism for the beneficial effects of blood transfusion in human transplantation. Ann Surg 1984;199:79-86.
101. Leivestad T, Flatmark A, Hirschberg H, Thorsby E. Effect of pretransplant donor specific transfusions in renal transplantation. Transplant Proc 1982;14: 370-3.
102. Korinkova P, Vorlicer J, Majsky A. A study of granulocyte cytotoxins and detection of granulocyte allospecific antigens. Transfusion 1982;22:379-83.
103. McCarty MF. A gene al strategy for the use of allogeneic lymphocyte infusions in the treatment of disorders characterized by impaired helper or suppressor T-cell function: autoimmune diseases and the acquired immunodeficiency syndrome (AIDS). Med Hypotheses 1985;16:189-206.
104. Saha K, Mittal MM, Maheswari HB. Passive transfer of immunity in leprosy patients by transfusion of lymphocytes from lepromin positive healthy donors. J Ind Med Ass 1976;66:93-8.

PLATELET FUNCTIONS AND PLATELET TRANSFUSION

J.W. ten Cate, M.H.J. van Oers

Platelets are required to maintain optimal hemostasis under normal conditions and in particular following trauma or surgical intervention.

Thrombocytopenia and/or thrombocytopathy may be associated with spontaneous hemorrhages or excessive bleeding following trauma. Spontaneous hemorrhage includes easy bruisability, epistaxis, gingival bleeding, menorrhagia and occasionally bleeding from the digestive and urogenital tract. Severe thrombocytopenia is associated with petecchiae.

Thrombocytopenia and thrombocytopathy occur in myriads of clinical conditions, in particular in severe desease states such as acute leukemia, sepsis, multiple trauma and shock. Bleeding problems are regularly encountered in such patients. The increasing availability of platelet concentrates has contributed to effective control of hemorrhage in particular in patients with thrombocytopenia on the basis of defective production, as for example in acute leukemia.

At present it is less clearly documented whether platelet transfusions have contributed to control hemorrhage effectively in other severe clinical conditions accompanied by enhanced platelet turnover.

In this chapter the following issues will be discussed briefly:

1. Function of platelets in hemostasis.
2. Laboratory techniques used to assess platelet function, particularly with respect to transfused platelets and their hemostatic effectiveness.
3. Survey on platelet concentrate transfusion in the Academic Medical Center, Amsterdam.
4. Essential requirements for a prospective study on the safety and efficacy of platelet concentrate transfusion.

It is not the aim to present a complete review of the literature concerning several of these issues, but rather to stimulate the discussion of future clinical studies evaluating the various aspects of platelet concentrate transfusion.

Function of platelets in hemostasis

Following the infliction of a wound platelets accumulate at the site of the lesion and adhere to exposed collagen tissue. Adhesion of platelets requires plasma proteins, such as factor VIII-von Willebrand factor and intact platelet surface glycoprotein structures, such as glycoprotein Ib which is essential for the interaction with factor VIII-von Willebrand factor which bridges platelets with collagen tissue. Other platelet surface glycoproteins, (IIb and IIIa) are essential for platelet aggregation. Defective glycoprotein structures or deficiency of the factor VIII-von Willebrand factor results in abnormal hemostasis and prolonged bleeding. Following platelet adhesion platelets are activated and undergo a conformational transformation 'shape change' with formation of pseudopodes and secretion of substances from the platelet granules. ADP, ATP and serotonin are secreted from the dense bodies. These substances and thromboxane A_2 (TXA_2) liberated from activated platelets induce aggregation of platelets in the vicinity of the vascular lesion. The locally accumulated platelets form the hemostatic plug which results in the arrest of bleeding.

The hemostatic plug is stabilized by fibrin which is the end-product of the activated coagulation cascade. Adequate fibrin formation requires an intact coagulation system. Inherited or acquired deficiencies of clotting factors will lead to delayed fibrin formation, unstable hemostatic plug formation and thus resulting in rebleeding.

Hence, effective primary hemostasis requires platelets with an intact surface receptor (glycoprotein) system, an intact storage pool of pro-aggregatory substances within the platelet granules and an intact metabolism for energy dependent processes such as secretion.

Platelet function tests

The most important test for the assessment of the hemostatic capacity of (transfused) platelets is the bleeding time. Several bleeding time techniques have been described in the literature. However, only two techniques have been standardized properly [1,2].

The most sensitive test is the one designed by Mielke et al [1]. Small incisions are made in the forearm skin following inflation of a sphygmomanometer cuff to a pressure of 40 mm mercury around the upper arm. The blood oozing from the superficial skin lesions is collected into filter paper at regular intervals and the time recorded. This test is a modification of Ivy's method [2] in which small standardized puncture wounds are produced.

All other bleeding time techniques, including Duke's earlobe method, are less reliable and cannot be recommended.

In vitro techniques include measurement of platelet adhesion to glass or collagen surfaces and of platelet aggregation using the turbidimetric method of Born [3].

Measurement of platelet adhesion generally provides no specific information. The platelet aggregation method allows the analysis of responses of platelets to specific stimuli, such as ADP, serotonin, arachidonic acid and collagen. Abnormal platelet aggregation may be due to a variety of platelet defects, e.g. defects of the surface glycoproteins, deficiency or defects of essential enzymes such as cyclo-oxygenase or thromboxane synthetase, and deficiency of the granular contents ('storage pool disease'). It should be noted that a normal result of platelet aggregation tests does not exclude partial storage pool deficiency.

Measurements of platelet storage pool contents may therefore provide additional useful information. The available assays comprise enzymatic assays for ADP/ATP, a fluorimetric assay for serotonin and radioimmunoassays for platelet beta-thromboglobulin and platelet factor-4.

The bleeding time test and the platelet increment following platelet transfusion are the tests most frequently used in the quality control of platelet suspensions, although of course the platelet increment is not a measure of the hemostatic effectiveness of these platelets.

Prior to transfusion platelets are stored: depending upon the circumstances the pH decreases, whereas both plasma lactate levels and the pCO_2 increase. These changes may result in loss of platelet viability and function.

In recent years several improved storage conditions have been described in order to preserve platelet viability, for example by the use of bags with increased permeability for gas. This has resulted in increased increments of platelets following transfusion. Survey of the literature in this respect revealed that hemostatic effectiveness of improved platelet concentrates was either investigated in volunteers or in patients with stable thrombocytopenia (Tabel 1).

Table 1. Platelet transfusion study.

Author	Population studied
Lazarus, 1981 [4]*	Stable thrombocytopenic patients
Murphy et al, 1982 [5]	Normal volunteers Patients with thrombocytopenia secundary to acute leukemia
Lazarus et al, 1982 [6]	Stable thrombocytopenic patients
Rock et al, 1984 [7]	Normal volunteers Stable thrombocytopenic patients
Snyder et al, 1984 [8]	Normal volunteers
Moroff et al, 1984 [9]	Neonates with destructive thrombocytopenia
Simon et al, 1984 [10]	Patients undergoing coronary bypass surgery

* Reference.

Only two studies provide data on patients with increased platelet turnover or destruction [9,10].

Obviously, data obtained in volunteers or in clinically stable patients do not necessarily provide information relevant for thrombocytopenic patients in intensive care untis with traumatic and/or septic complications. These patients who frequently suffer from bleeding problems are transfused with platelets although objective data on the hemostatic efficacy of platelet concentrate transfusion under these complicated clinical conditions are lacking. Transfusion is mainly based on the assumption that platelets showing hemostatic efficacy under stable clinical conditions will be effective here as well. However, concurrent disseminated intravascular coagulation with enhanced platelet turnover and/or antibiotic treatment which may induce platelet defects may abolish the desired hemostatic effect of platelet transfusion. In order to obtain an impression of the efficacy control of platelet transfusion in our hospital we performed a retrospective survey of data available in the hospital computer system over the year 1985 and the first six months of 1986.

Survey on platelet concentrate transfusion

Platelet concentrate transfusion data could be obtained from four defined areas, i.e. platelet concentrates used during surgery, concentrates given at the intensive care unit (involving postoperative and medical patients in high risk situations) and transfusion in the various 'wards', where the majority of the transfusions were performed in hematological patients (Table 2).

Table 2. Consumption of platelet concentrates (units) Academic Medical Center 1985-1986(1/2).

Location	1985-I*	1985-II*	1986-I*
During surgery	176	260	180
Intensive care unit	1607	1478	1012
'Wards' (total)	4204	5780	3571
Hematology ward	2971	4965	2379

* I refers to first half year; II to second half year.

Analysis of the intensive care data revealed that most transfusions were given to patients following major abdominal surgery, cardiopulmonary bypass surgery and to medical patients (Table 3).

Table 3. Consumption of platelets (units) in the intensive care unit.

Location	1985-I*	1985-II*	1986-I*
Abdominal surgery	395	532	462
Cardiopulmonary bypass surgery	343	424	240
Neurosurgery	208	0	64
Vascular surgery	56	104	64
Medical patients	605	378	94

* I refers to first half year; II to second half year.

For obvious reasons bleeding times are almost never performed in hematological patients, therefore the efficacy data were analysed in 68 consecutive intensive care patients for 1986-I. Bleeding time data were provided by the data-base of the hospital computer system and matched with the patients transfused with platelet concentrates.

In these 68 patients bleeding times were performed in 19 only. Prior to platelet transfusion the bleeding time was prolonged in 16 patients and remained so in 9 patients following transfusion.

Because these bleeding time data were obtained neither from a rigid quality control programme nor from a study protocol, our results provide only a weak indication of a possible reduced hemostatic efficacy in this category of patients. No data regarding clinical efficacy were available. It can be concluded that platelet transfusion is not submitted to quality control, which is urgently required (in general). However, this demands an adequate trial design with adequate techniques and hospital staff.

Trial design

Any study regarding the safety and efficacy of platelet transfusion in high risk patients, in particular in those patients admitted to an intensive care unit should at least be a prospective one. Regarding efficacy predefined endpoints should be established such as quantitative assessment of blood loss, and eventually morbidity and or mortality. The effect of platelet transfusion on the bleeding time could be used as an acceptable substitution endpoint.

A pilot study should provide some indication of the efficacy. When the efficacy seems to be reduced a randomized study should be feasible which however requires extensive ethical considerations.

Until the results of such a stucy are available, we are not certain whether platelet transfusion in intensive care patients with all complications of disseminated intravascular coagulation and of platelet defects inducing medication is justified.

Acknowledgement

We acknowledge the accurate assistance of Els Bertelsman for the data collection.

References

1. Mielke CH, Kaneshiro MM, Maher IA, Weiner JM, Rapaport SI. The stanard normal Ivy bleeding time and its prolongation by aspirin. Blood 1969;34:204-15.
2. Ivy AC, Nelson D, Buchet G. The standardization of certain factors in the cutaneous 'venostasis' bleeding time technique. J Lab Clin Med 1941;26:1812-6.
3. Born GVR. Aggregation of blood platelets and its reversal. Nature 1962;194: 927-9.
4. Lazarus HM, Kaniecki-Green EA, Warm SE, Aikawa M, Herzig RH. Therapeutic effectiveness of frozen platelet concentrates for transfusion. Blood 1981;57:243-8.
5. Murphy S, Kahn RA, Holme S, et al. Improved storage of platelets for transfusion in a new container. Blood 1982;60:194-200.
6. Lazarus HM, Herzig RH, Warm SE, Fishman DJ. Transfusion experience with platelet concentrates stored for 24-72 hours at 22°C. Transfusion 1982;22:39-43.
7. Rock G, Sherring VA, Tittley P. Five-day storage of platelet concentrates. Transfusion 1984;24:147-52.

8. Snyder EL, Ferri PM, Smith EO, Ezekowitz MD. Use of an electromechanical infusion pump for transfusion of platelet concentrates. Transfusion 1984;24: 524-7.
9. Moroff G, Friedman A, Robkin-Kline L, Gautier G, Luban NLC. Reduction of the volume of stored platelet concentrates for use in neonatal patients. Transfusion 1984;24:144-6.
10. Simon TL, Akl BF, Murphy W. Controlled trial of routine administration of platelet concentrates in cardiopulmonary bypass surgery. Ann Thor Surg 1984; 37:359-64.

DISCUSSION

C.P. Engelfriet and J.C. Chermann

S. Murphy (Philadelphia): I wonder if either dr. Moore or prof. Engelfriet could give us some idea about the quantitative relationship between lymphocyte contamination and the ability to induce a unanimous response that is to be dealt with as techniques are developed to make lymphocyte depleted platelets. To what extend does that has to be done to achieve the results of suppressing immunization?

S.B. Moor (Rochester): I do not know how much of a dose-relationship there is between the lymphocyte content of a platelet concentrate, or a renal transplant for example and its ability to induce an immune response to HLA antigens. I have an intuitive reaction to the question: It is not an all or non phenomenon. Secondly, there probably is a concentration or dose of immunizing lymphocytes below which one does not see immunization.

C.P. Engelfriet (Amsterdam): I do not think there is a real answer to the question. If it is true that class II positive cells are the main cells to induce alloimmunizations, then monocytes and B-cells are the most important. But as far as I know there have been no studies to show that the removal of these cells exclusively will prevent alloimmunization better than anything else.

S.B. Moore: There have been a number of experimental studies looking at the coating of the class II antigen site by monoclonal antibodies in an attempt to demonstrate that the presence of the class II antigens on the antigen presenting cell was necessary, but those studies tend to give an all or none phenomenon. In other words, in the absence of the coating one saw the presentation of antigens. In the presence of the antibody one could abbrogate it. The question of the number of cells that one would have to block to prevent the reaction has to my knowledge not been investigated.

C.P. Engelfriet: The number of cells, so far studied, is the total number of leukocytes. So there is no real answer to the question.

C.Th. Smit Sibinga (Groningen): Prof. Engelfriet could you give us some further insight in what the actual mechanism is believed to be in the inactivation of antigenicity of white cells present in platelets when treated with UV light?

C.P. Engelfriet: Well, dr. Slichter has actually done the experiment with her colleagues. Perhaps she would like to answer the question.

S.J. Slichter (Seattle): UV-irradiation of blood cells apparently does not interfere with the expression of either class I or class II MHC antigens. It is hypothesized that UV-irradiation interferes with the function of antigen-presenting cells possibly by impairing the release of Interleukin I. Failure of UV-irradiated lymphocytes to stimulate in mixed lymphocyte culture may be an 'in vitro' correlate to select the required UV dose to prevent alloimmune recognition of blood products following transfusion.

C.Th. Smit Sibinga: Does that mean that a plea is coming forward for UV-irradiation of platelet concentrates in an attempt to further reduce sensitization or reaction?

S.J. Slichter: Unfortunately, there are some practical problems with UV-irradiation. Specifically, it may be difficult to deliver an effective dose, because of the poor penetrance of UV-irradiation. For our dog platelet transfusion experiments, presented by dr. Engelfriet, the donor dog's platelet concentrate was placed in an open Petri dish and agitated with a stir bar while the cells were exposed to UV-irradiation. Obviously, such an open system is not applicable to platelet transfusion therapy for patients. However, we are now conducting experiments on UV irradiating platelet concentrates through a standard blood bag while the platelets are agitated on a platform rocker. In normal volunteers, the MLC reactivity of UV-irradiated lymphocytes in the platelet concentrates are being evaluated as well as the ^{51}Cr survival of UV-irradiated platelets. It will probably be possible to effectively UV-irradiate platelets, but the real problem is that most thrombocytopenic patients also require red cell transfusions. Delivering an effective UV-dose to a large volume of red cells may be a substantially more difficult task. Thus, there are clearly practical problems to be solved before UV-irradiation can be used clinically.

P.C. Das (Groningen): Dr. ten Cate, you made a very original, very critical and very constructive presentation. May I take one or two points that you suggested. During that study you did not take into consideration how old the platelets were: Were they 2 days old, were they 5 days old, or what was the period of storage. That might affect the results that you have had. I mention this, because the tendency at the moment in the Blood Bank world is to prolong the shelf-life by producing new plastics and thinner plastics.

J.W. ten Cate (Amsterdam): The main question was: What is the hemostatic effectiveness of the platelets used in our hospital in this particular category of patients in the intensive care unit. Secondly, it is a retrospective study, the data are highly incomplete. I could have taken into account the age of the platelet concentrates, but that would deliver us not with any data of importance, because the surveillance was extremely limited.

C.Th. Smit Sibinga: But probably you could add this point to your list of criteria for setting up a prospective study and add another point. One of the things that worries us very much is what actually is the practice of transfusing platelets at the bed-side. This is usually out of our scope. We leave it to the competence of the clinician and the nursing staff, but if you carefully look at what happens in a ward you see that the practice in transfusing platelets is not always optimal, which eventually influences the clinical efficacy.

S. Murphy: The extrapolation from laboratory data to general clinical practice is done on a wide scale and very effective compounds such as penicillin have never been subjected to randomized trials. In the context of an intensive care, I have the feeling that transfused platelet concentrates contribute only marginally to the final outcome of the patient. So, platelet transfusion in bleeding patients with thrombocytopenia, should be investigated in more depth. I personally believe that the studies that are in the literature of fresh and stored platelets correcting the bleeding time of thrombocytopenic patients demonstrate the efficacy of the stored product. Finally, I think the bleeding time is not a very good technique for doing what you are proposing to do. If for example I have a patient with leukemia and a platelet count of 5,000 and raise his platelet count to 30,000, that in a major way prevents the possibility of spontaneous bleeding, but I do not think it will change his bleeding time.

J.W. ten Cate: Well, you raised similar issues as I did: Improvement of the platelet concentrate has been tested and should be tested in patients with stable thrombocytopenia. Your second remark regarding the sample size of eventual trials is totally dependent upon the contribution you want to be given to the reduction of mortality or morbidity by platelet concentrate transfusion. It is most uncertain, so you have to make an estimate. I agree entirely; a prior sample size assessment is complicated. Your third point was the increment of platelets. I think it is empirical and it is valid for your hematology patients. But I am not so sure that this is relevant for totally different patient categories, e.g. patients with sepsis.

S. Murhpy: Well, I am not in the least confident about when we should transfuse hematology patients. What I am confident about is that a patient with hypoplastic thrombocytopenia is probably going to be quite stable at a platelet count of 30,000. While at 2,000 he would not be. Yet the bleeding time is well over 20 minutes in both situations.

S.B. Moore: I agree with both speakers that the criteria for the use of platelet transfusions have not really been looked at closely enough. In our institution, where we do quite some cardiac surgery, the use of platelet concentrates has increased by some 300% over 10 years. The number of cases has increased, but only by 50% in that time. Secondly, the type of cases has not significantly changed, and the mortality has not changed. So I am convinced that we are using far too many platelets for patients who really do not need them. Apart from the fact altogether that we have to establish criteria for patients who have hematologic disorders and thrombocytopenia, we just simply do not have enough platelets derived from our donor population to cover all of the demands from clinicians for platelets. If we are going to use them, we should use them for patients who in fact absolutely need them.

J. Seidel (Hannover): The Blood Bank in our vicinity has the policy to activate platelet concentrates before giving them to the patients by simply putting them into the freezer for about 30 minutes to give them a cold shock. They argue that that would activate the platelets and procure a very good hemostatical effect.

C.Th. Smit Sibinga: Dr. Seidel, in your presentation you listed two techniques of which to the best of my knowledge one has been abandoned already years ago: Filtration leukapheresis. Is it still in use in your Centre or is that a misunderstanding.

J. Seidel: It is not in use in our Centre, but it is still in Germany.

C.Th. Smit Sibinga: When you spoke about blood salvaging intraoperatively, you showed a slide about the fundamental technique. It is known from work in Groningen (prof. Wildevuur) that specifically the suction causes most of the trouble, reason why a controlled suction device was developed to try to reduce the damaging effect. It was shown that specifically the suction is very causative for complement activation in this type of blood salvaging. Could you comment on that?

J. Seidel: Not exactly, because this technique of measuring aggregation activity is very recent in our laboratory and we have not done the study yet. But that is being planned and probably within the next months we can provide some data.

II. CLINICAL ASPECTS
A. Presence of cells

PLATELET TRANSFUSION

S. Murphy

In 1952, Hirsch and Gardner described the first extensive series of patients treated by 'platelet transfusion' [1]. In fact, whole nonanticoagulated blood from thrombocytotic patients with polycythemia vera was transferred with siliconized syringes to the circulation of thrombocytopenic patients. The authors made observations which continue to dominate the philosophy of platelet transfusion therapy today. First, in 11 transfusions in patients with marrow failure and normal spleen size, immediate mean in vivo recovery of platelets infused was 67% and subsequent survival was 5-6 days. Second, in 6 patients with chronic idiopathic thrombocytopenic purpura (ITP) mean recovery was essentially the same, 52%, but survival time was shorter, 2-4 days. Thirdly, as several of the patients were repeatedly transfused, recovery and survival were progressively reduced undoubtedly due to alloimmunization.

In the mid-1950s, one would have assumed, as the authors did, that platelet lifespan was 5-6 days and wondered why in vivo recovery was only 67% rather than 100%. In the early 1960s, Aster and Jandl perfected the technique for measuring platelet kinetics after labelling of the cells with ^{51}chromium [2]. They clearly established that one-third of the total body platelet mass is sequestered in a splenic pool, which is, nonetheless, in free communication with a circulating pool which contains the other two-thirds. This physiologic splenic pool explains the 67% recovery. However, the ^{51}chromium technique suggested that platelet survival time was 8-10 days, raising questions about Hirsch and Gardner's 5-6 day figure.

This issue and many others were addressed by Slichter in her 1980 review of platelet transfusion therapy [3]. Using ^{51}chromium labelling, she found that platelet survival in normal individuals was 9.6 days while it was 5.2 days in patients with thrombocytopenia related to defective production and platelet counts $<70{,}000/\mu l$. She hypothesized that platelets normally interact with the vascular endothelium. When the platelet count is normal, the percentage of circulating platelets involved in this process is very small. However, in thrombocytopenic patients, vascular consumption may be proportionately much larger. Therefore, as predicted by Hirsch and Gardner, vigorous platelet support in such patients would require transfusions twice weekly.

In subsequent studies by Hanson and Slichter, this fixed vascular requirement for platelets was examined quantitatively [4]. Using data from platelet kinetic measurements in patients with bone marrow hypoplasia, they developed a model which predicted a maximum platelet life span of 10.5 days, and a fixed requirement for 4,700 platelets/μl of blood per day, or about 18% of the normal rate of platelet turnover which was 26,000 platelets/μl of blood per day. In patients with severe thrombocytopenia, approximately 20,000 platelets/μl, this fixed vascular requirement was 84% of daily platelet turnover.

These theoretical considerations have great relevance for the practice of platelet transfusion therapy. Hypoplastic patients with platelet counts in the range of 5,000-15,000/μl, probably have greater platelet production than one would think with a platelet mean survival close to two days. Thus they meet their daily requirement, 4,700/μl/day, and, if otherwise stable, have no spontaneous bleeding. Slichter has supported this concept experimentally by showing that stool blood loss increases only slightly when the platelet count is in the range of 5,000-10,000/μl, and becomes markedly elevated only when the platelet level is less than 5,000/μl [3]. However, one would reason that spontaneous bleeding might be seen at higher platelet levels of 5,000-20,000/μl, if there were other factors which might predispose to bleeding such as extreme leukocytosis, sepsis, platelet dysfunction due to drugs and as carbenicillin, or an anatomical lesion such as gastrointestinal ulceration.

In spite of these considerations, the standard of practice in the United States commonly calls for prophylactic platelet transfusion whenever the platelet count falls below 20,000/μl particularly in patients who are receiving chemotherapy for malignancies. This practice probably arose because of physician anxiety but may have originated with data obtained before the availability of platelet transfusions from the article of Gaydos et al. published in 1962 [5]. In children with acute leukemia, they correlated the frequency of hemorrhage with platelet counts. Minor bleeding such as petechiae, ecchymoses, and epistaxis were increasingly common as platelet counts fell below 50,000/μl. Gross forms of hemorrhage such as hematuria, melaena, and hematemesis only began to appear at levels below 20,000/μl. However, there was no real threshold and such gross hemorrhage was seen on 2-4% of days in the range of 5,000-20,000/μl, and on 10-30% of days in the range of 0-5,000/μl. In fact, the authors actually concluded that thrombocytopenia alone is rarely responsible for hemorrhage, but that precipitating events such as those listed above, that alone would also fail to cause hemorrhage, may result in hemorrhage when coupled with thrombocytopenia. Thus, that study in fact provided little support for prophylactic transfusion in the range of 5,000-20,000/μl.

Only two studies have addressed this issue in a controlled, prospective fashion, and one of these was published only as a letter to the editor of Lancet [6]. Neither supported prophylactic transfusion. Murphy et al. randomized 56 children with acute leukemia to one of two regimens of platelet transfusions [7]. The prophylactic group received platelets whenever the platelet count fell below 20,000/μl irrespective of clinical events. The therapeutic group was transfused only for the occurrence of significant bleeding such as epistaxis not controlled by initial packing, gross gastrointestinal or urinary tract bleeding, any central nervous system bleeding, or any bleeding episode felt to be life-threatening. The time to first serious bleeding episode was significantly longer in the prophylactic group, but this result required the use of twice as many platelets as used in the therapeutic group and the survival curves of the two groups could not be distinguished. The analysis suggests that the vast majority of patients who bleed in the absence of prophylactic transfusion can recover after a therapeutic transfusion.

It is worth pointing out in retrospect that it is essentially impossible to prove efficacy for prophylactic platelet transfusion during the initial induction therapy for acute leukemia. If it is true that patients with platelet counts in the range of 5,000-20,000/μl, bleed significantly on only 3% of days [5] (once per month) and if the majority of these bleeds can be stopped by therapeutic platelet transfusion without serious sequelae [7], one might expect an irreversible event on approximately 0.3% of days (once every 10 patient-months). If prophylactic transfusion prevented all of these irreversible events (which is doubtful) and if the period of thrombocytopenia for each leukemia induction is approximately one month, one would have to have two treatment arms of 150 patients each to have only a 70% chance of detecting a difference at the level, $p<0.05$. If prophylactic therapy was effective half the time, one would need 660 patients in each group to have a 90% chance of detecting the difference at the level, $p<0.05$.

There are obvious economic disadvantages to rigid programs of prophylactic platelet transfusion. Are there other disadvantages? Now that random and single donor platelets are easily available, the major problem in providing platelet support is the development of alloimmunization and refractoriness to platelet transfusion. One would assume that reduction in the number of platelet transfusions given would, at least, delay the onset of alloimmunization. However, in the one study that addressed this issue, there was no such dose-response relationship [8]. Amongst 106 newly diagnosed patients with acute leukemia receiving initial induction therapy, the rate of alloimmunization was 38% with no relationship between the number of platelet transfusions given and the rate or severity of alloimmunization. In a subsequent study it was shown that patients who did not become alloimmunized during induction did not become alloimmunized during subsequent management [9]. Thus, very liberal use of platelets does not appear to increase the alloimmunization rate. However, it would be a welcome addition to the literature if other groups were to study their patients in an effort to confirm or refute these conclusions.

Nonetheless, I feel that platelet transfusions are overused in the management of hypoplastic thrombocytopenia, at least in the United States. Their increasingly easy availability has contributed to this. Perhaps, we can now reduce prophylactic therapy knowing that platelets are readily available if needed. Cost-benefit analysis supports this approach. I favor a modification of the protocol of Gmur et al. who recommended platelet transfusion for:

1. Morning platelet count <5,000/μl;
2. Morning platelet count of 5,000-10,000/μl, with new hemorrhage or fever >38°C; or
3. Major bleeding [10].

I would add to criterion #2: extreme leukocytosis, administration of drugs known to interfere with platelet function, and a known anatomical lesion likely to produce major hemorrhage. To use this approach, platelet counting must be accurate. This is best accomplished by using the procedure of Gaydos et al. [5] who performed counts by phase microscopy on patients whose platelet counts were less than 50,000/μl by using 1:20 dilution and counting 50 squares rather than a 1:100 dilution and counting only 10 squares as in the routine method [11]. Taking extra care to obtain accurate platelet counts undoubtedly is more cost effective than administering unnecessary platelet transfusions.

The 1952 article of Hirsch and Gardner [1] demonstrated that platelet survival time was short in ITP. This is now known to be due to immune destruction. This has led to the view that platelet transfusions are useless in ITP since the transfused platelets will be destroyed as fast as the patient's own platelets. In fact, a recent report [12] showed that platelets can be effective in ITP confirming what was clear in the 1952 article. Carr et al. [12] showed that 42% of platelet transfusions in ITP resulted in immediate post-transfusion increments of 20,000/μl or more. Next day platelet counts remained elevated in 39% of these transfusions. I do not recommend any form of prophylactic platelet transfusion in ITP, but a platelet infusion may be helpful in the rare patient who has life-threatening bleeding or who must go for surgery of tissues which are highly vascular or inflamed.

As mentioned above, the major, current problem in platelet transfusion therapy is the development of alloimmunization and refractoriness to platelets after exposure to multiple units of random-donor platelets. These patients can often be managed with platelets from single donors selected by HLA typing, platelet cross matching, or both [13,14]. Not infrequently, however, management is unsatisfactory, and it would be far preferable to prevent alloimmunization from occurring. Two approaches have been studied, use of leukocyte-depleted products and initiation of therapy with single-donor platelets from the beginning.

In 1981, Eernisse and Brand suggested that alloimmunization to platelets resulted from infusing contaminating leukocytes [15]. This concept received theoretical backing with observations suggesting that immunization against HLA antigens required both class-I and class-II antigens and that class-II antigens must be presented by viable lymphocytes. Since platelets and red cells lack class-II antigens, transfusion with only these elements might never immunize. In a 1981 study [16], retrospective analysis of 28 patients transfused with routine methods prior to 1974 indicated that 26(93%) became refractory to random-donor platelets. After 1974, 68 patients were given only red cells filtered so as to remove 97% of the leukocytes and platelets which were depleted of leukocytes by centrifugation. Of these, only 16(24%) became refractory. Therefore, in this study which used historical controls, reduction in leukocyte contamination of transfusion products appeared to reduce the incidence of alloimmunization. In 1983, Schiffer et al. [17] reported a prospective, randomized trial comparing standard platelet concentrates with leukocyte-depleted platelet concentrates finding that 42% of the controls and 20% of patients receiving leukocyte-depleted platelets became alloimmunized. Although the difference was suggestive, it was not significant statitically ($p = 0.071$). The authors pointed out that Eernisse and Brand had achieved a 10-fold greater reduction in leukocyte contamination than they had been able to achieve.

Gmur et al. took a different approach [10]. In a prospective study, they randomized patients with newly diagnosed acute leukemia to receive either random, multiple-donor platelet concentrates or single-donor platelets which were not matched in any way. The patients receiving single-donor platelets became refractory less frequently, after a longer period of time, and after a higher number of transfusions. Finally, in a prospective but not randomized study, Murphy et al. treated all of their patients with acute leukemia with single-donor platelets from the beginning and found that leukocyte depletion of the single-donor products reduced the incidence of alloimmunization [18].

Table 1 shows some of the problems in interpreting data in this complex field. Routine, random-donor platelet transfusion produced a 93% incidence of refractoriness in reference 16 while it was 52% and 42% in references 10 and 17 respectively. Leukocyte contamination was 5-10 fold higher in reference 16. The experimental group in reference 10 and the control group in reference 18 both received single-donor platelets which were not leukocyte-depleted from the start of treatment. The incidences of refractoriness were 15% and 48% respectively although the levels of leukocyte contamination of the products were similar. Thus, similar protocols produce widely different results in different centers. Furthermore, the ability of centers to achieve leukocyte depletion varies. Reference 16, which indicated benefit, achieved a 400-fold reduction while reference 17, which did not indicate benefit, achieved only a 4-fold reduction. With this variation from center to center, we will have to be quite cautious in our interpretations.

In their influential 'sounding board' article published in 1982, Schiffer and Slichter reviewed their reasons for recommending that thrombocytopenic patients receive pooled platelet concentrates from random donors as their initial source of platelet support, with single-donor platelets from selected compatible donors used only when refractoriness to random-donor platelets had been documented [19]. Four years later, this is still the most common approach in the United States. However, one anticipates that techniques will continue to evolve to allow rapid procurement of a leukocyte-depleted, therapeutic dose of platelets from a single donor. It may then be appropriate to use such products as routine initial support for selected patients who will require long periods of support. It will be of great interest to see how these issues evolve in the years ahead.

Table 1.

Reference	Product	Leukocyte depletion	Refractoriness incidence (%)	Leukocyte/platelet ratio ($\times 10^{-3}$)*
10	random-donor	no	52	1.89
	single-donor	no	15	9.09
16	random-donor	no	93	8.13
	random-donor	yes	24	0.02
17	random-donor	no	42	0.88
	random-donor	yes	20	0.22
18	single-donor	no	48	14.39
	single-donor	yest	16	0.86

* Calculating by dividing the leukocyte content of the product by the platelet content of the product and multiplying by 1000. The number represents the number of leukocytes per 1000 platelets.

References

1. Hirsch EO, Gardner FH. The transfusion of human blood platelets with a note on the transfusion of granulocytes. J Lab & Clin Med 1952;39:556-69.
2. Aster RH. Splenic platelet pooling as a cause of 'hypersplenic' thrombocytopenia. Trans Assoc Amer Physicians 1965;78:362-73.
3. Slichter SJ. Controversies in platelet transfusion therapy. Ann Rev Med 1980;31: 509-40.
4. Hanson SR, Slichter SJ. Platelet kinetics in patients with bone marrow hypolasia: Evidence for a fixed platelet requirement. Blood 1985;66:1105-9.
5. Gaydos LA, Freireich EJ, Mantel N. The quantitative relation between platelet count and hemorrhage in patients with acute leukemia. N Engl J Med 1962;266: 905-9.
6. Solomon J, Bofenkamp T, Fahey JL, Chillar RK, Beutler E. Platelet prophylaxis in acute non-lymphoblastic leukemia. Lancet 1978;i:267.
7. Murphy S, Litwin S, Herring LM et al. Indications for platelet transfusion in children with acute leukemia. Am J Hematol 1982;12:347-56.
8. Dutcher JP, Schiffer CA, Aisner J, Wiernik PH. Alloimmunization following platelet transfusion: The absence of a dose-response relationship. Blood 1981;57: 395-8.
9. Dutcher JP, Schiffer CA, Aisner J, Wiernik PH. Long-term follow-up of patients with leukemia receiving platelet transfusions: Identification of a large group of patients who do not become alloimmunized. Blood 1981;58:1007-11.
10. Gmur J, von Felten A, Osterwalder B et al. Delayed alloimmunization using random single platelet transfusions: A prospective study in thrombocytopenic patients with acute leukemia. Blood 1983;62:473-9.
11. Brecher G, Schneiderman M, Cronkite EP. Reproducibility and constancy of platelet count. Am J Clin Path 1953;23:15-26.
12. Carr JM, Kruskall MS, Kaye JA, Robinson SH. Efficacy of platelet transfusions in immune thrombocytopenia. Am J Med 1986;80:1051-4.
13. Duquesnoy RJ, Filip DJ, Rodey GE, Rimm AA, Aster RH. Successful transfusion of platelets 'mismatched' for HLA antigens to alloimmunized thrombocytopenic patients. Am J Hematol 1977;2:219-6.
14. Kickler TS, Braine HG, Ness PM, Koester A, Bias W. A radiolabeled antiglobulin test for crossmatching platelet transfusions. Blood 1983;61:238-42.
15. Claas FHJ, Smeenk RJT, Schmidt R, van Steenbrugge GJ, Eernisse JG. Alloimmunization against the MHC antigens after platelet transfusions is due to contaminating leukocytes in the platelet suspension. Exp Hematol 1981;9:84-9.
16. Eerniss JG, Brand A. Prevention of platelet refractoriness due to HLA antibodies by administration of leukocyte-poor blood components. Exp Hematol 1981;9: 77-83.
17. Schiffer CA, Dutcher JP, Aisner J, Hogge D, Wiernik PH, Reilly JP. A randomized trial of leukocyte-depleted platelet transfusion to modify alloimmunization in patients with leukemia. Blood 1983;62:815-20.
18. Murphy MF, Metcalfe P, Thomas H et al. Use of leukocyte-poor blood component and HLA-matched-platelet donors to prevent HLA alloimmunization. Brit J Haematol 1986;62:529-34.
19. Schiffer CA, Slichter SJ. Sounding board. Platelet transfusions from single donors. N Engl J Med 1982;307:245-8.

PROSPECTIVE SELECTION OF COMPATIBLE PLATELET DONORS FOR ALLOIMMUNIZED PATIENTS BY AN ELISA PLATELET CROSS-MATCH ONLY*

K. Sintnicolaas, W. Sizoo, R.L.H. Bolhuis

Introduction

Alloimmunization to platelets frequently occurs in multitransfused patients and represents a major problem in platelet supportive therapy [1,2]. The provision of compatible platelets for alloimmunized patients remain difficult for the blood bank. Compatible platelet donors are usually selected based on HLA-compatibility between donor and recipient. Drawbacks of this approach are: a) a large HLA-typed donor panel is required that needs continuously updating and is therefore very expensive; 2) a significant percentage (13-31%) of HLA-matched platelet transfusions does not result in satisfactory post-transfusion platelet increments [3-6].

Another approach is to select platelet donors from the random donor population using a platelet cross-match test only. This requires an assay for the detection of antiplatelet alloantibodies that is sensitive, rapid and can be performed on preserved donor cells. We have recently developed a microplate platelet-ELISA that meets these criteria [7]. Here, we describe our initial experience with transfusions of ELISA cross-match compatible platelets to alloimmunized patients.

Materials and methods

Patients

Eight patients with acute leukemia were studied. All patients were alloimmunized as indicated by refractoriness to random donor platelets and the presence in the serum of antiplatelet alloantibodies. At the time of transfusion there were no other factors present known to interfere with platelet increments (e.g. fever, sepsis, splenomegaly, massive bleeding, disseminated intravascular coagulation).

* Supported by a grant from the Josephine Nefkens Foundation.

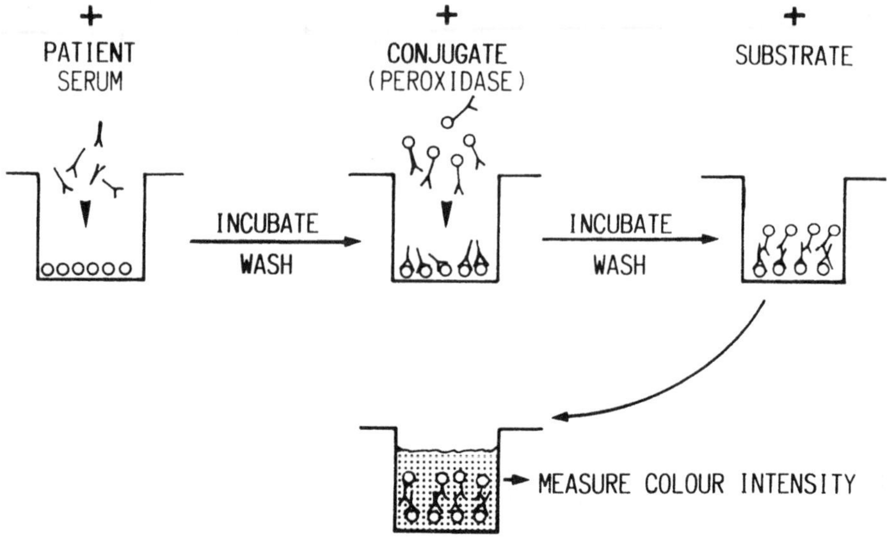

Figure 1. Schematic representation of the ELISA for the detection of antiplatelet alloantibodies.

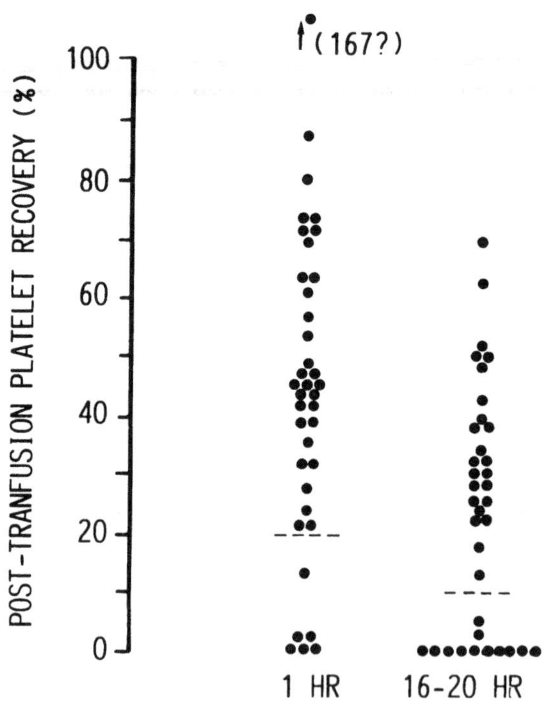

Figure 2. One hour and 24 hour post-transfusion platelet recoveries following the transfusion of ELISA-cross-match negative platelets into alloimmunized recipients. The dashed horizontal lines indicate the lower level of a successful transfusions.

Platelet ELISA

For compatibility testing a microplate ELISA was used where platelets were coated onto the plastic to form a solid phase as detailed elsewhere [7.] In brief, platelets were isolated from donor blood and resuspended in EDTA-PBS at $200 \times 10^9/l$ (Fig. 1). Platelets (5×10^6) were coated onto the wells of a microtiter plate. After washing with PBS-Tween (0.05% v/v), fifty μl of undiluted serum were added and incubated for 60 minutes at 37°C. After washing, 100 μl of $F(ab')_2$-fragments of goat-anti-human IgG conjugated to horseradish peroxidase diluted in PBS-Tween-BSA (4%) were added and incubated for 30 minutes at 37°C. Tween was added since it reduces non-specific binding of serum-IgG to the plastic. Enzymatic activity was measured using orthophenylenediamine as substrate. The reaction was stopped by adding 50 μl 4N H_2SO_4. Optical densities (OD) of the wells were read by an automated micro-ELISA-reader (Titertek, Multiscan MC) at 492 nm (against 620 nm, dual wave length).

Calculation of results

All tests were performed in triplicate and mean values were used for further calculations. The platelets from a single donor were coated onto the wells of an individual plate, and 10 negative control and 1 positive control sera were run in parallel. The test result was expressed as the ratio of the OD value of a test serum to the mean of the OD values of 10 negative control sera. A ratio of 1.5 or more was considered to be positive. Calculations were performed using a microcomputer on-line with the ELISA-reader.

Donor selection

Platelets from plateletapheresis donors were coated onto microtiter plates and stored in the freezer. When a patient developed alloantibodies, the patient serum was tested using the ELISA against a number of available ABO compatible donors. Usually 15-30 donors were tested. Donors with a negative test were used for transfusion.

Platelet collection and transfusions

Platelets were collected by plateletapheresis with the Haemonetics V-50 I autosurge cellseparator with a median platelet yield of 4.8×10^{11} (range 0.2-9.1) and a median leukocyte contamination of 1.6×10^8 (range 0.03-36.4). For evaluation of the transfusion results, a blood platelet count was done in triplicate just prior to, at one hour and at 20 hours following transfusion. The in vivo recovery of the platelets was calculated by use of the following formula:

$$\text{Recovery (\%)} = 100 \times \frac{\text{platelet increment} \times \text{blood volume}}{\text{number of platelets transfused}}$$

Blood volume [1] was estimated to be 2.5 times body surface area (m^2).

Results

For 8 alloimmunized patients platelet donors were selected from the random donor population by the ELISA platelet cross-match. It appeared that most sera reacted with 30-70% the donors tested. Thirty-six platelet transfusions obtained from donors with a negative ELISA cross-match, were administered to 8 patients. In Figure 2 the post-transfusion platelet recoveries are shown. A satisfactory 1 hour post-transfusion recovery (>20%) [8] was obtained in 30 out of 36 (83%) transfusions. In 6 out of these 30 transfusions the survival of the transfused platelets was significantly reduced as indicated by a 20 hours post-transfusion platelet recovery of less than 10%. Thus 24 out of 36 (69%) transfusions of ELISA cross-match negative platelets to alloimmunized patients were associated with a successful transfusion response.

Discussion

Most reports on the value of a platelet cross-match for donor selection for alloimmunized recipients have been performed retrospectively on platelet transfusions from HLA-matched donors. This study differs in that we have prospectively selected compatible random donors using a platelet cross-match only. This approach does not use HLA typing as a selection criterion. A surprising finding was that for all alloimmunized patients tested, negative cross-matches were obtained with 30-70% of the donors tested.

Thus, even with a small donor pool we were able to find cross-match-negative donors for all patients tested. Similar results have been reported using a platelet radioactive antiglobulin test (PRAT) [9].

The optimal study design to evaluate the precise value of a platelet cross-match assay is to compare the test result with the transfusion outcome using single donor platelets. Using this approach we found that the transfusion of ELISA cross-match-negative platelets to alloimmunized patients resulted on 24 out of 36 occasions (67%) in a successful transfusion response. In 6 additional transfusions the 1 hour recovery was satisfactory, although the platelet survival was significantly reduced. In another study [9] alloimmunized patients were transfused with a mixture of cross-match-negative platelets with a 92% success rate. However, this figure may not be directly compared with our's as the use of mixtures of platelets might not give an accurate estimate of the value of the cross-match, e.g. when only a subpopulation of the mixture does not behave according to the cross-match prediction, this might not sufficiently influence the post-transfusion recovery to result in a transfusion failure.

Thus, based on the available data a meaningful comparison between the ELISA and the PRAT cannot be made and only studies using single donor transfusions will allow a correct evaluation of the value of platelet cross-match assay.

In conclusion, the platelet ELISA allows rapid platelet cross-matching. Two-thirds of transfusions of cross-match-negative platelets to alloimmunized patients resulted in a successful transfusion response.

References

1. Tejada F, Bias WB, Santos GW, Zieve PD. Immunologic respons of patients with acute leukemia to platelet transfusions. Blood 1973;42:405-12.
2. Dutcher JP, Schiffer CA, Aisner J, Wiernik PH. Alloimmunization following platelet transfusion: The absence of a dose-response relationship. Blood 1981;57: 395-8.
3. Duquesnoy RJ, Filip DJ, Rodey GE, Rimm AA, Aster RH. Successful transfusion of platelets 'mismatched' for HLA antigens to alloimmunized thrombocytopenic patients. Am J Haemat 1977;2:219-26.
4. Brand A, van Leeuwen A, Eernisse JG, van Rood JJ. Platelet transfusion therapy. Optimal donor selection with a combination of lymphocytotoxicity and platelet fluorescence tests. Blood 1978;51:781-8.
5. Pegels J, Bruynes E, Engelfriet C, von dem Borne AEG Kr. Serological studies in patients on platelet- and granulocyte-substitution therapy. Br J Haemat 1982; 52:59-68.
6. Bonacossa IA, Perchotte M-RY, Olchowecki JK, Schroeder ML. Role of lymphocytotoxicity and Staph-Protein A assays in platelet donor selection. Curr Stud Haematol Blood Transf 1986;52:58-64.
7. Sintnicolaas K, van der Steuyt KJB, van Putten WLJ, Bolhuis RLH. A microplate ELISA for the detection of platelet alloantibodies; comparison with the platelet immunofluorescence test. Br J Haemat 1987;66:363-7.
8. van der Velden KJ, Sintnicolaas K, Löwenberg B. The value of a ^{51}Cr platelet lysis assay as cross-match test in patients with leukemia on platelet transfusion therapy. Br J Haemat 1986;62:635-40.
9. Freedman J, Hooi C, Garbey MB. Prospective platelet cross-matching for selection of compatible random donors. Br J Haemat 1984;56:9-18.

WHITE BLOOD CELL TRANSFUSIONS IN THE IMMUNO-COMPROMISED PATIENTS

A.B. Glassman, P.R. Madyastha

Introduction

Over the past two decades, there has been increased interest in support of the immunocompromised patient. Aggressive chemo and radiation therapy have increased the number of patients who have decreased cellular and humoral immunologic responses. These patients have to be supported by a variety of blood products. Specific interest in this discussion will be directed to the use of granulocytes and monocytes/macrophages in the treatment of the immunocompromised patient. General indications for the use of granulocytes include patients with documented granulocytopenia (counts of less than 500/μl), granulocyte dysfunctions, such as those patients with chronic granulomatous disease and the variety of other causes of neutropenia which can occur (Table 1). Generally, patients who have counts higher than 500 granulocytes/μl have a higher resistance to infection [1]. Granulocytes can be provided

Table 1. General indications for granulocyte transfusions.

1. Patients* with neutropenia and strong clinical or bacteriological evidence of infection unresponsive to antibiotics.
2. Patients with documented granulocytopenia and severe infections.
   a. transfusion should begin within 24 hours of the onset of infections in patients with granulocyte counts of $<100/\mu$l;
   b. transfusion should start in patients with granulocyte counts $<500/\mu$l but $>100/\mu$l if their infection is not improved within 48 hours.
3. Patients with granulocyte dysfunctions.
4. Patients not responding to antibiotic therapy.
5. Patients with fever of unknown origin unresponsive to antibiotics but granulocyte transfusions are generally ineffective.

* The patient should have reasonable expectations of producing adequate granulocytes if the acute infectious episode is successfully treated.

by infusing collected peripheral granulocytes using centrifugal devices and harvesting the equivalent of the number of white cells that would be present in 16-20 single units of blood. Another mechanism for providing granulocyte function would be to collect peripheral stem cells and transfuse the monocyte/macrophages that could be obtained [2,3]. Because of problems with granulocyte antigen matching, subsequent development of antibodies against specific granulocytes [4] and the short half-life of peripheral granulocytes, this therapy cannot be given indefinitely. When successful, the use of peripheral stem cells or monocyte/macrophages can result in the production of granulocytes from the stem cells that are present.

Since providing granulocytes or stem cells presents certain problems, the candidate for granulocyte transfusions should be evaluated and the probability that eventual recovery from the particular neutropenic episode should be substantiated. In those patients in whom bone marrow function is not expected to recover, the stem cells are preferred. The infectious agents that are phagocytized by granulocytes include bacteria (*Haemophilus influenzae, Streptococcus pneumonia, Staphylococcus aureus* and other staphylococcal species), fungi particularly *Candida albicans*, variety of parasites and some viruses, particularly the vesicular stomatitis virus. Parts of these activities (Table 2) are related to the ability of the human polymorphonuclear leukocyte to recognize mannose on the surface of the organism and actively phagocytize that organism. Another way in which phagocytosis is induced, is by the alternative pathway activation of the complement system. This is particularly true when one looks at the fixation of C3 and opsonization of *Staphylococcus aureus* in the presence of normal serum.

Table 2. Role of granulocytes and macrophages (G/M).

1. To be effective, transfused G/M must encounter the infecting organisms.
2. Initially, they enter infected tissue by first adhering to vascular endothelium.
3. Subsequently, they emigrate from the blood stream by chemotaxis.
4. Eventually, they recognize, engulf and kill microorganisms through a variety of intracellular processes.

Objectives

The objectives of this paper are:
1. to discuss the role of granulocytes in the immunocompromised patient;
2. to explore the role and indications of granulocytes in the therapy of the immunocompromised patient;
3. to evaluate the circumstances and indications for the use of monocytes/stem cells in the treatment of the immunocompromised patient; and
4. to explore the therapeutic use of granulocytes or monocytes in adult and pediatric patients.

Granulocytes in the treatment of infection

Transfused granulocytes are thought to function reasonably normal after transfusion if they are obtained fresh and infused rapidly into the patient. Granulocytes can be prepared by cytapheresis. This requires expensive equipment, competent nurses and/or medical technologists and the supervision of a transfusion medicine physician. It takes about 2-4 hours of donor's time in order to collect sufficient granulocytes for therapy. Early in the history of granulocyte therapy, better yields were obtained from patients with chronic myelogenous leukemia [5,6], but a variety of considerations have curtailed the use of these patients. In order to increase the granulocyte yield from normal donors, vigorous exercise and/or the use of steroids 1-4 hours prior to the leukapheresis procedure has been recommended [7,8]. Donors for peripheral granulocytes must meet all other criteria for blood donors (Table 3). Because

Table 3. Protocol followed for the selection of donors.

1. Members of the family are most often sought. Whenever not available, unrelated volunteers are used.
2. All donors should meet the standard requirements and criteria for whole blood donation.
3. Potential donors should have a normal CBC, platelet count and serum albumin.
4. Donors are screened for ABO and Rh compatibility.
5. Leukoagglutinins and lymphocytotoxic antibodies should be absent.
6. A complete history and physical examination are done.
7. Although HLA matching is controversial, typing is done for data collection purposes.
8. Steroids or hydroxyethyl starch is used to increase the granulocyte yield.

of problems with HLA and granulocyte antigen considerations, family donors are most often recommended. Thus far known and identified granulocyte antigens are shown in Table 4. Criteria for granulocyte use should be carefully

Table 4. Granulocyte specific antigens

Specific to neutrophils	Common to all granulocytes
NA1	HGA-3
NA2	9A
NB1	GA, GB, GC
NB2	GR1, GR2
NC1	Cold (G)
ND1	Group 1-3
NE1	Group 1-5

Antigen Mart is present in granulocytes, lymphocytes, monocytes, but not in platelets and erythrocytes [37]. Antigen CNl [38] (neutrophil specific) is present in 31% blacks and <2% whites [Madyastha et al, unpublished]. Four additional and unnamed neutrophil specificities (Lalezari [39]) are not listed.

defined. These include a documented infection unresponsive to adequate combined antibiotic therapy and continued fever and/or clinical infection after the addition of an anti-fungal agent for a minimum of 48 hours. The primary concern remains neutropenia with the granulocyte count of less than 500/μl.

It is extremely costly to provide granulocytes for patients, even for a relatively short length of time [9]. Granulocyte transfusions have not proven effective in patients with localizing infections or with infectious agents other than bacteria. The patient receiving granulocyte transfusions should have a prognosis such that his survival from the acute infection could be expected to result in a satisfactory quality of life for some period of time. The use of granulocytes in children is less stringent. Children are thought to have a much reduced granulocyte reserve in their bone marrow and neonatal medicine specialists recommend prompt use of granulocytes in the neonatal low-birth-weight infant [10,11]. It should be recognized that a significant portion of neonatal granulocytopenia may be associated with antibodies against granulocytes [12-14] and antigens associated with it [15]. In these instances, it is extremely important that these antibodies be identified so that proper granulocytes can be used for greater clinical effect. The clinical response that is evaluated includes reduction in size or the site of infection; for instance, if the patient had pneumonia, clearing of the pneumonia or clearing of the bacteremia at specific sites of infection. Attempts at measuring granulocyte effectiveness by elevations in the peripheral granulocyte count or radiolabeling of the granulocytes are ineffective [16,17]. The number of granulocytes that are infused are too few to give more than a 10 percent rise in peripheral granulocyte count. Labeling of granulocytes with radioisotopes is expensive, time consuming and at best gives only partial information as to the effectiveness of these granulocytes. Indium-111 labeling of granulocytes has been used as a diagnostic test for finding abscesses [18], but is not useful in determining therapy.

Clinical use of granulocytes

Granulocytes must be transfused as soon as possible after collection. In any case, the usual standard is within 24 hours. Granulocytes do not function well after refrigeration. It is recommended that granulocytes be kept at room temperature for a minimal period of time without agitation prior to infusion [19]. The duration, (the number of days) for which granulocyte transfusions should be given remains controversial. It has been recommended that granulocyte concentrates be given daily for at least 4-6 days or until bone marrow recovery occurs. Granulocytes are infused through a standard blood filter. If a patient is a potential recipient for bone marrow, he/she should not receive granulocyte transfusion from the potential bone marrow donor. While granulocyte antigens can be determined and granulocyte antibodies can be assayed for in the laboratory [20-22], this is not a usual clinical procedure. It is recommended that a minimum of $1.5\text{-}2.5 \times 10^{10}$ granulocytes be infused in order to have an adequate dose [23,24]. The granulocytes should be given on the basis of donor red blood cells ABO compatibility. In order to give a sufficient number of granulocytes, approximately 200-400 ml will be required. Various procedures result in varying amounts of red cell contamination of the granulocytes. Leukapheresis requires differential centrifugation and the addition of hydroxyethyl starch (HES) so that better separation can be obtained [25]. Pediatric patients, particularly low-birth weight infants, can be treated with the equivalent number of granulocytes presenting a single unit of whole blood. The number of granulocytes in this case would be 5.7×10^9 cells [26].

Adverse reactions

Adverse reactions to granulocytes are fairly common [27] (Table 5). It has been stated in the literature that as many as 50-60% of all granulocyte recipients will have some sort of transfusion reaction [82]. These include pulmonary reactions which may be related to leukoagglutinins, pre-existing infection, e.g. bacterial pneumonia, fluid overload in patients with marginal cardiovascular reserve or the release of endotoxins after interaction with granulocytes and complement. Febrile and allergic reactions are very common. These are usually mild and may be treated through the use of non-steroidal anti-inflammatory agents, use of meperidine to decrease shaking chills and/or the use of antihistamine [29]. Aspirin is to be avoided because of its concurrent adverse effects on platelet activity. Many of these patients will also have thrombocytopenia and the aspirin may exacerbate the bleeding tendency. Occasionally, steroids may be given prior to granulocyte transfusions particularly if there have been significant and severe respiratory reactions.

Table 5. Complications of granulocyte transfusions.

1. Immunological
   - Graft versus host disease
   - Recipient alloimmunization
   - Febrile non-hymolytic transfusion reactions
2. Transmission of infections
   - CMV
   - Hepatitis
   - HIV
   - Malaria
   - Toxoplasmosis
3. Transfusion associated toxic reactions
   - Hypopyrexia
   - Dyspnea
   - Shaking chills
   - Hypertension
   - Wheezing
   - Pulmonary infiltrates
4. Related to medication for transfusion reactions
   - Allergy
   - Acute pulmonary stress
   - Platelet, granulocyte dysfunctions

A major problem following granulocyte transfusions, particularly in patients with marked immunosuppression is graft vs. host reaction [30,31]. Graft vs. host disease (GVH) is secondary to transfusion of lymphocytes to these immunocompromised patients. The transfused lymphocytes then undergo blast transformation and are active against the cells of the recipient. Manifestations of graft vs. host disease include gastrointestinal, skin, and pulmonary manifestations. There are recommendations that granulocyte concentrations be irradiated with at least 1,500 rad prior to transfusion in the severely immunocompromised patient to decrease the incidence of GvHD [32,33].

Granulocyte transfusions have not been found effective for fungal or viral infections. It is of note, however, that there have been reports of severe pulmonary infiltration and acute respiratory stress secondary to the infusion of granulocytes in patients who are receiving amphotericin B [34]. The reason for this complication is not known, but is well recognized and should be respected and remembered for those that are contemplating granulocyte therapy.

There has been a decreased use of granulocyte transfusions over the past three years in our institution. Only one instance of granulocyte transfusions in an adult has been performed over the past two years. Granulocyte transfusions are still used although less frequently in the neonatal intensive care unit in our institution. The total number of granulocyte transfusions given at the Medical University of South Carolina last year was down to one patient for a total of 11 transfusions.

Stem cells and monocyte collections and use

The use of stem cells and/or monocytes/macrophages from the circulating blood is an area of increasing interest. It has been estimated that the equivalent of one-half the number of cells from a bone marrow transplant can be collected from circulating peripheral stem cells by the use of centrifugal leukapheresis apparatus. The dose for peripheral stem cells in an adult is not yet settled upon, but probably should be in the range of 3×10^9 [35]. It is thought to be well within the capabilities of leukapheresis apparatus to collect sufficient stem cells from an adult to provide the equivalent of a bone marrow transplant quantity to a low-birth-weight neonate. Peripheral stem cells collected in this way must be given as soon after being obtained as possible. They cannot be stored in the refrigerator. They must be stored at room temperature without agitation and used as quickly as possible with infusion through a standard blood filter. The use of microaggregate filters may remove sufficient number of stem cells to decrease the effective dose. As with peripheral granulocytes, proper ABO and Rh grouping as well as an antibody screen, hepatitis B surface antigen and human immunodeficiency virus testing should be done. The donor should meet all the criteria that a normal blood donor otherwise would. The use of HES in the separation of stem cells has been advocated but experience over long term is lacking as to whether this would have an adverse affect on the subsequent function and ability of these stem cells to produce granulocyte colonies. The use of stem cells or monocyte transfusions brings up the problem of HLA and granulocyte antigen testing as was mentioned under peripheral granulocytes. Prospective donors should not have been previous granulocyte donors to the same patient as there may be a sensitization to the leukocyte antigens or a sensitization to the granulocyte antigens. The use of corticosteroids to increase peripheral counts does not seem to be necessary or effective when collecting peripheral stem cells. Overall, the clinical utility of stem cells is in its early infancy as far as evaluation is concerned. It would seem as though it would be cost effective and optimal if sufficient numbers of stem cells or monocytes could be collected from a prospective donor by a leukapheresis procedure [35]. This would avoid the cost of hospitalization for obtaining bone marrow material from these prospective donors. Whether the long range problems identifying and obtaining adequate stem cells from the peripheral blood and documentation of their function as colony forming cells remains for the future.

Summary and conclusions

The immunocompromised patient for the purpose of granulocyte transfusion is one with granulocytopenia of less than 500 neutrophils/μl. An infected immunocompromised patient is one who has been treated with appropriate antibiotics and antifungal agents without a clinical response. In those instances, the use of granulocytes may be indicated. This is a costly procedure and has potential adverse clinical problems of severe pulmonary reactions and the development of antibodies by the recipient. Most clinical services now believe that the infected granulocytopenic patient should be treated vigorously with a wide range of antibiotics. The cost effectiveness of the use of granulocytes is such that it would require $200,000 or more per year to sustain a granulocytopenic patient [9]. This does not take into account the fact that many recipients would be refactory because of the development of antibodies long before this money would be expended. There are difficulties in obtaining donors, matching for HLA and granulocyte antigens, as well as the difficulty in storing granulocytes. Granulocytes and stem cells must be obtained and used very soon after they are procured. Obtaining stem cells or monocytes from the peripheral blood may be a possible alternative for bone marrow transplantation in the future. The use of granulocytes in the pediatric neonatal group remains the primary indication, today. Generally, there has been decreased use in adults with a continued interest for granulocytes in the neutropenic child. Granulocytes, monocytes and stem cells may be useful for treatment of the infected immunocompromised patient. Procurement, storage, donor-recipient matching and cost of these products remain problems that must be examined and evaluated.

References

1. BodeyGP, Buckley M, Sathe US, Freireich EJ. Quantitative relationships between circulating leukocytes and infection in patients with acute leukemia. Ann Intern Med 1966;64:328-40.
2. Goldman JM, Catovsky D, Hows J, Spiers ASD, Galton DAG. Cryopreserved peripheral blood cells functioning as autografts in patients with chronic granulocytic leukemia in transformation. Brit Med Journal 1979;1:1310-3.
3. Djerassi I, Kim JS, Suvansri U. Harvesting of human monocytes (macrophages) as by - product of filtration leukapheresis. Proc Amer Ass Cancer Res 1973;14:103.

4. Goldstein IM, Eyre HJ, Terasaki PI, Henderson ES, Graw RG. Leukocyte transformations: Role of leukocyte alloantibodies in determining transfusion response. Transfusion 1971;11:19-24.
5. Schwarzenberg L, Mathe G, Amiel JL. Study of factors determining the usefulness and complications of leukocyte transfusion. Am J Med 1967;43:206-13.
6. Freireich EJ, Levin RH, Whang J et al. The function and fate of transfused leukocytes from donors with chronic myelocytic leukemia in leukopenic recipients. Ann NY Acad Sci 1964;113:1081-9.
7. Shoji M, Vogler WR. Effects of hydrocortisone on the yield and bactericidal function of granulocytes collected by continuous flow centrifugation. Blood 1974;44: 435-43.
8. Soderlund I, Engstedt L, Paleus S, Unger P. Induction of leukocytosis by means of hydrocortisone and/or muscular excercise. In: Goldman J, Lowenthal RM (eds). Leukocytes: Separation, collection and transfusion. London: Academic Press 1975:97-103.
9. Rosenshein MS, Farewell VT, Price TH, Larson EB, Dale DC. The cost effectiveness of therapeutic and prophylactic leukocyte transfusions. N Engl J Med 1980;302:1058-62.
10. Erdman SH, Christensen RD, Brandley PP et al. The supply and release of storage neutrophils: A developmental study. Biol Neonate 1982;41:132-7.
11. Christensen R, Anstall HB, Rothstein G. Review. Deficiencies in the neutrophil system of newborn infants, and the use of leukocyte transfusions in the treatment of neonatal sepsis. J Clin Apheresis 1982;1:33-41.
12. Lalezari P, Radel E. Neutrophil specific antigens: Immunology and clinical significance. Sem Hematol 1974;11:281-90.
13. Levine DH, Madyastha PR. Immune neonatal neutropenia. Am J Perinatol 1986;3:231-3.
14. Madyastha PR, Glassman AB, Groves WE, Levine DH, Davidson R. A computerized system for the identification of alloimmune neutropenia in neonates. Comp Meth Progr Biomed 1985;20:241-7.
15. Madyastha PR, Glassman AB, Levine DH. Incidence of neutrophil antigens on human cord neutrophils. Am J Repro Immunol 1984;6:124-7.
16. Thakur ML, Lavender JP, Arnot RN, Silvester DJ, Segal AW. Indium-III-labelled autologous leukocytes in man. J Nucl Med 1977;18:1014-21.
17. Weiblen BJ, Forstrom L, McCullough J. Studies of the kinetics of Indium-III-labelled granulocytes. J Lab Clin Med 1979;94:246-55.
18. Segal AW, Arnot RN, Thakur ML, Lavender JP. Indium-III-labelled leukocyte for localization of abscesses. Lancet 1976;ii:1056-8.
19. McCullough J, Weiblen BJ, Peterson PK, Quie PG. Effect of temperature on granulocyte preservation. Blood 1978;52:301-10.
20. Lalezari P, Pryce SC. Detection of neutrophil and platelet antibodies in immunologically induced neutropenia and thrombocytopenia. In: Rose NR, Friedmann H (eds) Manual of clinical immunology. Washington, DC: American Society of Microbiology 1980:744-9.
21. Madyastha PR, Kyong CU, Darby CP, Genco PV et al. Role of neutrophil antigen NA1 in an infant with autoimmune neutropenia. Am J Dis Child 1982;136: 718-21.
22. Ducos R, Madyastha PR, Warrier RP, Glassman AB, Shirley LR. Neutrophil agglutinins in idiopathic chronic neutropenia of early childhood. Am J Dis Child 1986;140:65-8.
23. Higny DJ, Burnette D. Granulocyte transfusion. Current status. Blood 1980;55: 2-8.

24. Winton EF, Moffitt S, Vogler WR, Mallard HE, Lawson DH, Malcom LG, Monfagne ML. Influence of quantity of granulocytes transfused on response. In: Cytapheresis and plasma Exchange: Clinical indications. New York: Alan R. Liss 1982:75-91.
25. Mishler JM, Hadlock DC, Fortuny IE, Nicora RA, McCullough JJ. Increased efficiency of leukocyte collection by the addition of hydroxyethyl starch to the continuous flow centrifuge. Blood 1974;44:571-81.
26. Buchholz DH, Schiffer CA, Wiernik PH et al. Granulocyte harvest for transfusion: Donor response to repeated leukapheresis. Transfusion 1975;15:96-106.
27. Schiffer CA, Aisner J, Daly PA, Schimpff SC, Wiernik PH. Alloimmunization following prophylactic granulocyte transfusion. Blood 1979;54:766-74.
28. Morse EE, Freireich EJ, Carbone PP, Bronson W, Frei E. The transfusion of leukocytes from donors with chronic myelogenous leukemia to patients with leukopenia. Transfusion 1966;6:183-92.
29. Higby DJ, Burnett D, Ruppert K, Henderson ES, Cohen E. Granulocyte transfusions: Experience at Rosewell Park Memorial Institute. In: The granulocytes: Function and clinical utilization. New York: Alan R. Liss 1977:293-304.
30. Ford JM, Lecey JJ, Cullen MH, Tobias JS, Lister TA. Fatal graft-versus-host disease following transfusion of granulocytes from normal donors. Lancet 1976;ii: 1167-9.
31. Rosen RC, Huestis DW, Corrigan JJ jr. Acute leukemia and granulocyte transfusion: fatal graft-vs-host reaction following transfusion of cells obtained from normal donors. J Pediatr 1978;93:268-70.
32. McCullough J, Benson S, Yunis E, Quic P. Effect of blood bank storage on leukocyte function. Lancet 1969;ii:1333-7.
33. Button LN, de Wolf WC, Newburger PE, Jacobson MS, Kevy SV. The effects of irradiation on blood components. Transfusion 1981;21:419-26.
34. Wright DG, Robichaud KJ, Pizzo P, Deisserothe AB. Lethal pulmonary reactions associated with the combined use of amphotericin B and leukocyte transfusions. N Engl J Med 1981;304:1185-9.
35. Djerassi I, Kim JS, Suvansri U, Cicsielka W, Lohrke J. Filtration leukapheresis: Principles and techniques for harvesting and transfusion of filtered granulocytes and monocytes. In: Goldman JM, Lowenthal RM (eds). Leukocytes: separation, collection and transfusions. London: Academic Press 1975:123-36.
36. Djerassi I, Kim JS, Suvansri U. Harvesting of human monocytes (macrophages) as by-product of filtration leukapheresis. Proc Amer Ass Cancer Res 1973;14:103.
37. Lalezari P. Granulocyte antigen systems. In: Engelfriet CP, van Loghem JJ, von dem Borne AEG Kr (eds). Immune-hematology. Amsterdam: Elsevier Science Publ. BV 1984:33-43.
38. Kline WE, Press C, Clay ME, McCullough JJ. Studies of sera defining a new granulocyte antigen. Transfusion (Abst) 1982;22:428.
39. Madyastha PR, Glassman AB, Levine DH et al. Identification of new neutrophil antigen (CNI) more prevalent among American Blacks. Transfusion (Abst) 1983; 23:426.

IMMUNIZATION WITH ANTIGEN-BOUND ANTIBODY: AN EXPERIMENTAL APPROACH TO PREVENTION OF SENSITIZATION TO ALLOGENEIC BLOOD CELLS

P. Terness, C. Süsal, G. Opelz

Introduction

As no two humans, except identical twins, have the same genetic makeup, a blood transfusion exposes a patient to numerous 'foreign' antigens. Antibodies may develop to any of the donor blood components, days, weeks, or months after transfusion [1]. Antibodies may cause adverse reactions and lower the therapeutic effect of transfused blood components.

In the majority of recipients of multiple random donor platelet transfusions, the degree of alloimmunization increases with the number of transfusions while platelet survival becomes progressively shorter. According to Shulman [2] platelet antibodies can be detected in 5% of patients who received one to 10 transfusions, in 24% who received 25-50 transfusions, and in 80% who received more than 100 transfusions.

Even if platelet transfusions are matched for HLA antigens, a recipient may still develop antibodies to other incompatible antigens. For example, with repeated transfusions of HLA-A and -B compatible thrombocytes, transfusions became inefficient in approximately 25% of cases [3].

It can be concluded that alloimmunization represents the most important long-term complication of platelet transfusion.

Alloimmunization is also a major problem in leukocyte transfusion. The majority of patients with multiple granulocyte transfusions will develop anti-granulocyte antibodies [4] which frequently causes transfusion reactions [5]. Brittingham and Chaplin have shown that, in patients with leukoagglutinins, the transfusion of blood fraction containing more than 90% of the buffy coat produced a severe febrile reaction, whereas the transfusion, from the same bottle of blood, of red cells and plasma containing less than 10% of the buffy coat caused no reaction [6].

In experiments in dogs it was shown that injection of non-matched granulocytes into sensitized granulocytopenic recipients results in no cell migration to skin chambers, markedly decreased granulocyte recovery, and accompanying fall in platelet counts [7].

A special problem is the sensitization of kidney graft recipients by pretransplant blood transfusion. Following random-donor transfusions, a small but significant number of patients develop broadly reacting lymphocytotoxic antibodies [8,9]. With donor-specific transfusions, which are often administered to potential recipients of related-donor transplants, the risk of significant humoral sensitization is much higher. In most statistics, approximately one-third of the recipients are reported to develop antibodies against the donor

[10,11]. If antibodies are produced against the potential kidney donor (positive cross-match), the transplant cannot be performed because of a high risk of hyperacute antibody-mediated graft rejection [12].

Our goal was to develop a clinically relevant method of suppression of cytotoxic antibody response to allogeneic blood components. In experiments in rats we were able to show that pretreatment of animals with allogeneic blood cells that were coated with homologous or heterologous antibodies resulted in a suppression of antibody responses to subsequent transfusions [13-15]. While other models of antibody feedback inhibition [16-19] mainly addressed the specific primary antibody response or kidney graft survival, we focused on the suppression of antibody responses to repeated booster transfusions from specific or third party donors.

Preparation of antigen-bound antibody

Allogeneic rat blood cells were incubated at room temperature with recipient-anti-donor serum or monoclonal antibody (homologous), or with rabbit anti-rat lymphocyte serum (ALS heterologous). Excess antibody was washed out after incubation and cells were injected i.v. [13].

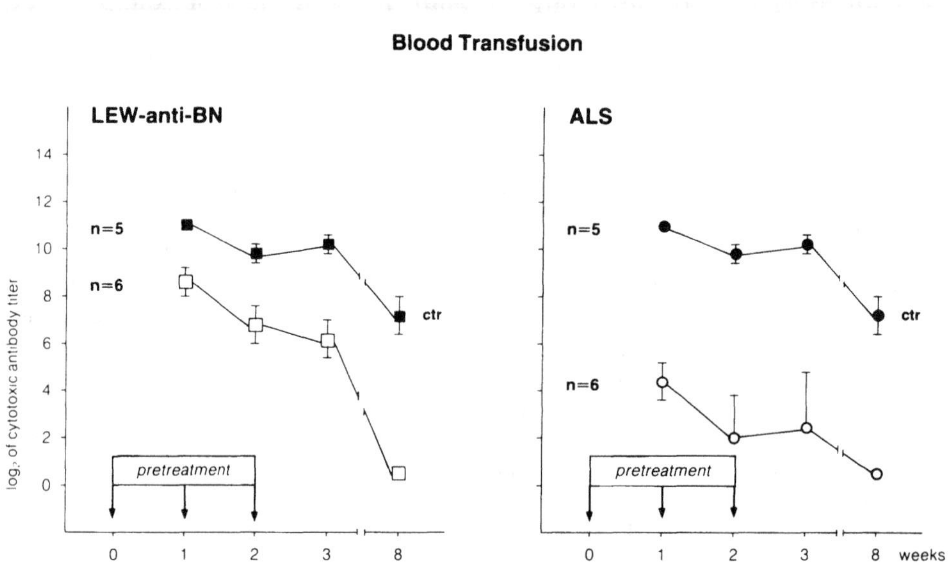

Figure 1. LEW rats were transfused three times with antibody-coated BN blood cells (1 ml BN blood + 0.05 ml LEW-anti-BN serum or 0.025 ml ALS). Controls were transfused with 1 ml BN ($p<0.01$). Cytotoxic antibody titers (means ± SD) are shown.

Immunization with antigen-bound antibody

Strong incompatible donor-recipient combinations were used (BN→LEW, DA→LEW, WF→LEW, DA→AO). Whole blood, leukocyte (mononuclear cells), or thrombocytes were transfused.

Lymphocytotoxic antibodies were determined by an immunofluorescence microcytotoxicity technique [13]. Anti-thrombocyte antibodies were determined by a platelet complement fixation microtechnique [20].

Graft-versus-host (GvH) reaction was measured in a popliteal lymph node weight assay as described by Ford et al. [21].

Suppression of antibody response to allogeneic blood

When LEW rats were transfused three times with LEW-anti-BN- or ALS-coated blood cells the antibody response became progressively lower, reaching an almost complete suppression in the ALS-group (Fig. 1).

Suppression in the LEW-anti-BN group could be made stronger by increasing (4-10×) the amount of LEW-anti-BN serum [13].

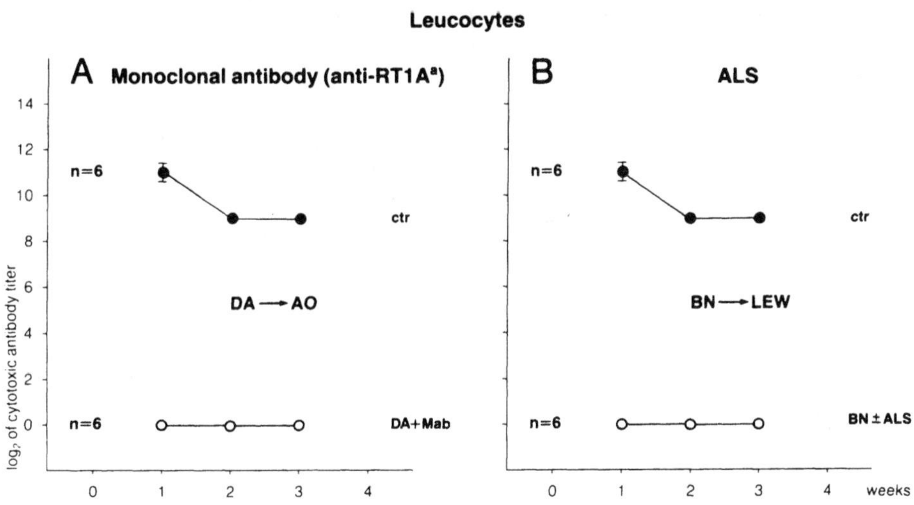

Figure 2. (A) AO rats were transfused on day 0 with 5×10^6DA leukocytes preincubated with 2.5-5 μg of three monoclonal anti-RT 1A^a antibodies. Controls were transfused with 5×10^6 DA leukocytes only.
(B) LEW rats received 5×10^6 BN leukocytes pretreated with 0.1 ml ALS; controls received leukocytes only.

Completely suppressed antibody response to allogeneic leukocytes

In one experiment (Fig. 2A) AO recipients received a transfusion with DA leukocytes preincubated with three different AO-anti-DA (class I MHC antigen) monoclonal antibodies. In another experiment (Fig. 2B) LEW rats were transfused with BN cells coated with ALS. Controls consisted of animals transfused with untreated leukocytes. No anti-leukocyte antibodies could be detected in any preconditioned group.

Complete suppression of anti-thrombocyte antibody response

LEW rates were immunized three times with BN leukocytes preincubated with ALS. Controls were injected with untreated leukocytes. Three weeks later the animals received one transfusion of BN platelets.

Following the pretreatment of animals with antibody-coated leukocytes subsequent thrombocyte-transfusion did not elicite an antibody response (neither anti-leukocyte, nor anti-transfusion) (Fig. 3).

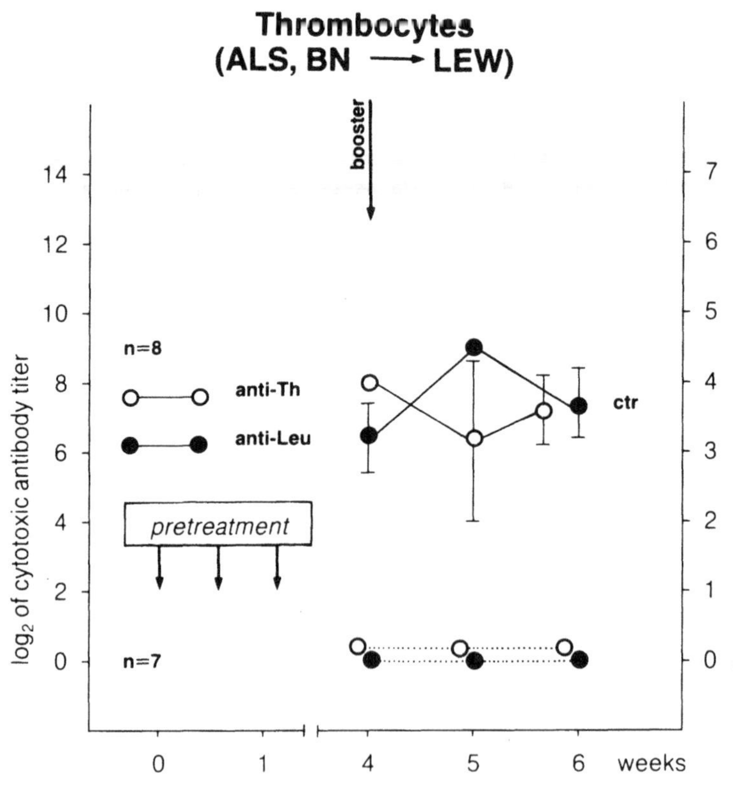

Figure 3. LEW rates were immunized three times with 5×10^6 BN leukocytes only (controls) or leukocytes preincubated with 0.05 ml ALS. Three weeks later animals were boosted with 10^9 BN thrombocytes. Titers of cytotoxic anti-leukocyte antibody and scores of platelet complement fixation reaction (means ± SD) are shown.

Even with repeated booster transfusions the suppression is not abrogated

The question was raised whether suppression of the antibody response in preconditioned animals persists after repeated booster transfusions with untreated cells (Fig. 4).

Our experiments showed that the suppression, once induced could not be abrogated by repeated boosters. Suppression was almost complete in the ALS group. The weaker suppression seen in the LEW-anti-BN group might be due to the smaller amount of antiserum. In previous experiments [13] we showed that the suppressive effect was dose-dependent within certain limits. A total suppression of secondary antibody response was achieved by increasing the amount of LEW-anti-BN serum to 0.2 ml (see Fig. 6A)(in the experiment present in Fig. 4 only 0.05 ml were used).

There is no general immunization schedule for prevention of sensitization

In our experiments the pretreatment had to be adjusted to the antigen (whole blood, leukocytes, thrombocytes) to which suppression was induced, as well as to the strain combination.

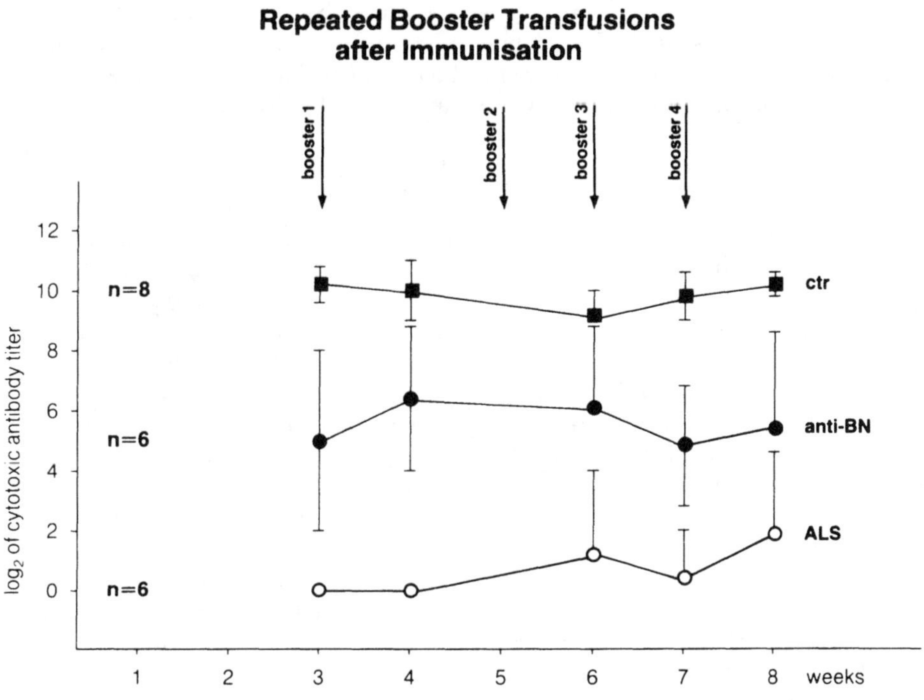

Figure 4. One week after three transfusions of 1 ml BN blood preincubated with 0.05 ml LEW-anti-BN serum or 0.025 ml ALS, LEW rats were boosted repeatedly with 1 ml BN blood. Controls were transfused with BN blood only. Mean cytotoxic antibody titers ± SD are shown (<0.01).

Table 1. Transfer of suppressive activity with serum.

Days after serum transfer	**Pretreatment of LEW rats**	
	Normal LEW serum + BN blood (n=6)	**Suppressive serum + BN blood (n=6)**
7	10.5±0.5	2.2±1.9
14	9.5±0.5	0.7±1.6
21	8.7±0.5	1.2±1.8

Suppressive serum was obtained from LEW rats which were pretreated with antibody-coated cells (1 ml BN cells + 0.2 ml LEW-anti-BN serum)(means of log2 of cytotoxic antibody titers ± SD are given; $p < 10^{-3}$).

The parameters which proved influential on the degree of suppression for a given antigen and strain combination were: dose and origin of antibody and immunization schedule.

With respect to whole blood transfusions, good suppression was obtained both with homologous and heterologous antiserum, whereas in the platelet transfusion model only ALS (heterologous) seemed to work well.

When immunizing animals only once with ALS-coated cells [13], weak or no suppression was achieved. When injecting the same immunogen three times [14] a drastic suppression was induced. With LEW-anti-BN serum the effect was as strong after one immunization as after three.

Active suppression or lack of antibody response?

We were concerned that unresponsiveness was a simple lack of antibody response rather than a real suppression. The injected allogeneic cells coated by antibody might have been lysed in the recipient. It seemed also possible that exogenous antibodies had masked antigens so that they 'could not be seen' by the rescipient's immune system or that transfused cells had rapidly deviated into the macrophage system.

The following findings argue against a simple lack of antibody response:

1. Transfer of suppressive activity with serum or cells (Tables 1,2). These findings show that a suppressive factor and suppressive cells are involved in the mechanism of unresponsiveness. These results are not compatible with a simple lack of antibody response.

2. Reduced GvH activity in preconditioned animals. If lack of antibody response by antigen destruction (or a similar mechanism) were the explanation for the observed unresponssiveness, pretreated animals would have presented the same GvH reaction as untreated animals. As shown in Figure 5 this was not the case.

3. Prolonged kidney graft survival in pretreated animals. We observed [22] in a strongly incompatible donor-recipient combination (BN→LEW) that transfusion with antibody-coated donor cells leads to a significant prolonga-

Table 2. Transfer of suppressive activity with spleen cells.

Days after cell transfer	Pretreatment of LEW rats		
	Controls no pretreatment	(BN + anti-BN)×3 (n=6)	(BN + ALS)×3 (n=8)
7	10.1±0.6	7.7±0.5	8.0±0.5
14	8.7±1.0	5.8±1.1	6.1±0.6
21	6.6±1.0	1.0±2.2	4.2±2.1

LEW rats were pretreated with antibody-coated BN cells (1 ml BN blood, 0.2 ml LEW-anti-BN, 0.025 ml ALS) and 5×10^7 spleen cells were transfused into syngeneic animals (log2 of cytotoxic antibody titers ± SD; $p<0.01$).

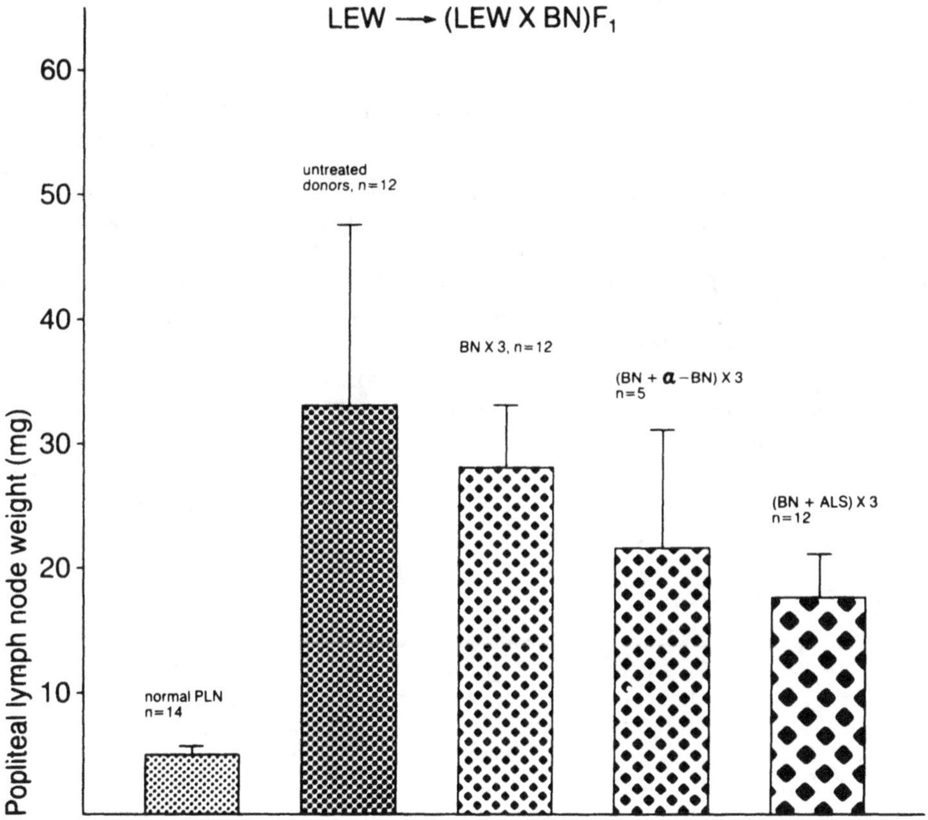

Figure 5. Donor LEW rats were immunized with 1 ml untreated or antibody-pretreated BN blood (0.2 ml LEW-anti-BN serum or 0.025 ml ALS). One week later spleen cells were tested in a GvH assay in hybrid (LEW×BN)F1 rats. ALS-coated cells induced a strong suppression ($p<10^{-4}$), anti-BN coated cells induced a weaker suppression (significant when compared to untreated controls, $p<0.05$) of Gvh.

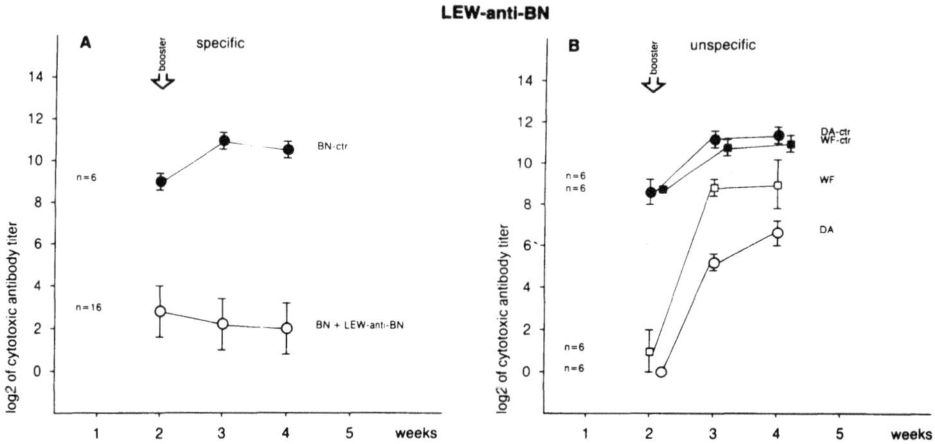

Figure 6. LEW rats were transfused first with 1 ml BN blood pretreated with 0.2 ml LEW-anti-BN serum. Controls received untreated BN blood. Animals were boosted thereafter with either 1 ml BN (A) or DA or WF blood (B). Suppression was strongest with the specific BN booster, but a significant reduction was also seen with DA or WF ($p < 4 \times 10^{-3}$). Means of log2 of antibody titers ± SD are given.

tion of kidney graft survival (median survival time 67 days, untreated controls 9 days). If a lack of exposure to antigen had occurred, the preconditioned group would have had the same kidney graft survival as the untreated group.

4. Suppression of secondary antibody response after immunization with antibody-coated cells. The persistence of unresponsiveness even after repeated boosters with allogeneic cells (Fig. 5) can only be explained by an active suppressive mechanism.

We conclude that an active immunologic suppression is induced by immunization with antigen-bound antibody.

Specificity of suppression

The question was raised whether suppression was specific or nonspecific. For instance, if LEW rats are immunized with antibody-coated BN cells, can suppression be induced only to BN antigens or does the suppression extend to third party cells?

It was shown by others [23,24] that injection of allogeneic cells on whom only some antigens were coated, induced an unresponsiveness both to antibody-coated and uncoated antigens.

In our experiments LEW rats injected with BN cells coated with anti-BN antibody were boosted with unrelated third party cells (DA, WF)(Fig. 6B). A partial but significant suppression was noted of the response to both DA and WF cells. It seems possible that by modifying the immunization schedule

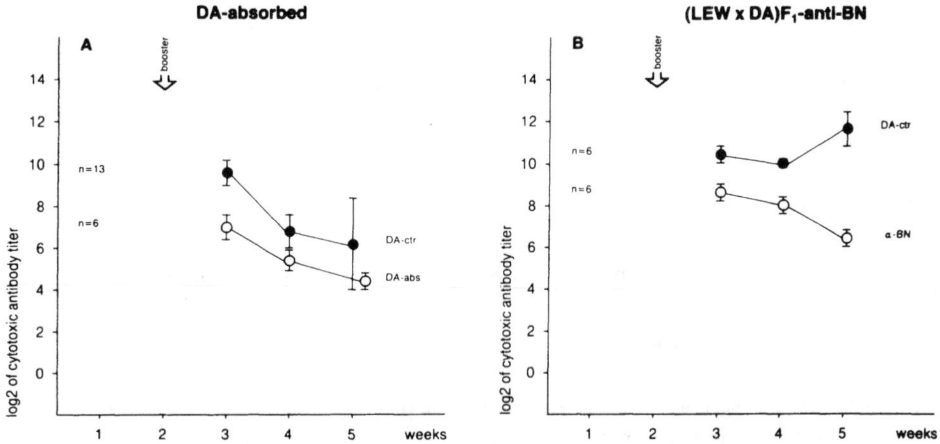

Figure 7. (A) LEW rats were injected with 0.1 ml BN blood preincubated with 0.1 ml DA-absorbed LEW-anti-BN serum or BN blood only (controls) and boosted two weeks later with 0.1 ml DA blood. Cytotoxic antibody titers were significantly suppressed in antibody-coated cell preconditioned animals ($p<3\times10^{-3}$).
(B) 1 ml BN blood cells were incubated with 0.2 ml (LEW×BN)F1-anti-BN serum. This serum had no cross-reactivity with DA cells. Antibody-coated BN cells were injected into LEW rats. Controls were injected with untreated BN blood. Two weeks later animals were boosted with DA blood. The antibody response was reduced in preconditioned animals as compared to controls ($p<2\times10^{-3}$).

a complete suppression could be induced also against third party cells. If further experiments would confirm this, a suppression induced with cells from donor 'A' could be extended to cells from donor 'B' under certain circumstances.

A further question concerns the specificity of exogenous antibody used for induction of suppression. Is it possible to induce a suppression against donor 'B' using an 'anti-A antibody' which does not cross-react with cells 'B'?

Heyman and Wigzell [25] immunized mice with sheep red blood cells (SRBC) and different anti-SRBC monoclonal antibodies. Some of the antibodies cross-reacted with goat red blood cells (GRBC), others did not. The anti-SRBC and anti-GRBC responses were suppressed in parallel regardless of whether or not the monoclonal reacted with GRBC.

Our LEW-anti-BN serum cross-reacted both with DA and WF cells. To test the role of specificity of exogenous antibody a non-cross-reactive anti-BN antibody was produced.

In the experiment shown in Figure 7A the anti-DA activity of our cross-reacting LEW-anti-BN antibody was absorbed out. Using that antibody, a weak but significant suppression against DA cells was found. The experiment is not conclusive since, even after extensive absorption, minute undetectable amounts of anti-DA antibody might have persisted. To eliminate this possibility an anti-BN antibody was produced immunizing (LEW×DA)F1 hybrid rats with BN cells. By definition, this antibody could not cross-react with DA cells. In the experiment shown in Figure 7B a significant suppression of anti-DA activity was achieved with this antibody.

Although the suppression achieved with these non-cross-reactive antibodies was not strong, the results prove that it is possible to induce suppression with an antibody that has no activity against third party donor cells.

Mechanism of suppression

Which could be the mechanism mediating suppression in this model?

Antigen-reactive cell opsonization

A mechanism of antibody-mediated immune suppression which could partly explain our data is the 'antigen-reactive cell opsonization' (ARCO) proposed by Hutchinson and Zola [26]. According tot his hypothesis, the recipient's lymphocytes (antigen-reactive cells) react with the determinant of the injected antigen that is not occupied by exogenous antibody. The exogenous antibody attached to the antigen binds the macrophages via its Fc portion. This binding leads to an activation of macrophages and to the subsequent destruction of recipient lymphocytes attached to the antigen.

Fc-dependent B cell inactivation

Another model of immunoregulation by antibody was proposed by Sinclair and Chan [27]. They suggested that the recipient's B cells interact with the free determinants of donor antigen (not covered by the exogenous antibody). The exogenous antibody which is bound to other determinants on the same antigen would inactivate the recipient's B cells. This inactivation would be induced by binding of the antibody's Fc portion to the Fc-receptor of B cells.

Both hypotheses do not require specific antibody for induction of suppression, which is in line with the results obtained in our experiments.

Anti-idiotypic antibodies

A mechanism which must be considered is mediation of suppression by anti-idiotypic antibodies.

It has been shown that anti-idiotypic antibodies administered to mice can suppress B cell activity [28-31]. Similarly, it was shown in man that anti-idiotypic antibodies can inhibit immunoglobulin synthesis of normal [32-34] and malignant [35] lymphocytes in vitro.

Whereas induction of anti-idiotypic antibodies might serve as a hypothesis for specific suppression in our experiments, it is difficult to conceive that the observed suppression against third party donors would be produced by anti-idiotypic antibodies.

Nonspecific suppressive serum factor

Based on our findings we proposed a further mechanism whereby suppression might be induced by treatment with antigen-bound antibody.

Before considering this mechanism it will be helpful to review some of our findings:

1. Pretreatment of rats with antigen-bound antibody produced suppression to subsequent boosters with the same antigen. Pretreatment under the same conditions with either antigen or antibody resulted in a weak or no suppression. That means that the induction of suppression is related in some way to the binding of antibody to antigen.

2. The specificity of suppression does not seem to be limited by the specificity of antibody or antigen by which it was induced.

3. The suppressive activity can be better transferred by serum than by cells. This finding suggests that a suppressive serum factor is involved.

These results raised the question whether an unspecific factor induced by antigen-bound antibody could be responsible for mediation of suppression.

If binding of immunoglobulin (Ig) to antigen is a precondition for the effective induction of suppression, let us examine what happens when antibody binds to antigen.

It is known that binding of Ig to antigen may trigger biological activities like complement activation or phagocytosis [36-41]. Consequently there is a difference with functional implications between bound and unbound Ig.

There is evidence that antigen binding induces a conformational change in the Fc region of antibody. Mota et al [42] showed that antigen-antibody binding exposes a new binding site for protein A of *Staphylococcus aureus* (SpA). As SpA binds to the Fc part of Ig, the conformational change must take place in that region.

The new site of Ig created by antigen binding seems to be immunogenic. Brown and Bekisz [43] induced anti-human IgG antibody by immunizing rabbits with antigen bound Ig. Rabbits had been made tolerant against unbound human IgG before immunization. The raised antibodies reacted only with antigen-bound IgG (not with unbound). They recognized a neoantigen in the IgG structure which appeared following antigen binding.

Nemazee and Sato [44] described monoclonal antibodies that had binding specificity for autologous Ig bound to antigen. These antibodies arose as a natural response to a new antigenic determinant present in the antibody-antigen complex recognized as 'foreign' by the immune system.

We raised the question whether anti-neo-Ig antibody could be involved in the mediation of unspecific suppression induced by antigen-antibody complexes as seen in our experiments.

Some of our findings support this hypothesis:

1. The serum of LEW rats pretreated with BN cells + anti-BN antibody suppressed not only anti-BN (specific) but also anti-DA and anti-WF activity (unspecific). It seems that this serum contains an unspecific suppressive factor. With respect to BN- and DA-suppression chromatographic separations have shown that the suppressive factor is contained in the IgG fraction.

2. Preliminary results have shown that serum of rats pretreated with antigen-bound rat Ig contains an antibody which binds to antigen-bound rabbit Ig. If one admits the existence of anti-neo-Ig antibody, such unspecific binding to antigen-bound Ig across species can be explained. Brown and Bekisz [43] demonstrated that their rabbit anti-human neo-IgG bound to immune complexes of human IgG with various antigens. The specificity of anti-neo-IgG was not limited to the antigen or to the antibody it was induced with.

3. Preliminary data obtained in hybrid rats are concordant with the hypothesis of an unspecific regulatory factor induced by antigen-bound antibody. Hybrid (LEW×BN)F1 rats were immunized with BN cells coated with LEW-anti-BN antibody. In this system both injected cells and antibody were derived from parental animals and must consequently be accepted as 'self' by F1 recipients. Under these conditions either anti-idiotypic antibodies or antibodies against an 'antigenically modified' Ig (induced by binding of Ig to antigen) could be raised. If anti-idiotypic antibodies were induced, the serum of pretreated animals would specifically suppress the anti-BN response. If an unspecific factor were induced, it would suppress the antibody response against third party cells.

To test the latter possibility serum of immunized hybrid rats was transferred into syngeneic recipients. The recipients were injected concomitantly with DA blood cells (unrelated third party cells). The anti-DA antibody response was suppressed approximately 35% as compared to controls.

These data cannot be considered definitive. It is possible, for instance, that specific suppression induced by IgG would be mediated by anti-idiotypic antibodies while unspecific suppression would be an 'IgG effect' as described in humans [45], regardless of whether or not the animals were pretreated with antigen-bound antibody.

In our model the possibility must also be considered that treatment with immune complexes induces suppressive lymphokines. It is known that B lymphocytes secrete regulatory factors including not only those capable of enhancing but also of suppressing further B cell Ig production. Suzuki et al [46] described a lymphokine termed suppressive B cell factor that is released by B cells after binding of immune complexes. The factor suppresses the proliferation of B cells. A similar lymphokine capable of suppressing a human polyclonal antibody-forming cell response was described by Pisko et al. [47]. The factor was produced by B lymphocytes after stimulation with heat-aggregated IgG, a model for immune complexes.

Alternative, suppressive T cells [48], natural killer cells [49,50], or monocytes/macrophages [51] may all be involved in the suppression of antibody response by immune complexes.

Why are some antibodies suppressive and others are not?

It seems that some characteristics of the exogenous antibody play a role in the induction of suppression.

Brüggemann and Rajewsky [52] have shown that antibody feedback inhibition depends on the affinity of exogenous antibody for antigen. In general the antibodies with the highest affinity inhibit best. Similar results were reported by Heyman and Wigzell [25].

The number of antigenic sites recognized by antibody on the foreign cell was shown to correlate with the degree of suppression [25]. This finding is in accordance with our own data. We found that by incubating allogeneic cells with one monoclonal antibody a partial suppression was achieved; incubating the cells with 3 monoclonal antibodies with related specificities (anti-MHC class I), i.e. increasing the density of antibodies on the cell surface, a complete suppression was induced.

While antibody affinity and density on the cell surface seems to be important, it was shown that antibody induced suppression is not dependent on a particular Ig subclass [25,52,53].

We could imagine a model of feedback inhibition of antibody synthesis depending on the density and affinity of endogenous antibody.

It was shown that as immunization proceeds the affinity of secreted antibodies continuously increases [54]; it can be assumed that the density of antibodies on the cell surface also increases. In other words, endogenous antibodies gain properties which are known to confer suppressive capacity. Such high affinity antibodies may 'down regulate' further antibody production perhaps by an induction of suppressive serum factors (lymphokines, suppressive IgG, etc.).

The hypothesis advanced here is in accordance with our previous finding [55] that repeated transfusions of rats with allogeneic blood led to a successive decrease of antibody production. After 15 transfusions no antibody titer could be detected.

As already discussed several hypotheses can be used to explain the induction of suppression by antigen-bound antibody. It is possible that antigen-bound antibody exerts its suppressive effect at several levels and that various hypotheses explain part of a complex mechanism of interactions.

Conclusions

1. Primary antibody response can be suppressed by coating the blood cells with antibodies prior to transfusion.
2. Even with repeated booster transfusions the induced suppression is not abrogated.
3. The immunization schedule for induction of suppression must be adjusted to the type of allogeneic cells and to the donor-recipient combination.
4. An active suppression and not a lack of antibody response is induced by immunization with antigen-bound antibody.
5. Injecting third party cells following immunization with antibody-coated donor cells still shows a partial but significant suppression.
6. The mechanism of suppression requires further elucidation. ARCO [26], Fc-dependent B cell inactivation [27], anti-idiotypic antibodies, or the induction of unspecific suppressive factors (lymphokines, IgG) all must be considered.

References

1. Holland PV. Other adverse effects of transfusion. In: Petz LD, Swisher SN (eds). Clinical practice of blood transfusion. New York, Edinburgh, London, Melbourne: Churchill Livingstone 1981:797-803.
2. Shulman NR. Immunological considerations attending platelet transfusion. Transfusion 1966;6:39-49.
3. Tomasulo PA. Management of the alloimmunized patient with HLA-matched platelets. In: Schiffer CJ (ed). Platelet physiology and transfusion. A technical workshop. New Orleans, Louisiana: Am Assoc Blood Banks 1978:69-81.
4. Thompson JS, Burns CP, Herbick. Stimulation of granulocyte antibodies by granulocyte transfusion. Blood 1977;50(Suppl):303.
5. Schiffer CA, Aisner J, Daly PA, Schimpff SC, Wiernik PH. Alloimmunization following prophylactic granulocyte transfusion. Blood 1979;54:766-74.
6. Brittingham TE, Chaplin H. Febrile transfusion reactions caused by sensitivity to donor leukocytes and platelets. J Amer Med Assoc 1957;165:819-25.
7. Appelbaum FR, Trapani RJ, Graw RG. Consequences of prior alloimmunization during granulocyte transfusion. Transfusion 1977;17:460-4.
8. Opelz g, Graver B, Mickey MR, Terasaki PI. Lymphocytotoxic antibody responses to transfusions in potential kidney transplant recipients. Transplantation 1981;32:177-83.
9. Moore SB, Sterioff S, Pierides AM, Watts SK, Ruud CM. Transfusion-induced alloimmunization in patients awaiting renal allografts. Vox Sang 1984;47:354-61.
10. Salvatierra O, Vincenti F, Amend W et al. Deliberate donor-specific blood transfusions prior to living related renal transplantation. Ann Surg 1980;192:543-52.
11. Salvatierra O, Amend W, Vincenti F et al. Pretreatment with donor-specific blood transfusions in related recipients with high MLC. Transplant Proc 1981;13: 142-9.
12. Patel R, Terasaki PI. Significance of positive crossmatch test in kidney transplantation. N Engl J Med 1969;280:735-9.
13. Terness P, Opelz G. Suppression of antibody response to transfusions in rats by preconditioning with antibody-coated cells. Transplantation 1985;40:389-93.
14. Terness P, Süsal C, Opelz G. Suppression of antibody-response to allogeneic blood in rats: a model for preventing sensitization to donor-specific transfusion. Transplant Proc 1985;17:2409-13.
15. Terness P, Kisiel U, Süsal C, Opelz G. Prevention of sensitization by transfusion with antibody-coated cells: specificity of suppression and transfer with serum or spleen cells. Transplant Proc 1987 (in press).
16. Fabre JW, Batchelor JR. Prevention of blood transfusion-induced immunization against transplantation antigens by treatment of the blood with antibody. Transplantation 1975;20:473-9.
17. Möller G, Wigzell H. Antibody synthesis at the cellular level: antibody-induced suppression of 18S and 7S antibody response. J Exp Med 1965;121:969-89.
18. Uhr JW, Baumann JB. Antibody formation. I. The suppression of antibody formation by passively administered antibody. J Exp Med 1961;113:935-57.
19. McKearn TJ, Weiss A, Stuart FP, Fitch FW. Selective suppression of humoral and cell-mediated immune responses to rat alloantigens by monoclonal antibodies produced by hybridoma cell lines. Transplant Proc 1979;11:932-5.
20. Colombani, D'Amaro J, Gabb B, Smith G, Svejgaard A. International agreement on a microtechnique of platelet complement fixation (Pl. C Fix.). Transplant Proc 1971;3:121-6.

21. Ford WL, Burr W, Simonsen M. A lymph node weight assay for the graft-versus-host activity of rat lymphoid cells. Transplantation 1970;10:258-66.
22. Schiffl R, Terness P, Opelz G. Prolongation of rat kidney graft survival by preconditioning with antibody-coated cells. Transplant Proc 1985;17:2414-8.
23. Milton JD. Immunosuppressive effect of murine alloantibody given only partial H-2 cover. Transplantation 1980;29:339-41.
24. Greenbury CL, Moore DH. Non specific antibody-induced suppression of immune response. Nature 1968;219:526-7.
25. Heyman B, Wigzell H. Immunoregulation by monoclonal sheep erythrocyte-specific IgG antibodies: suppression is correlated to level of antigen binding and not to isotype. J Immunol 1984;132:1136-43.
26. Hutchinson IV, Zola H. Antigen-reactive cell opsonization: a mechanism of antibody-mediated immune suppression. Cell Immunol 1978;36:161-9.
27. Sinclair NRSC, Chan PL. Regulation of the immune response. IV. The role of the Fc-fragment in feedback inhibition by antibody. Adv Exp Med Biol 1971;12:609-15.
28. Consenza H, Kohler H. Specific suppression of the antibody response by antibodies to receptors. Proc Natl Acad Sci USA 1972;69:2701-5.
29. Hart DA, Wang AL, Pawlak LL, Nisonoff A. Suppression of idiotypic specificities in adult mice by administration of anti-idiotypic antibody. J Exp Med 1972;135:1293-1300.
30. Kelsoe G, Reth M, Rajewsky K. Control of idiotope expression by monoclonal anti-idiotope antibodies. Immunol Rev 1980;52:75-88.
31. Rothstein TL, Margolies MM, Gefter ML, Marshak-Rothstein A. Fine specificity of idiotope suppression in the A/J anti-azophenylarsonate response. J Exp Med 1983;157:795-800.
32. Mudawwar F, Awdeh Z, Ault K, Geha RS. Regulation of monoclonal immunoglobulin G synthesis by anti-idiotypic antibody in a patient with hypogammaglobulinemia. J Clin Invest 1980;65:1202-9.
33. Geha RS, Comunale M. Regualtion of immunoglobulin E antibody synthesis in man by anti-idiotypic antibodies. J Clin Invest 1983;71:46-54.
34. Koopman WJ, Schrohenloher RE, Barton JC, Greenleaf E. Suppression of in vitro monoclonal human rheumatoid factor synthesis by anti-idiotypic antibody. J Clin Invest 1983;72:1410-9.
35. Bona CA, Fauci AS. In vitro idiotypic suppression of chronic lymphatic leukemia lymphocytes secreting monoclonal immunoglobulin M anti-sheep erythrocyte antibody. J Clin Invest 1980;65:761-7.
36. Borsos T, Rapp HJ. Complement fixation on cell surfaces by 19S and 7S antibodies. Science 1965;150:505-6.
37. Cohen S. The requirement for association of two adjacent rabbit IgG antibody molecules in the fixation of complement by immune complexes. J Immunol 1968;100:407-13.
38. Silverstein SC, Steinman RM, Cohn ZA. Endocytosis. Ann Rev Biochem 1977;46:669-722.
39. Leslie RGQ. Macrophage handling of soluble immune complexes. Ingestion and digestion of complexes at 4, 20 and 37°C. Eur J Immunol 1980;10:323-33.
40. Basten A, Miller JFAP, Sprent J, Pye J. A receptor for antibody on B-lymphocytes. I. Method of detection of functional significance. J Exp Med 1972:135:610-26.
41. Leslie RGQ, Alexander MD. Cytophilic antibodies. Curr Top Microbiol Immunol 1979;88:25-104.

42. Mota G, Moraru I, Sjöquist J, Ghetie V. Protein A as a molecular probe for detection of antigen induced conformational change in Fc region of rabbit antibody. Mol Immunol 1981;18:373-8.
43. Brown EJ, Bekisz J. Neoantigens appear in human IgG upon antigen binding: detection by antibodies that react specifically with antigen-bound IgG. J Immunol 1984;132:1346-52.
44. Nemazee DA, Sato VL. Enhancing antibody: a novel component of immune response. Proc Natl Acad Sci USA 1982;79:3828-32.
45. Imbach P, d'Apuzzo V, Hirt A, et al. High-dose intravenous gammaglobulin for idiopathic thrombocytopenic purpura in childhood. Lancet 1981;i:1228-32.
46. Suzuki T, Miyama-Inaba M, Masuda T, Uchino H, Murakami A, Tanaka H. Suppressive B-cell factor (SBF) produced by FcRγ-bearing B cells; suppression of B, but not non-B-cell proliferation. Immunology 1983;50:149-157.
47. Pisko EJ, Foster SL, White RE, Panetti M, Turner RA. Suppression of a pokeweed mitogen-stimulated plaque-forming cell response by a human B lymphocyte-derived aggregated IgG-stimulated suppressor factor: suppressive B cell factor (SBF). J Immunol 1986;136:2141-50.
48. Pantel JP, Medof ME, Oger JF, Kuo HH, Arnason BGW. Generation of suppressor cells by aggregated human globulin. Clin Exp Immunol 1981;43:351-6.
49. Arai S, Yamamoto H, Itoh K, Kumagai K. Suppressive effect of human natural killer cells on pokeweed mitogen-induced B cell differentation. J Immunol 1983; 131:651-7.
50. Abruzzo LV, Rowley DA. Homeostasis of the antibody response: immunoregulation by NK cells. Science 1983;222:581-5.
51. Metzger Z, Hoffeld JT, Oppenheim JJ. Macrophage-mediated suppression. I. Evidence for participation of both hydrogen peroxide and prostaglandins in suppression of murine lymphocyte proliferation. J Immunol 1980;124:983-8.
52. Brüggemann M, Rajewsky K. Regulation of antibody response against hapten-coupled erythrocytes by monoclonal antihapten antibodies of various isotypes. Cellular Immunology 1982;71:365-73.
53. McKearn T, Fitch FW, Smilek DE, Sarmiento M, Stuart FP. Properties of rat anti-MHC antibodies produced by cloned rat-mouse hybridomas. Immunol Rev 1979;47:91-115.
54. Eisen HN, Siskind GW. Variations in affinities of antibodies during the immune response. Biochemistry 1964;3:996-1008.
55. Lenhard V, Renner D, Hansen B, Opelz G. Suppression of antibody response and prolongation of skin graft survival by multiple blood transfusions in the rat. Transplantation 1985;39:424-9.

AUTOLOGOUS BONE MARROW TRANSPLANTATION IN ACUTE MYELOBLASTIC LEUKEMIA (AML): IN VITRO STUDIES TO DETECT MINIMAL DISEASE IN REMISSION MARROW

B. Löwenberg, R. Delwel

Introduction

Autologous bone marrow transplantation (ABMT) is a promising therapeutic modality which is currently under investigation in patients in first complete remission [1-4] as well as those who have attained a subsequent remission following relapse [5,6]. Current results from these studies suggest that remissions are durable in a significant proportion of patients with AML following consolidation with marrow ablative cytotoxic regimens and ABMT. The advantages of ABMT over allogeneic BMT are that donor selection is not needed and thus that the restrictions of the availability of HLA matched donors do not apply. In addition, the age limitations in ABMT are far less stringent, i.e., ABMT can probably be applied in recipients up to 60 years of age. The principal drawback of ABMT is the higher probability of relapse following transplantation and this accounts for most failures and mortality after ABMT in patients with AML. Relapse is attributed to (a) the absence of a graft-versus-leukemia effect in autotransplantation (which appears to protect against relapse after allogeneic marrow transplantation) and (b) the use of autologous bone marrow grafts containing residual leukemia. The latter factor implies that in the further development of ABMT it will be important to identify these residual AML cells and to remove them.

Efforts to detect minimal numbers of AML clonogenic cells (AML-CFU) in the marrow during complete remission depend on phenotypic properties which distinguish AML-CFU from normal marrow stem and progenitor cells. We and others have previously shown that AML-CFU represent a minority population among the total leukemic blast pool [7-9]. Among the phenotypically heterogeneous AML cells, the AML-CFU are typically the most immature subset of cells which give rise to maturing progeny during proliferation in vitro [9-11]. Earlier studies have established that the phenotypes of AML-CFU differ, but the differences correlate with the heterogeneous classes of normal progenitors as a function of maturity [20]. Although AML-CFU phenotypes show considerable variability when different cases of AML are compared, it is noteworthy that surface markers to distinguish AML-CFU from their normal counterparts have not been reported as yet.

We wished to investigate whether abnormal surface markers are expressed on the subset of clonogenic cells of AML and whether these differences provide clues for the diagnosis of minimal numbers of AML cells among normal marrow. In a systematic search for identifying discriminative markers between AML-CFU and normal hematopoietic precursor cells, we selected a combination of surface markers (i.e., three MCA and a fucose binding lectin), which are expressed as a consistent phenotype on early as well as late hematopoietic progenitors. These investigations were conducted with fluorescence activated cell sorting (FACS) of colony forming cells. We assessed the membrane marker expression not only by presence or absence of the marker but also by relative fluorescence intensity to measure the antigen density on the cell surface.

Materials and methods

The collection and processing of marrow and blood from patients with AML and from normal individuals [9], the colony assay for AML-CFU [12-14] and for normal myeloid progenitors (CFU-GM) [14], the use of indirect immunofluorescence [9,10], fluorescence activated cell sorting [15] and the application of the fucose binding lectin UEA (Ulex Europaeus Agglutinin) coupled to the fluorescent label FITC [15] have been described in detail. Vim-2 is a murine MCA (IgM7 which recognizes an antigen expressed on granulocytic cells (from myeloblasts to polymorphonuclear cells) and monocytes [16]. The mouse MCA My-10 (IgGl) is expressed on immature human marrow cells, including normal hematopoietic in vitro colony forming cells [17]. The MCA, RFB-1 (IgGl), reacts with immature progenitor cells of the granulocytic-monocytic cells, including colony forming units and terminal deoxynucleotidyl transferase-positive (TdT^+) cells in the marrow and thymus [18].

Results

Characterization of CFU-GM in normal marrow with four surface markers

We have previously reported that a varying proportion of Ficoll separated normal bone marrow cells are UEA positive. Normal CFU-GM are UEA negative or only weakly positive, i.e., they express receptors for the lectin UEA at only low density on the cell surface [15]. Normal marrow shows a bimodal Vim-2 fluorescence profile indicative of distinct Vim-2 positive and Vim-2 negative populations. CFU-GM are almost entirely recovered among the Vim-2 negative cells. The My-10 fluorescence histogram reveals a minor (approx. 5%) subset of highly reactive cells from which almost all CFU-GM are recoverable. Finally, normal marrow contains 20-50% RFB-1 positive cells and all CFU-GM are RFB-1 strongly positive. In summary, CFU-GM in normal marrow are characterized by the following surface phenotype: UEA −/+, My-10 + +, Vim-2 −, RFB-1 + +. Studies involved with other progenitor cells, confirmed the same phenotype for early (day 7) and late (day 14) CFU-GM, BFU-e and CFU-GEMM [20].

Characterization of AML-CFU with four surface markers

AML blasts from 20 cases of AML were labelled with the MCA My-10, RFB-1, Vim-2 and the lectin UEA and analyzed by FACS. The cells were sorted into three fractions of relative fluorescence intensity, i.e., negative (−),

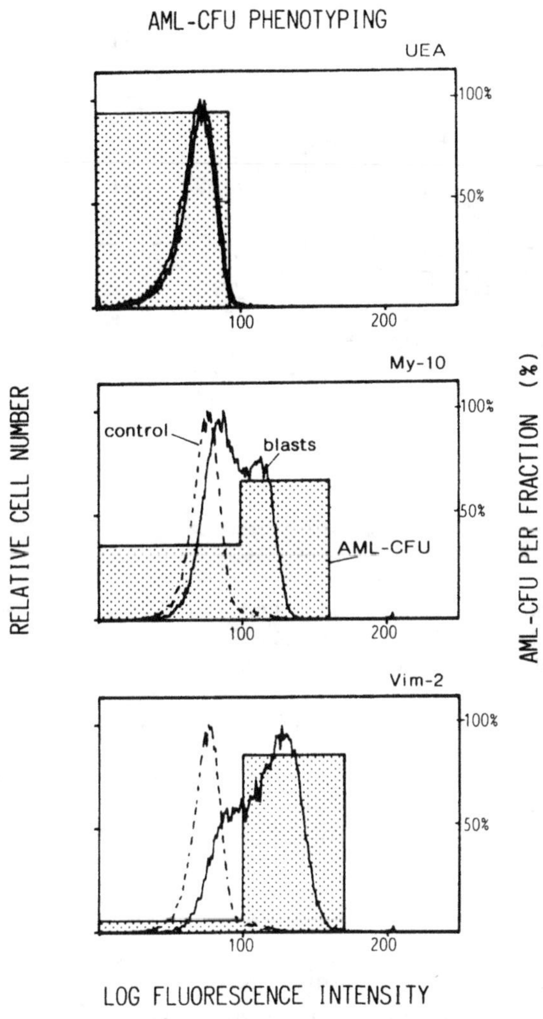

Figure 1. Cytofluorographic analysis of the leukemic blasts and AML-CFU in one patient with AML using three surface markers.

Following FACS of marker negative (−), weakly positive (+) and clearly positive (+ +) cells, the separated fractions were cultured in the colony assay in order to assess the surface phenotype of AML-CFU. The different panels indicate the data for each of the surface reagents.

Open histogram in each panel: distribution of AML blasts as a function of surface marker expression. Hatched histogram in each panel: distribution of AML-CFU relative to surface marker expression.

Table 1. Surface phenotypes of AML-CFU in 20 patients with AML.

Patient	FAB	Reactivity with surface markers: UEA	My-10	Vim-2	RFB-1	Patterns of reactivity	Number of markers different from normal
1	M2	+ +	+ +	–	+ +	A	2
2	M4	+ +	+ +	+	+ +		
3	M4	+ +	+ +	+	+ +	B	2
4	M4	+ +	+ +	+	+ +		
5	M4	+ +	+ +	+ +	+ +	C	2
6	M2	+	+ +	+ +	+ +	D	1
7	M1	–	+ +	+ +	+ +		
8	M1	–	+ +	+ +	+ +	E	1
9	M1	–	+ +	+ +	+ +		
10	M2	–	+ +	+ +	+ +		
11	M1	–	+ +	+ +	+	F	2
12	M4	–	+	+ +	+ +	G	2
13	M5	–	–	+ +	+ +	H	2
14	M2	–	–	+ +	+ +		
15	M1	–	–	+	+ +	K	2
16	M1			[illegible]	[illegible]		
17	M1	–	+ +	–	+ +	L	0
18	M2	–	+ +	–			
19	M2	–	+ +	–			
20	M2	–	+ +	–			
	normal[1]	–/+ [2]	+ + [3]	– [4]	+ + [5]	L	

The surface marker profile was established in the individual patients with FACS using the lectin UEA-FITC and three monoclonal antibodies (My-10, Vim-2, RFB-1) as illustrated in the example of Figure 1. Negative –; weakly positive +; strongly positive + +.

1. Reference data for normal hematopoietic precursor cells CFU-GM, BFU-e and CFU-GEMM.
2. 45-50% of normal precursors are UEA negative, 50% are UEA +, and less than 10% UEA + +.
3. Between 90-100% of normal progenitors.
4. Between 90-100% of normal progenitors.
5. 100% of normal progenitors.

weakly positive (+) and intensely positive (+ +) cells. These separated fractions were inoculated in colony culture to determine the distribution of AML-CFU as a function of antigen density expression in each of the cases. An example of a complete analysis of the binding abilities of AML blasts and AML-CFU to these reagents is given in Figure 1. It illustrates a case of AML in which the majority of AML-CFU were shown to be UEA –, My-10 + + and Vim-2 + +. Thus AML-CFU from this patient differ from CFU-GM (see above) by one marker, i.e., UEA. The results of the analogous analyses for the complete series of patients are compiled in Table 1. Ten classes of surface phenotypes were recognized depending on the composite antigenic configuration expressed on AML-CFU. In the table these are designated as A through L. In 16/20 patients two or at least one discrepant marker(s), based on the relative amount of surface binding to AML-CFU, were different from normal CFU-GM. This refers to the surface categories A through K. In contrast, in the four patients 17, 18, 19 and 20, AML-CFU phenotypes (profile L) were indistinguishable from their normal counterparts.

Conclusion

For demonstrating minimal residual AML in autologous bone marrow grafts one would wish to identify AML clonogenic cells and distinguish those from their normal counterparts. This would provide a basis for better qualification of these transplants in terms of malignant cell contamination as well as for the selective purging of these grafts.

No unique AML-associated surface markers have been reported. AML cells share differentation antigens with normal marrow cells. In the present study we have phenotyped the clonogenic cells in 20 cases of human AML (AML-CFU) with three MCA (monoclonal antibodies), My-10, Vim-2 and RFB-1 and the fucose binding lectin UEA. Using fluorescence activated cell sorting and colony culture of subpopulations with different fluorescence intensities, we did not only determine the abnormal presence or absence of these surface markers on AML-CFU, but also whether the expression was apparent at an abnormal (i.e., increased or decreased) density on the cell surface. Based on this approach, the surface profile was established in each of the individual cases of AML.

We demonstrate that AML-CFU phenotypes are highly variable and 10 combinations of phenotypes were distinguished. In 16 of these 20 cases, we were able to differentiate AML-CFU from the majority of the normal hematopoietic precursors, i.e., AML-GEMM, early (day 14) and late (day 7) CFU-GM and BFU-e. Only, in 4 cases AML-CFU phenotypes were identical to the normal counterparts as far as these four markers are concerned. Other studies involving monoclonal antibodies have previously indicated discrepancies as regards their reactivity with AML-CFU and CFU-GM. However, these approaches have usually been based on complement mediated lysis so that more subtle distinctions founded on relative binding abilities were not made.

We have defined a reference phenotype, which included 4 heterogeneous classes of normal precursors. The frequent discrepancies between the AML and normal precursors are striking. The fact that AML-CFU phenotypes were so diverse and so frequently dissimilar to the standard surface pattern of each of the types of normal progenitors, suggests that these polymorphic phenotypes of AML-CFU reflect abnormalities of differentiation. At the present time we can not distinguish between the two possibilities to explain this bizarre marker expression: i.e., AML-CFU present altered phenotypes as the result of malignant transformation or they correlate with expansions of precursors with essentially normal but unfrequent phenotypes.

The problem of the identification of minimal numbers of AML clonogenic cells in a remission bone marrow aspirate relates not only to the unfavourable quantitative ratio of AML versus normal cells, but also to the cross reactivity of the surface reagents with AML cells and diverse normal cell types. The experiments presented utilizing FACS allow for differentiating AML-CFU from the normal hematopoietic precursors by fluorescence intensity and thus open new possibilities for detecting minimal leukemia. These possibilities increase when surface markers are selected which indicate a stable phenotype for the different categories of normal hematopoietic precursors and which permit the identification of a high frequency of deviations in AML.

In order to successfully detect minimal numbers of AML cells, the marrow cell suspension needs to be processed so that a fraction is obtained from which contaminant normal precursors are removed and which is highly enriched for AML precursors. It is conceivable that this goal can be reached if advantage is taken of the disordered differentiation which characterizes most cases of AML as demonstrated in our studies. Attempts at detection can for instance be made by sorting My-10 postive cells in a first separation step, so that 95% of contaminant non leukemic marrow are removed. In a second step utilizing a discriminative marker the AML-CFU can be recovered and CFU-GM removed. This may result in the ultimate concentration of AML-CFU by 30-100 fold.

Preliminary data (not shown) indicate possibilities for detection of AML cells when they make up only 0.1-1% of a mixed normal marrow and AML cell preparation.

Acknowledgements

This work was supported by the Netherlands Cancer Society 'Queen Wilhelmina Fund'. The monoclonal antibodies My-10, Vim-2 and RFB-1 were kindly provided by Dr. C.I. Civin (Baltimore), Dr. W. Knapp (Vienna) and Dr. M.P. Bodger (London), respectively.

References

1. Burnett AK, Tansey P, Watkins R et al. Transplantation of unpurged autologous bone marrow in acute myeloid leukemia in first remission. Lancet 1984;i:1068-70.
2. Löwenberg B, Abels J, van Bekkum DW et al. Transplantation of non-purified autologous bone marrow in patients with AML in first remission. Cancer 1984; 54:2840-3.
3. Löwenberg B, Hagenbeek A, Sizoo W, de Gast GC, Verdonck LF. Bone marrow transplantation strategies in acute leukemia. Lancet 1984;ii:1400-1.
4. Burnett AK, McKinnon S. Autologous bone marrow transplantation in first remission AML using non purged marrow - update. In: Hagenbeek A, Löwenberg B (eds). Minimal residual disease in acute leukemia. Dordrecht: Martinus Nijhoff Publishers 1986:211-21.

5. Yeager AM, Kaizer H, Santos GW et al. Autologous bone marrow transplantation in patients with acute non-lymphocytic leukemia, using ex vivo marrow treatment with 4-hydroperoxycyclophosphamide. N Engl J Med 1986;315:141-7.
6. Hervé P, Tamayo E, Chan JY, Plouvier E, Flesch M, Peters A. Attempts to eliminate residual acute myeloid leukemia from autologous bone marrow grafts through in vitro chemotherapy. A review. In: Hagenbeek A, Löwenberg B (eds). Minimal residual disease in actue leukemia. Dordrecht: Martinus Nijhoff Publishers 1986:248-66.
7. Lange B, Ferrero D, Pessano S et al. Surface phenotype of clonogenic cells in acute myeloid leukemia defined by monoclonal antibodies. Blood 1984;64: 693-700.
8. Sabbath KD, Ball ED, Larcom P, Davis RB, Griffin JD. Heterogeneity of clonogenic cells in acute myeloblastic leukemia. J Clin Invest 1985;75:746-53.
9. Löwenberg B, Bauman JGS. Further results in understanding the subpopulation structure in AML: clonogenic cells and their progeny identified by differentiation markers. Blood 1985;66:1225-32.
10. Wouters R, Löwenberg B. On the maturation order of AML cells: a distinction on the basis of self-renewal properties and immunologic phenotypes. Blood 1984; 63:684-9.
11. Touw IP, Löwenberg B. Variable differentiation of human acute myeloid leukemia during colony formation in vitro. A membrane marker analysis with monoclonal antibodies. Brit J Haemat 1985;59:37-44.
12. Löwenberg B, Swart K, Hagemeijer A. PHA-induced colony formation in acute non-lymphocytic and chronic myeloid leukemia. Leuk Res 1980;4:143-9.
13. Löwenberg B, Hagemeijer A, Swart K. Karyotypically distinct subpopulations in acute leukemia with specific growth requirements. Blood 1982;59:641-5.
14. Swart K, Hagemeijer A, Löwenberg B. Acute myeloid leukemia colony growth in vitro: differences of colony forming cells in PHA-supplemented and standard leukocyte feeder cultures. Blood 1982;59:816-21.
15. Delwel HR, Touw IP, Löwenberg B. A fucose binding lectin (UEA) for characterizing acute myeloid leukemia progenitor cells. Blood 1985;68:41-5.
16. Majdic O, Bettelheim P, Stockinger H et al. M2, a novel myelomonocytic cell surface antigen and its distribution on leukemic cells. Int J Cancer 1984;33:617-23.
17. Civin CI, Strauss LC, Brovall C, Fackler MJ, Schwartz JF, Shaper JH. Antigenic analysis of hematopoiesis III. A hematopoietic progenitor cell surface antigen defined by a monoclonal antibody raised against KG-1a cells. J Immunol 1984;133:157-65.
18. Bodger MP, Francis GE, Delia D, Granger SM, Janossy G. A monoclonal antibody specific for immature human hemopoietic cells and T lineage cells. J Immunol 1981;127:2269-74.
19. Delwel R, Bot F, Touw IP, Löwenberg B. Exceptional phenotypes of progenitors in acute myelocytic leukemia (AML-CFU): possibilities for separating AML-CFU from normal marrow progenitors. Cancer Res 1987 (in press).
20. Griffin JD, Löwenberg B. Clonogenic cells in acute myeloblastic leukemia. 1986; 68:1185-95.

AUTOLOGOUS BONE MARROW TRANSPLANTATION IN SOLID MALIGNANCIES

P.O.M. Mulder, D.Th. Sleijfer, E.G.E. de Vries, P.H.B. Willemse, P.E. Postmus, J.L.M. Orie, C.Th. Smit Sibinga, M.R. Halie, N.H. Mulder

Introduction

The natural resistance of a fraction of cells in a tumor to a conventional dose of chemotherapy can partly be overcome by high dose (HD) chemotherapy [1]. HD chemotherapy may kill more tumor cells but could also cause long lasting or irreversible bone marrow aplasia.

Both animal research on the protective effect of autologous bone marrow infusion from lethal doses of chemotherapy and/or total body irradiation [2], and clinical experience [3] indicate that autologous bone marrow transplantation (ABMT) in man after intensive chemotherapy of malignant disease is feasible and could increase response rates.

The criteria for the use of ABMT have been formulated previously [4].

Of major importance are:

- The tumor should preferably respond to a standard dose of drugs to be used in HD.
- Dose escalation of that drug must be known to improve the tumor responsiveness.
- High drug levels should usually produce profound marrow depression persisting for periods of >2-3 weeks without severely affecting non-hematopoietic tissues.
- Autologous bone marrow should be collected before the institution of intensive chemotherapy and should be free of contaminating tumor cells.

Since 1981 we perform a program in the University Hospital, aimed at defining appropriate regimens of HD chemotherapy with ABMT in adult patients with disseminated solid tumors, and at evaluating the effect of such chemotherapeutic regimens in various tumor types.

Patients and procedures

Fifty-two patients have been treated. Their age ranged from 20 to 66 years, median 40 years.

The tumor types involved were:

- Breast cancer (5 patients) in complete remission after induction chemotherapy (methotrexate, 5-fluorouracil, adriamycin and vincristin) in women below the age of 45 years.

- Ovarian cancer (10 patients) in women below the age of 65 years who have failed standard chemotherapy (cisplatin, adriamycin and cyclophosphamide) with residual limited disease on diagnostic laparotomy (4 patients). Six other patients with bulky disease after standard treatment were entered in phase I studies.
- Germ cell tumors (14 patients) after failure on standard chemotherapy with cisplatin, bleomycin, vinblastine and/or etoposide. One patient was treated twice.
- Small cell lung cancer (18 patients) recurrent or progressive after standard chemotherapy with cisplatin, cyclophosphamide and etoposide, vincristin, adriamycin, procarbazine, BCNU and hexamethylamine. Nine patients were treated in a phase I study and also 9 patients were treated in a phase II study.
- Colon cancer (1 patient), no prior chemotherapy, treated in a phase I protocol.
- Malignant melanoma (1 patient). ABMT was tried following response to prior treatment with dacarbazine, bleomycin and vindesine.
- Carcinoma of unknown origin (3 patients), prior treatment included cisplatin, adriamycin and vinblastine, mitomycin and 5-fluorouracil. These patients were treated in phase I ABMT protocols.

Additional selection criteria were: no detectable tumor cells in marrow biopsies, smears and cultures, normal serum bilirubin and creatinin levels, no untreatable cardiac decompensation, a Karnofsky performance score above 60 and an informed consent after a standard information procedure. The study was approved by the local medical ethical committee.

Bone marrow collection: procedure in vivo and in vitro

Bone marrow was collected in the 52 patients by multiple punctures from the posterior iliac crest under local anesthesia with lidocain without narcosis after premedication with 100 mg meperidine and 20 mg diazepam i.m. [5]

The marrow was aspirated in 10 ml disposable syringes and collected in Hanks solution with hepes buffer and heparin, final concentration of heparin 150.000 IU/l. The marrow was centrifuged in a Haemonetics 30S® apheresis machine. After sedimentation of red blood cells in a 10% hydroxyethyl starch solution and concentration of nucleated cells to 200×10^6 cells per ml, cryopreservation followed.

A minimum number of 2×10^8 nucleated cells per kg body weight was collected. Recovery of nucleated cells, after separation of the buffy coat in the apheresis machine and purification of white cells by hydroxyethyl starch, was approximately 50%.

Cryopreservation and reinfusion

The nucleated cells are resuspended in autologous plasma, and 20% dimethylsulfoxide (DMSO) is added in a 1:1 solution. The marrow concentrate containing 100×10^6 nucleated cells/ml and 10% DMSO, is placed in 5 ml ampoules (Nunc). These are frozen in a Cryoson BV-4 liquid nitrogen controlled freezer at a rate of 1.0°C/min until −40°C. Ampoules are then transferred for storage in liquid nitrogen.

Granulocytic-macrophage colony forming units (CFU-GM) were determined in a two layer agar system using bone marrow obtained during collection, after separation, before freezing and after thawing, to evaluate the procedure in 6 patients. The CFU-GM are routinely measured in harvested marrow of all patients. Immediately prior to infusion, the cryopreserved bone marrow is thawed in a water bath at 40°C and aspirated in 50 ml syringes in a laminar flow cabinet. The thawed marrow is reinfused over a standard blood filter into a central venous (Hickman) catheter.

The DMSO is not washed out [6]. Patients receive 2 mg clemastine and 60 mg prednisolone i.v. prior to all infusions containing DMSO.

Chemotherapy regimens

Antitumor regimens consisted of combinations of two or more of the following drugs: cyclophosphamide 7 g/m², etoposide range 0.9 to 3 g/m², carboplatin 750 mg/m², mitoxantrone 30-45 mg/m², melphalan 210 mg/m² and dacarbazine 1.2 g/m². Two patients received total body irradiation in combination with teniposide 500 mg/m².

Transfusion support

During the aplastic period patients were reconstituted with autologous cryopreserved platelets, when platelets were below 15×10^9/l or in case of bleeding tendency. Thrombapheresis was done prior to ablative therapy with a Haemonetics V50® blood cell separator, using a platelet elutriation programme [7]. After centrifugation to remove red cells, DMSO 10% and autologous plasma were added. The final volume of about 100 ml with a concentration of 5% DMSO was frozen and stored in liquid nitrogen [8].

Results and discussion

The ultimate goal of this form of treatment is to provide a perspective of cure or at least prolonged survival for patients with apparent incurable cancers. Most of our patients have been treated in studies aimed at defining tolerable regimens, they were in an end stage of the disease. Usually only an indication of the activity of a regimen can be found in that situation.

Tumor response

Breast cancer

Two of four patients with breast cancer remained free of disease after more than 18 months. Two patients had a relapse after 4 and 8 months. One patient has only recently been treated and therefore not evaluable for response.

Ovarian cancer

Four patients with minimal disease had a complete response. Three of these patients are disease-free after 12, 13 and 33 months respectively. One patient relapsed and died after 26 months. One patient had bulky Sertoli-Leydigcell cancer of the ovary, which became operable after ABMT. She is without evidence of disease 11 months after surgery.

Germ cell tumors

One patient had a complete remission for 36 weeks. Two patients did not respond. Nine patients had a partial remission for a mean duration of only 11 weeks. Two patients died during treatment, without tumor detectable on autopsy.

Small cell lung cancer (SCLC)

In the phase I studies, using 7 g/m^2 cyclophosphamide and increasing dosages of etoposide, one patient had a partial remission of 9 months and one patient had a complete remission of 5 months. In the phase II study the regimen consisted of 7 g/m^2 cyclophosphamide and 1.5 g/m^2 etoposide (patients ≤ 50 years) or 0.9 g/m^2 (patients >50 years). Nine patients entered this study, six had a partial remission and two had a complete remission. The longest remission period was 12 months with a mean duration of remission of 5 months. One patient died of treatment-related toxicity.

From these results it is evident that HD chemotherapy has a high response rate, however this was not translated in an increased survival in SCLC and germ cell tumors with the regimens that we studied. In the literature the best results with HD chemotherapy have been described in malignant lymphoma [9] and childhood neuroblastoma [10]. Our results in ovarian and breast cancer indicate that some patients with these tumor types could also benefit from this form of treatment provided that it can be instituted in a situation with minimal disease.

Hematopoietic recovery

Recovery of the hematopoiesis after HD chemotherapy depends upon a number of factors. The quantity and quality of the marrow surviving chemotherapy are important, and therefore the nature of the drugs used. It has been established that high dose etoposide does not require marrow substitution [11]. However, if alkylating agents or radiotherapy are used in patients who have previously been extensively treated with chemotherapy, this is less sure.

Hematopoietic reconstruction was found to be accelerated with ABMT after high-dose melphalan [12] and nitrosurea [13], but this was not found in patients who received single agent HD cyclophosphamide [14].

We do not know if, after our conditioning regimen, autologous bone marrow reinfusion adds to the speed of hematopoietic recovery but we feel it is not ethically justified to omit reinfusion of bone marrow in a randomized study, especially because the harvesting procedure does not require general anesthesia, and is therefore barely a burden for the patient.

Animal studies showed a consistent engraftment when a minimum of 0.5×10^8 nucleated cells/kg bodyweight were infused [2]. In human subjects a minimum of two to four times the animal dose is given to secure engraftment potential. Into our patients a mean of 1.41×10^8 nucleated cells per kg bodyweight was reinfused (range 0.73-2.9).

The number of infused colony forming units in culture also has been found to influence the marrow reconstitutive capability especially neutrophil repopulating ability [15]. It is suggested that this correlation is only demonstrated for low numbers [16]. In our patients mean numbers of CFU-GM transfused were 40.09×10^3/kg bodyweight (SD 36.80). Patients were thrombopenic (less than 40×10^9/l) for a median of 14 days (range 9-28) and leukopenic (less than 1.0×10^9/l) for 15 days (range 11-22). We found no clear correlation between duration of thrombocytopenia or granulocytopenia and the number of nucleated cells or the number of CFU-GM infused.

In contrast to allogeneic bone marrow transplantation where the marrow is collected from a healthy donor, autologous marrow is harvested from heavily pretreated patients. We found no correlation between the number of nucleated cells obtained and the degree of pretreatment, as the highest numbers were found in 2 women who had received 6 courses of adriamycin, cisplatin and cyclophosphamide for ovarian cancer and a woman who was to receive a second course of ablative chemotherapy with cyclophosphamide and etoposide after failure of previous standard treatment with cisplatin, vinblastine and bleomycin.

If it is accepted that the infused marrow accelerates or garantees the recovery of hemopoiesis in patients treated with HD chemotherapy, it is essential that the optimal form of marrow recovery, storage and reinfusion are defined. The storage temperature is of influence on the viability of marrow. Human marrow CFU-GM declined to 15% after storage at 4°C after 72 hours [17]. It seems that marrow frozen in DMSO and stored in liquid nitrogen will stay biologically active indefinitely though no absolute proof is available. Changes in ambient temperature can decrease the engraftment potentials of marrow specimens even with present freezing methods and storage conditions. Problems related with allogeneic bone marrow transplantation such as HLA-incompatibility, delicate immunologic balance between graft rejection and graft-versus-host disease [18], immunosuppressive regimens, longstanding posttransplant immunodeficiency [19], (viral) infections transmitted by foreign graft, in vitro manipulations on graft T-lymphocytes prior to infusion are all avoided in autologous bone marrow transplantation and have therefore no influence on hematopoietic recovery.

Bone marrow reinfusion

The moment of bone marrow reinfusion is determined by the period required for elimination of the chemotherapeutic agents from the circulation and therefore depends on the chemotherapeutic regimen used.

Melphalan is cleared rapidly from the circulation [20]. We found that etoposide was only cleared after 6 days [21]. Carboplatin in the dosage used was found to be still present after 7 days. In the literature usually only marginal attention is being paid to the pharmacokinetic characteristics of the drugs used in HD regimens.

A number of features concerning the treatment of these patients have been further evaluated in our program.

We found that bone marrow can be procured under local anesthesia and meperidine/diazepam analgesia on an outpatient basis and that general anesthesia is not necessary. Fifty-two patients underwent 54 harvesting procedures.

For all 54 procedures the mean duration was 90 minutes (range 45-165 minutes). During and after the procedure, 3 units of leukocyte-free red blood cells were administered. In contrast, in 7 donors for allogeneic transplantation brought under general anesthesia the procedure took a mean of 160 minutes from the start of anesthesia.

All patients were evaluated for complications and acceptance of the harvesting procedure. Forty-four patients had no complications, 4 patients vomitted, 4 patients had a brief period of hypotension. Acceptance was excellent in 28 patients, reasonable in 21 and poor in 3. In one patient the procedure under local anesthesia was stopped and continued under general anesthesia.

A potential lethal effect of the marrow aplasia brought about by HD chemotherapy is the period of thrombocytopenia. The routine use of allogeneic platelets harbours the risk of sensitization and also of viral contamination. Both problems can be circumvented by the use of autologous platelets frozen before chemotherapy is instituted. We tried therefore to collect at least 4 thrombocyte concentrates from each patient by apheresis prior to chemotherapy. Those platelets are frozen under protection with DMSO. We studied in 12 patients whether washing of the platelets to remove DMSO, influenced platelet recovery after reinfusion. In a prospective cross-over study with washed and unwashed platelets the mean numbers of platelets infused were respectively 247 and $309 \times 10^9/l$ [6].

The increment in thrombocyte levels in the patient was the same in both situations (11.7 and $13.5 \times 10^9/l$). There was no side effect of DMSO containing platelet infusion, so we decided that washing out of the cryoprotective agent was not required. No bleeding episodes occurred in any of the patients who received autologous cryopreserved platelets, indicating their viability.

The use of allogeneic blood products in severely immune suppressed patients implicates a risk of graft-versus-host disease (GvHD). As GvHD is not usually seen in patients receiving chemotherapy we did not institute irradiation of allogeneic blood products in the first 25 patients. In 4 patients this was found to lead to histological signs in the skin of graft-versus-host disease [22]. All of these patients had symptoms (erythema of the skin and/or diarrhea) that can in retrospect be ascribed to GvHD). We therefore advocate irradiation of all allogeneic blood products infused in these patients.

Conclusion

The curative perspective of high-dose chemotherapy for resistant neoplasms is no longer limited by hematopoietic toxicity. Trials on the most effective drug combinations to the most suitable tumors are underway in many centers. Long-term survivors have been seen in our treatment modality only in ovarian and breast cancer patients, and not in patients with small cell lung cancer and germ cell tumors. Decontamination procedures of bone marrow with tumor cells will become of importance as soon as long-term remission emerge with these treatment modalities, indicating cure or control of primary disease localizations.

References

1. Lazarus HM, Herzig RH, Wolff SN et al. Treatment of metastatic malignant melanoma with intensive melphalan and autologous bone marrow transplantation. Cancer Treat Rep 1985;69:473-7.
2. Gorin NC, Herzig G, Bull MI, Graw RG. Long-term preservation of bone marrow and stem cell pool in dogs. Blood 1978;51:257-65.
3. Thomas ED, Buckner CD, Clift RA. Marrow transplantation for acute non-lymphoblastic leukemia in first remission. N Engl J Med 1979;300:597-9.
4. Deisseroth A, Abrams RA. The role of autologous stem cell reconstitution in intensive therapy for resistant neoplasms. Cancer Treat Rep 1979;63:461-71.
5. De Vries EGE, Vriesendorp R, Meinesz AF, Mulder NH, Postmus PE, Sleijfer DTh. No narcosis for bone marrow harvest in autologous bone marrow transplantation. Blut 1984;49:419-21.
6. Arnaud F, Orie JML, Mulder NH et al. Bone marrow separation, purification and cryopreservation: application for autologous bone marrow transplantation (ABMT). Int J Art Org 1985;8:209-14.
7. Elias MK, Oenema B, Scholten JT, Das PC, Smit Sibinga CTh. Surge pump plateletapheresis: a method for effective depletion of white cells from machine collected single donor platelets. Plasma Ther Transf Ther 1985;6:381-96.
8. von Bartheld M, Arnaud F, Das PC, Smit Sibinga CTh. Cryopreservation of platelet concentrate: a comparison of DMSO and glycerol systems. In: Smit Sibinga CTh, Das PC, van Loghem JJ (eds). Blood transfusion and problems of bleeding. The Hague/Boston/London: Martinus Nijhoff Publishers 1982:89-95.
9. Philip T, Biron P, Maraninchi D et al. Massive chemotherapy with autologous bone marrow transplantation in 50 cases of bad prognosis non-Hodgkin's lymphoma. Brit J Haemat 1985;60:599-609.
10. De Kraker J, Voute PA. The effect of high dose melphalan with autologous bone marrow transplantation in neuroblastoma patients with advanced disease. In: McVie JG, Dalesio O, Smith IE (eds). Autologous bone marrow transplantation and solid tumors. Raven Press 1984:153-6.
11. Postmus PE, Mulder NH, Sleijfer DTh, Meinesz AF, Vriesendorp R, de Vries EGE. High-dose etoposide for refractory malignancies: a phase I study. Cancer Treat Rep 1984;68:1471-4.
12. McElwain TJ, Hedley DW, Burton G et al. Marrow autotransplantation accelerates haematological recovery in patients with malignant melanoma treated with high dose melphalan. Br J Cancer 1979;40:72-80.

13. Scheef W, Klein HO, Brock N et al. Controlled clinical studies with an antidote against the urotoxicity of oxazophophorines: Preliminary results. Cancer Treat Rep 1979;63:501-5.
14. Smith IE, Evans BD, Harland SJ, Millar JL. Autologous bone marrow rescue is unnecessary after very-high-dose cyclophosphamide. Lancet 1983;i:76-7.
15. Spitzer G, Verma DS, Fisher R et al. The myeloid progenitor cell – its value in predicting hematopoietic recovery after autologous bone marrow transplantation. Blood 1980;55:317-23.
16. Hartmann O, Beaujean F, Bayet S et al. Hematopoietic recovery following autologous bone marrow transplantation: Role of cryopreservation, number of cells infused and nature of high-dose chemotherapy. Eur J Cancer Clin Oncol 1985;21: 53-60.
17. Millar JL, Smith IE. The viability of marrow stored at 4°C. In: McVie JG, Dalesio O, Smith IE (eds). Autologous bone marrow transplantation and solid tumors. Raven Press 1984:9-12.
18. Patterson J, Prentice HG, Brenner MK et al. Graft rejection following HLA matched T-lymphocytes depleted bone marrow transplantation. Brit J Haemat 1986;63:221-30.
19. Shiobara S, Harada M, Mori T et al. Difference in posttransplant recovery of immune reactivity between allogeneic and autologous bone marrow transplantation. Transplant Proc 1982;15:429-33.
20. Gouyette A, Hartmann O, Pico GI. Pharmacokinetics of high-dose melphalan in children and adults. Cancer Chemother Pharmacol 1986;16:184-9.
21. Holthuis JJM, Postmus PE, van Oort WJ et al. Pharmacokinetics of high dose etoposide (VP 16-213). Proc Am Ass Clin Oncol 1986:5(abstract 113).
22. Postmus PE, Mulder NH, Elema JD. Graft versus host disease in autologous bone marrow transplantation. Cancer 1987 (in press).

DISCUSSION

M.R. Halie and S.B. Moore

S.F. Leitman (Bethesda): Dr. Mulder, four of your patients developed posttransfusion GvHD. Two fo the patients were treated with total body irradiation. Did both of the irradiated patients develop GvHD or were the GvHD patients treated with chemotherapy alone?

P.O.M. Mulder-Dijkstra (Groningen); There were only two patients who were treated with total body irradiation and teniposide. Graft-versus-Host disease did not occur in these two patients.

S.F. Leitman: These are the first reported cases of posttransfusion GvHD in breast and ovarian solid tumor patients. However, the chemotherapy they received was much more aggressive than standard chemotherapy for these tumors.

Dr. Sintnicolaas, the platelets that you used on your microplate were preserved. Were they cryopreserved?

K. Sintnicolaas (Rotterdam): Yes, the platelats were cryopreserved in DMSO.

J. Ord (Brentwood): Dr. Sintnicolaas, I am interested to know how many of your ELISA negative patients, who have a negative ELISA cross-match, gave a cytotoxic positive test. The reason I ask this question is because in our experience the ELISA test is relatively insensitive for HLA-antibodies.

K. Sintnicolaas: We had in the patients with a good transfusion response one out of the 24 with a positive lymphocytotoxic cross-match. But we also performed lymphocytoimmunofluorescence and there were more positive reactions, I think 4 or 5.

J. Ord: You would ignore the cytotoxic positive reaction if the ELISA test was negative. Is that your conclusion?

K. Sintnicolaas: Yes.

S.B. Moore (Rochester): Dr. Mulder, I was fascinated by the description of the four cases of mild transfusion induced GvHD, because of the fact that the experience in the literature with transfusion induced GvHD is almost invariably fatal. I am wondering if you like to comment on that.

P.O.M. Mulder-Dijkstra: All these patients have died. They also had progression of the tumor, but they died of GvHD.

G. Sciorelli (Milan): Dr. Terness, I was very impressed by your data. What is the percentage of pooled red cells that you have to reinfuse after antibody treatment to induce the suppression.

P. Terness (Heidelberg): The animals were pretreated once or 3 times with antibody coated cells and then they received repeatedly about 1 ml untreated blood cells. We could repeatedly transfuse them with strongly incompatible cells without any antibody response. The antibody response was completely suppressed in some models.

G. Sciorelli: How many cells did you coat with antibody for every injection?

P. Terness: If we used leukocytes, we coated 5 million of leukocytes. If we used whole blood to pretreat animals, we used an amount of 1 ml whole blood and coated the cells with antibodies.

P.C. Das (Groningen): Dr. Löwenberg, does purging of the bone marrow influence disease-free survival? How about engraftment?

B. Löwenberg (Rotterdam): I showed the in vitro methodology and an ongoing trial using autologous bone marrow. This trial is carried out with non-purged bone marrow. In fact the slow repopulation data are based on non-purged bone marrow. This is by itself very interesting. Repopulation from the autograft in patients with AML is significantly delayed as compared to patients with ALL or patients with solid tumors. This is now becoming clear from several studies and it points out, that we have to separately consider the effect of purging on repopulation. It is suggested that the disease by itself (AML) has a relationship to delayed regeneration.

P. Rebulla (Milan): Dr. Sintnicolaas, why do you chose the 20% recovery as a measure of effective transfusion? In our experience leukemia patients without HLA antibodies have a recovery which is well above 20% if they receive random platelets. Their actual recovery is in the range between 40 and 60 of expected. So, we should try to better define what is an effective platelet transfusion as far as the recovery is concerned.

K. Sintnicolaas: Well, it is very difficult to say what the precise limit is of the level below which you can call transfusion a failure and above which you can call it a success. The data in the literature mostly expressed as corrected count increments are comparable to this 20% when you compare the formula's. We have based this upon literature data and on non-sensitized patients, who received platelet transfusions. I agree that most transfusions will have recoveries about 40 to 50%, but it is a wide range one can observe in non-sensitized patients.

II. CLINICAL ASPECTS
B. Absence of cells

CLINICAL USE OF LEUKOCYTE POOR RED CELL CONCENTRATES

J.Th.M. de Wolf

Leukocytes present in blood components are associated with some more or less important transfusion complications: The production of alloantibodies directed against HLA and/or leukocyte specific antigens can be the cause of febrile non-hemolytic transfusion reactions (FNHTR) and of refractoriness to platelet transfusion; immunocompetent leukocytes transfused to severely immunodeficient patients may react against the tissues of the recipient and may develop graft-versus-host disease (GvHD). Finally, substantial clinical evidence exists for the transmission of cytomegalovirus by leukocytes.

We will discuss the clinical relevance of these complications and the necessity for transfusing leukocyte depleted blood to prevent these. Since there are better ways to prevent GvHD (irradiation) and CMV infection (CMV negative blood), these subjects will not be discussed.

Febrile non-hemolytic transfusion reaction (FNHTR) is defined by the following criteria: Temperature rise of 1°C or more during or within four hours following transfusion; normalisation of the temperature within 48 hours; no other causes of fever such as infectious disease and no signs of hemolytic transfusion reaction.

The reported *incidence* of FNHTR ranges from 1.6-3.8% [1,2], in the early 1960s to 0.4-0.73% [3,4] in the 1980s. To identify the different causes Decary et al. [3] analysed non hemolytic reactions following the transfusion of 26,318 units of blood components on 5,030 occasions giving an incidence per unit of 0.73%. The highest incidence of reactions was associated with white cell infusions (6.49%). The second highest incidence was with concentrated red cells (1.06%). Patients who had been transfused but who did not manifest any reaction were used as a control group.

With the use of a lymphocytotoxicity test with a prolonged incubation time, significantly more antibodies were detected in pretransfusion specimens from reactors (reactors: 51/101 positive, controls: 17/57 positive). In posttransfusion specimens from reactors, more antibodies were detected than in the pretransfusion specimens, however this higher incidence was not statistically significant. Other tests to detect antibodies included: Indirect immunofluorescence tests on lymphocytes and platelets, the leukocyte agglutination test and an ELISA test for platelet antibody. Three or four randomly selected donors were used with the application of all these tests; antibodies were detected in 66% of the reactors and in 30% of the controls.

The fact that not in all cases antibodies were detected may be explained by the small number of donors used in the tests and therefore antibodies directed against antigens of low frequency were not demonstrated.

Thulstrup [5] investigated sera from 274 patients with FNHTR and demonstrated leukocyte agglutinating antibodies in 48.9% and lymphocytotoxic antibodies in 54%. Matching of the sera of 39 of these patients with leukocytes and platelets of the donors whose blood actually caused the reaction, demonstrated incompatibility in all cases. In 26 cases sera were tested against control cells from donors whose blood had not caused reactions, a positive result was only found in one. De Rier et al. [6] looked for antibodies against leukocytes and platelets in the sera from forty patients with FNHTR. They used an immunofluorescence test on platelets, granulocytes and lymphocytes, as well as a leukocyte agglutination test and a lymphocytotoxicity test. With these tests antibodies were found in all forty sera when tested against the cells of at least nine donors. If only lymphocytotoxicity and platelet suspension immunofluorescence test were used, antibodies could be detected in 39 of 40 sera. Most frequently HLA antibodies were detected but also platelet specific antibodies were quite frequent: at least 25%; the least frequent were granulocyte specific antibodies (10%).

Menitove [4] reported 253 FNHTR after transfusion of 99,658 units of blood (0.5%); 144 of the reacting patients were transfused with RCC's. Only 21 (15%) had a second reaction. Therefore, it seems reasonable to wait with precautions until the patient has had three consecutive FNHTR. Perkins [7] thoroughly studied eight patients with recurrent FNHTR and found that although the sensitivity of each patient differed with respect to the number of incompatible white cells which could be tolerated without reaction, infusion of less than 0.25×10^9 leukocytes caused no reaction in any of them; that is, if blood depleted for more than 95% of the leukocytes is transfused, febrile reactions did not occur in these eight patients.

There are several ways to remove leukocytes from blood: Centrifugation, washing, sedimentation, freezing and thawing, and the use of specific leukocyte depletion filters. The shelf life of blood processed by these methods is 24 hours. Leukocyte depletion ranges from 80-100%, red cell loss varied from 10-40%. Microaggregate blood filters (MABF) remove 46-84% of the white cells [9], especially granulocytes. Combined with centrifugation they remove 74-91% of the leukocytes. The efficiency varies directly with the shelf life of the unit.

The use of MABF reduces the incidence of FNHTR by 77%. If MABF is combined with centrifugation the reduction is 98%. The advantages of the use of MABF above the other leukocyte depleting techniques are the lower costs and the simplicity: It can be used at the bedside. Therefore, if a patient has experienced three febrile reactions after transfusion of blood products one should initially use microaggregation blood filters for the prevention of FNHTR. If this appears to be insufficient, blood should be depleted of leukocytes by filtration with a specific leukocyte depleting filter, saline washing or freezing and thawing.

In summary: In the literature there is ample evidence that FNHTR are induced by leukocyte alloantibodies. In the case that a patients experiences a FNHTR it must be considered, whether specific measures should be taken to prevent such a reaction.

The development of refractoriness to platelet transfusion (alloimmuniation) is the second complication associated with the transfusion of leukocytes.

When poor posttransfusion platelet increments occur at two or more consecutive occasions in the absence of fever, infection, sepsis, disseminated intravascular coagulation, bleeding and splenomegaly, patients are considered refractory to platelet transfusion [10]. Acceptable posttransfusion count increments are: A percentage recovery at 1 hour of 30 and at 24 hour of 20 [11], corrected increment (ci) of 7.5×10^3 at 1 hour and 4.5×10^3 at 24 hour [12] or corrected count increment (cci) of 10×10^3 at 1 hour and of 7.5×10^3 at 24 hour [13].

Daly et al. [13] demonstrated a close correlation between a poor one hour cci and the presence of lymphocytotoxic antibodies in the patient. When these patients were given HLA-matched platelets a significantly better posttransfusion platelet increment was noticed.

A poor 24 hour increment was seen in patients with fever, infection, bleeding and DIC, indicating a poor platelet survival. From thalassemic and kidney transplant patients transfused with leukocyte poor blood products it is known that this can reduce the incidence of alloimmunization.

Sirchia et al. [14] transfused 11 thalassemic children over a period of 10 years with 12-129 units of leukocyte free red cells per patient (buffy coat deprived red cells were filtered through a specific leukocyte depleting filter, followed by two additional centrifugations). A control group of 13 thalassemic children were transfused with 49-108 buffy coat deprived red cell transfusions each. No patient treated with leukocyte free red cell transfusions produced antilymphocyte, antigranulocyte or antiplatelet alloantibodies, whereas 69% of control patients were immunized.

Fisher et al. [15] transfused 24 previously non-transfused patients awaiting renal transplantation at 14-day intervals three times 2×10^{10} platelets. Twelve patients received platelet suspensions contaminated with 15×10^6 leukocytes per transfusion. The other twelve received suspensions with less than 5×10^6 leukocytes per transfusion. Five patients in the first and none in the second group developed lymphocytotoxic antibodies. Studies in leukemic patients concerning the reduction effect of leukocyte poor blood products on alloimmunization are not consistent.

Eernisse et al. [12] showed in a retrospective study, using leukocyte depleted blood products, a reduction in alloimmunization from 93 (26/28) to 24% (16/68). Red blood cells were depleted of leukocytes with the use of a specific leukocyte depleting filter. With an additional centrifugation of pooled platelet concentrates the leukocyte contamination was reduced to 5×10^6/concentrate.

Schiffer et al. [16] performed a prospective study in acute non-lymphocytic leukemia patients. The patients received frozen, deglycerolized red blood cells and platelet concentrates with 0.12×10^8 leukocytes/unit in the leukocyte depleted group and 0.65×10^8 leukocytes/unit in the control group; 42% of the control group (13/31) and 20% (5/25) of the patients receiving leukocyte depleted platelets became alloimmunized. The difference was not statistically significant ($p=0.071$). Furthermore, 19% of the control group and 16% of the leukocyte depleted group required HLA-matched donors during remission induction because of poor count increments.

Of the patients who had not been previously transfused or pregnant 33% of the control group and 27% of the leukocyte depleted group became alloimmunized. This difference is not significant. Murphy et al. [17] also studied prospectively the effect of leukocyte poor blood products on alloimmunization. Leukocyte poor red cells were prepared using a specific leukocyte depleting filter; the maximum accepted leukocyte count per unit was 8×10^6. The mean leukocyte contamination of platelet concentrates in the control group was 5.38×10^9, in the leukocyte depleted group $0.07\text{-}0.22 \times 10^9$ per concentrate. A third group received leukocyte poor HLA-matched platelet concentrates. As a result 48% (15/31) in the control group and 16% (3/19) in the leukocyte depleted group developed HLA antibodies ($p=0.02$), and none in the HLA-matched group; 23% in the control group and 5% in the leukocyte depleted group became refractory to platelet transfusion and needed HLA-matched platelet transfusion.

In summary, although not proven for all categories of patients it seems very suggestive that transfusion of leukocyte poor or leukocyte free blood products reduces or prevents alloimmunization. Concerning red blood cells, it is very costly and time consuming to prepare leukocyte free red cells in the way Sirchia [14] does. In this context the following studies might be of interest: Oh et al. [18] transfused 6 groups of rhesus monkeys three times with whole blood. Group A received fresh blood, B received 1-week old blood, C received 2-week old blood, D received 3-week old blood, E received 4-week old blood and F received 1-week old platelet suspension. One week following each transfusion serum was tested for lymphocytotoxicity. The results showed that the longer blood was stored the less was its immunogenicity, especially after storage for more than 3 weeks. Dzik et al. [19] investigated changes in mononuclear subpopulations in whole blood stored under standard Blood Bank conditions. During the first week of storage the percentage of viable cells bearing T-lymphocyte markers, declined from 66% to 29%. When whole blood was stored at room temperature (22°C) these changes did not occur. Light et al. [20] also studied the effect of storage on the cellular characteristics of blood. They found a rapid disappearance of T-cells and other cells bearing HLA-antigens especially after storage of 17 or more days. Functional analysis of the cells revealed virtual disappearance of MLC and mitogen responsiveness. For these reasons we think it is worthwhile to examine the effect of transfusion of RCC's stored for more than 3 weeks in combination with leukocyte free platelet transfusion on the incidence of alloimmunization in leukemic patients.

References

1. Ahrons S, Kissmeyer-Nielsen F. Serological investigations of 1358 transfusion reactions. Dan Med Bull 1968;15:259-62.
2. Kevy SV, Schmidt PJ, McGinnis MH, Workman WG. Febrile, non-hemolytic transfusion reactions and the limited role of leuko-agglutinins in their etiology. Transfusion 1962;2:7-16.
3. Decary F, Ferner P, Girvidoni L et al. An investigation of nonhemolytic transfusion reactions. Vox Sang 1984;46:277-85.
4. Menitove JE, McElligott MC, Aster RH. Febrile transfusion reaction: What blood component should be given next? Vox Sang 1982;42:318-21.
5. Thulstrup H. The influence of leukocyte and thrombocyte incompatibility of non-hemolytic transfusion reactions. Vox Sang 1971;21:233-50.
6. De Rier MA, van der Plas-Dalen CM, Engelfriet CP, von dem Borne AEG Kr. The serology of febrile transfusion reactions. Vox Sang 1985;49:126-34.
7. Perkins HA, Payne R, Ferguson J, Wood M. Nonhemolytic febrile transfusion reactions. Vox Sang 1966;11:578-600.
8. Meryman HT, Hornblower M. The preparation of red cells depleted of leukocytes. Transfusion 1986;26:101-6.
9. Wenz B. Microaggregate blood filtrations and the febrile transfusion reaction. Transfusion 1983;23:95-8.
10. Kelton JG, All AM. Platelet transfusion – a critical appraisal. In: Schiffer CA (ed). Clinics in oncology. London: WA Saunders Publ. 1983;2:549-87.
11. Slichter SJ. Controversies in platelet transfusion therapy. Ann Rev Med 1980; 31:509-40.
12. Eernisse JG, Brand A. Prevention of platelet refractoriness due to HLA-antibodies by administration of leukocyte-poor blood components. Exp Haemat 1981;9:77-83.
13. Daly PA, Schiffer CA, Aisner J, Wiernik PH. One hour posttransfusion increments are valuable in predicting the need for HLA-matched preparations. JAMA 1980;243:435-8.
14. Sirchia G, Rebulla P, Mascaretti L et al. The clinical importance of leukocyte depletion in regular erythrocyte transfusions. Vox Sang 1986;51(suppl.1):2-8.
15. Fisher M, Chapman JR, Ting A, Morris PJ. Allo-immunization to HLA antigens following transfusion with leukocyte-poor and purified platelet suspensions. Vox Sang 1985;49:331-5.
16. Schiffer CA, Dutcher JP, Aisner J, Hogge D, Wiernik PH, Reilly JP. A randomized trial of leukocyte-depleted platelet transfusion to modify allo-immunization in patients with leukemia. Blood 1983;62:815-20.
17. Murphy MF, Metcalfe P, Thomas H et al. Use of leukocyte-poor blood components and HLA-matched platelet donors to prevent allo-immunization. Brit J Haemat 1986;62:529-34.
18. Oh JH, McClure HM. Lymphocytotoxic antibodies induced by fresh blood, stored blood, and platelets in rhesus monkeys. Transplant Proc 1982;14:410-2.
19. Dzik WH, Neckers L. Mononuclear cell-surface antigens during storage of banked blood. Transplant 1984;38:67-71.
20. Light JA, Metz S, Oddenino K et al. Donor-specific transfusion with deminished sensitization. Transplant 1982;34:352-5.

MANAGEMENT AND PREVENTION OF CYTOMEGALOVIRUS INFECTION

T.H. The, W. van der Bij

Introduction

Cytomegalovirus (CMV), a member of the family of *Herpesviridae*, is commonly spread in man. Infectious CMV is excreted in the saliva, urine, breastmilk, cervix and semen, also by apparently healthy individuals. This is the main reason for its ubiquitous nature.

CMV infections in experimental animals and natural infections in man have clearly demonstrated an intricate and close relationship between CMV and immunological response in the host. While a virus specific immune response is mounted to limit the virus spread, CMV infection is also likely to cause a serious depression of hosts' immune response. The resultant effect in healthy immunocompetent individuals is usually an asymptomatic seroconversion or a mononucleosis. However, active CMV infection may be associated with significant morbidity and mortality in patients with a deficient (cellular) immune system, such as premature newborn infants, congenital and acquired immunodeficiency syndromes, malignant diseases treated with intensive chemotherapy and irradiation, and immunosuppressed organ-transplant and bone marrow transplant recipients.

The essential role of cell mediated immunity has been well recognized in bone marrow transplant recipients who developed CMV infection. Patients with CMV infections who developed CMV specific cytotoxicity lymphocyte responses survived, but patients who failed to generate these responses generally died of CMV infection [1]. In addition, patients with fatal infection had depressed levels of natural killer cell and antibody-dependent killer cell activity before and during their CMV infection, while patients who survived did not. Thus, a correct evaluation of the crucial phase of the intricate relationship between CMV induced immunosuppression and host immune response is most important in the management of patients at risk.

It is important to note that a significant number of these infections is transmitted by blood transfusions and organ transplantations, especially when seronegative recipients receive organs from seropositive donors. These individuals acquire a so-called primary CMV infection and because a pre-existing immunity is not yet present the clinical symptoms in this group are more pronounced than in recipients who are already CMV-seropositive and have built up virus-specific memory T cells. However, this statement is relative because secondary CMV infections, caused by reinfections with other CMV strains or reactivation of latent CMV infections can also cause serious clinical problems in patients depending on their cellular immunocompetence under the given immunosuppressive therapy. Therefore, transfusion transmitted CMV infections are becoming increasingly important. This article will deal with the importance of early and reliable diagnostic techniques in the management and prevention of serous infections.

CMV-replication and viral antigens

The human CMV is a highly species-specific, double-stranded DNA virus with a large genome of 235 kB with a coding capacity of at least 70 proteins. Infection of fetal fibroblasts with AD169, one of the laboratory strains of

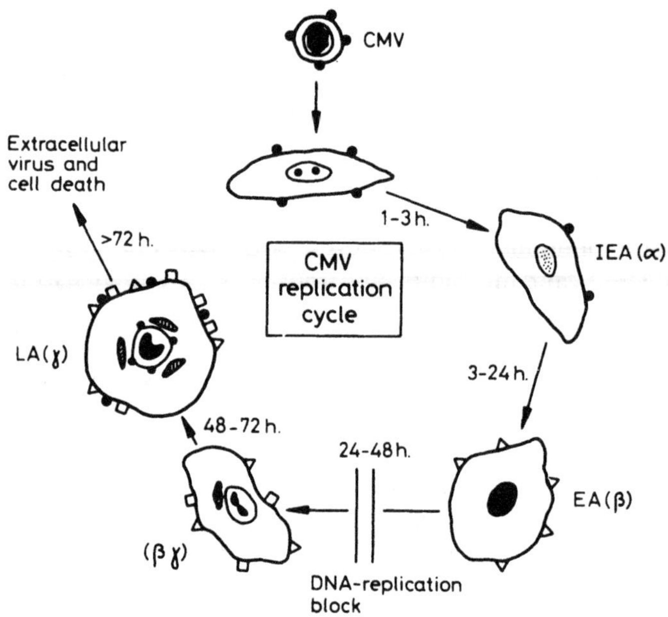

Figure 1. Distinct phase in the replication cycle of human cytomegalovirus – CMV = cytomegalovirus enveloped virion particle: IEA (α) = immediate early antigens, appearing diffusely in the nucleus within one hour after entry of CMV into the cell; EA (β) = early antigens induced at about 3 hours after infection which predominantly accumulate in the nucleus in the absence of viral DNA-replication (△) early membrane antigens; ($\beta\gamma$) = after onset of viral DNA-synthesis, which occurs about 24 hours after infection, nuclear inclusions are formed but infectious virus cannot be demonstrated yet (□) late membrane antigen; LA (γ) = late antigens, present in the nucleus as large nuclear inclusions and in the Golgi-region, being a predominant site of viral envelopment; (▲ , □) prominent expression of membrane antigens; (●) (possible) expression of viral envelope antigens or virus particles bound to the cell surface.

CMV, is a widely used system to have the CMV-specific antigens at one's disposal for diagnostic and immunological studies. After infection several CMV encoded antigens and induced host cell proteins appear intracellularly and on the surface membrane. Based on blocking of host cell metabolism and on patterns and localization of immunofluorescence with human sera three distinct phase of the infectious cycle can be defined, marking the emergence of immediate early, early and late antigens (IEA, EA and LA) (Fig. 1). The final result of the 'teamwork' of these subsequent phases is the release of new infectious viral particles and death of the host cell [2].

Detection of CMV in blood

Cytomegalovirus is transmittable by blood transfusions and especially leukocyte transfusions. These observations support our notion that we are dealing with a cell-associated virus and therefore the question arises whether CMV could be detected in certain cell types. Although for many years it is known that the virus can be transmitted by transfusions with blood from CMV-seropositive donors, viral cultures from blood cells derived from buffy coat from these donors were negative. It is important to note that infectious virus could only be isolated from leukocytes from patients with an *active* CMV infection.

Interestingly, Schrier and Oldstone [3] reported that HCMV specific messenger RNA is detectable in the CD4+ subpopulation of T lymphocytes in latently infected healthy subjects. The foregoing results indicate that CMV might be present in an incomplete form as CMV-DNA in certain lymphocytes from healthy individuals with a latent infection. The results of studies in patients after kidney transplantation have shown that positive virus isolation from the buffy coat (CMV-viremia) is related to those acute CMV infections with overt symptoms of disease. Using CMV specific monoclonal antibodies against immediate early antigens (CMV-IEA), prepared in our laboratory, we recently succeeded in showing these antigens in blood leukocytes from patients with an active CMV infection [4]. These CMV-IEA positive cells were only detected during the onset of disease in relation with the period of clinical symptoms of CMV infection and that these cells have the morphology of polymorphonuclear leukocytes and monocytes. Very rarely lymphocytes were positive which were T cells and not B lymphocytes. In a prospective longitudinal study in patients after organ transplantation the emergency of CMV-antigen positive blood leukocytes reached a peak, decreased and disappeared thereafter at the moment of the appearence or rise of virus-specific circulating antibodies. CMV antigens appeared, on average, nine days before a significant rise of antibody levels. The test was positive in patient groups with a primary as well as a secondary CMV infection. The test is virus-specific and of clinical relevance for the early and rapid diagnosis (within a few hours) of an active CMV infection and its possible therapeutic consequences. The essential steps of its method are presented in Table 1.

Table 1. Method of CMV antigen detection in blood leukocytes.

- Isolation of peripheral blood leukocytes
- Cytocentrifuge-preparations ($\geqslant 100 \times 10^3$ leukocytes)
- Indirect immunoperoxidase staining with:
  (three) monoclonal antibodies against CMV-IEA
- Detection and (semi)quantification of IEA positive leukocytes

Management of CMV infections

Especially in organ transplantation and bone marrow transplantation the management of CMV infections is difficult because the symptoms of infection resemble graft rejection and graft-versus-host disease. Therefore reliable and rapid methods are necessary for a correct diagnosis at the beginning of the disease because of the obvious important clinical implications with regard to the dosage of the immunosuppressive regime, which in cases of CMV infections has to be lowered, whereas graft rejections require high doses of these drugs. Diagnostic methods can be invasive in patients with pneumonitis, requiring lung biopsies for detection of the causative infectious agents. Evaluation of these difficult clinical situations could be aimed by following these patients with a sensitive serological method, a CMV-ELISA test. Seroconversions or significant rises, especially of IgM antibodies against CMV late antigens have been proved to be quite successful. Further improvement of diagnostic facilities is provided by rapid virus isolation methods from blood leukocytes developed by Griffiths et al. [5] using CMV-specific monoclonal antibodies applied on early virus isolates, and by our direct detection of virus-specific immediate early antigens in circulating blood leukocytes. For the patients with organ transplantation the diagnosis of acute infections implies a reduction or stopping of the immunosuppressive regimen in order to permit the host to recover from the CMV infection. Antiviral chemotherapy with dihydroxy-propoxy-methyl guanine and Foscarnet is applied increasingly in clinical trials, with varying success. In addition, treatment of patients with hyperimmune gammaglobulin fractions showed promising results [6,7].

Prevention of CMV infection

In patients belonging to the above mentioned high risk groups for serious CMV infections prevention and treatment of CMV infections is essential, and such a strategy is shown in Table 2.

Table 2. Prevention and treatment.

- Serological detection
- Selective use of 'CMV-negative' blood products
- Acceleration immune reconstitution, i.e. tapering of immunosuppression
- CMV immunoglobulins
- Antiviral chemotherapy

First, serotyping of recipients with a sensitive ELISA method for IgG anti-CMV-LA antibodies is needed to recognize CMV-seronegative from the positive individuals. Especially the seronegative ones need blood or blood cells and, if possible, also organs from CMV-seronegative donors. Prevention of secondary CMV infection may be partially achieved by using leukocyte-free blood in stead of whole blood for transfusion to CMV-seropositive recipients. In addition, the use of leukocyte depleted and stored blood in stead of fresh blood also reduces CMV infectivity.

References

1. Quinnan GV, Kirmani N, Esber E, et al. HLA-restricted cytotoxic T lymphocyte and nonthymic cytotoxic lymphocyte responses to cytomegalovirus infection of bone marrow transplantation. J Immunol 1981;126:2036-41.
2. Middeldorp JM. Diagnostic and immunological aspects of the antibody response to human cytomegalovirus infection. Acad Thesis, University of Groningen, 1985.
3. Schrier RD, Nelson JA, Oldstone MBA. Detection of human cytomegalovirus in peripheral blood lymphocytes in a natural infection. Science 1985;230:1048-51.
4. Van der Bij W, Torensma R, van Son WJ, et al. Expression of cytomegalovirus antigens in blood leukocytes and an early diagnostic marker of active infection. Submitted Transplantation.
5. Griffiths PD, Stirk PR, Ganczakowski M, et al. Rapid diagnosis of cytomegalovirus infection in immunocompromised patients by detection of early antigen fluorescent foci. Lancet 1984;ii:1242-5.
6. Winston DJ, Ho WG, Lin CH, Budinger MD, Champlin RE, Gale RP. Intravenous immunoglobulin for modification of cytomegalovirus infections associated with bone marrow transplantation. Am J Med 1984;30:128-33.
7. Condie RM, O'Reilly RJ. Prevention of cytomegalovirus infection by prophylaxis with an intravenous, hyperimmune, native, unmodified cytomegalovirus globulin. Am J Med 1984;30:134-41.

GRAFT-VERSUS-HOST DISEASE AND THE ROLE OF BLOOD PRODUCT IRRADIATION

S.F. Leitman, M.D.

Introduction

Antigenic differences between the donor and the recipient in a blood transfusion may lead to a variety of immunologic reactions following transfusion. Most frequently, this involves immunologic rejection of transfused red cells, white cells, or platelets. However, on rare occasions the reaction may occur in the opposite direction, and immunologically active lymphocytes in a transfused unit may generate a severe reaction against the recipient. This is known as a graft-versus-host (GvH) reaction. It has become clear that GvH reactions may occur whenever immunologically competent allogeneic lymphocytes are transfused into an immunocompromized host.

The aggressive and widespread use of chemotherapy, radiation therapy, and bone marrow transplantation in the treatment of neoplastic and non-neoplastic diseases has resulted in a large population of patients at risk of developing posttransfusion GvH disease. Increased demands have been placed on transfusion services to supply blood products from which all mitotically active lymphocytes have been removed. It now appears that the most efficient way to eliminate immunocompetent mononuclear cells from blood products is by exposure to ionizing radiation. In this review, the etiology of posttransfusion GvH reactions and the patient populations documented to be at risk of this disorder will be discussed. The efficacy of varying doses of irradiation on eliminating viable lymphocytes from blood products, and the potential for radiation-induced damage to other cell types in the irradiated unit will be reviewed.

Pathogenesis of graft-versus-host reactions

Animal systems have provided useful model for determining the etiology of graft-versus-host disease (GvHD). Newborn mice and lethally irradiated adult mice develop a fatal 'runting syndrom', characterized by weight loss, diarrhea, lymphoid atrophy, and hepatic necrosis following transfusions of heterologous spleen, lymph node, thymus, buffy coat, or bone marrow cells. [1,2]. Mature T lymphocytes carried in the donor inoculum have been shown to be the effector cells in this murine model of GvHD, whereas antigens of the major (H-2) histocompatibility locus act as the targets of the reaction [3,4] Spleen cells transplanted from neonatally thymectomized mice can reconstitute hematopoiesis in irradiated recipients without causing GvHD [5]. Elimination of mature T cells from murine donor marrow by pretreatment with monoclonal anti-T cell antibodies plus complement can prevent GvHD even in mice transplanted across major histocompatibility barriers [6]. Lethal GvHD has also occurred in irradiated mice receiving infusions of H-2 identical allogeneic lymphocytes; as few as 3×10^4 total T cells can cause GvHD in such donor-recipient pairs. Differences in minor (non H-2) histocompatibility antigens are assumed to be responsible for the reaction in such cases, although the precise identity of these target antigens is not known [7].

The occurrence of GvHD in man closely follows the pattern predicted by murine models. Donor T cell stimulation in response to the histocompatibility antigens of the host is thought to initiate the process [8]; Since extensive polymorphisms exist in both the major histocompatibility (HLA) locus of man as well as in minor, poorly described, tissue histocompatibility antigens, severe GvH reactions are common not only in recipients of HLA-incompatible marrow, but also in recipients of 'HLA-identical' sibling grafts. Currently, 30 to 60% of patients receiving marrow transplants from HLA-matched siblings will develop clinically significant acute GvHD, and 15-20% of transplanted patients will die of its complications [9].

The factors involved in determining which patients will develop acute GvHD following HLA-matched marrow transplantation, and in predicting the severity of their reactions, are not well defined. Older recipient age and sex-mismatched donor-recipient pairs, especially female-to-male transplants, have been associated with an increased occurrence of acute GvH reactions, whereas protective isolation has been shown to decrease their frequency and severity [10]. Systemic bacterial infection may both initiate and potentiate GvHD via the immunostimulatory effects of endotoxin. Circulating endotoxin released during Gram negative bacteremia has been shown to augment the response of T cells to alloantigen in vitro and enhance the reactivity of donor T cells to host antigens in vivo [11].

Treatment of established GvHD using immunosuppressive drugs such as corticosteroids, antithymocyte globulin, or cyclosporine is generally unsuccessful, and efforts have focused on prevention. Attempts to avert GvHD following bone marrow transplantation have followed two routes: treatment of the recipient with systemic immunosuppressives, and treatment of the donor marrow with agents that deplete it of T cells. Use of methotrexate or cyclosporine, alone or in combination with antithymocyte globulin, steroids or other drugs, may decrease the incidence and severity of acute GvHD if the agents are begun immediately after grafting and continued for 3 to 12 months [12-14], but they do not eliminate it entirely. In constrast, significant GvHD has been successfully avoided by depletion of mature T cells from donor marrow inoculum [15,16]. Several methods are available to accomplish this, including immunologic removal of T cells by incubation with monoclonal anti-T cell antibodies plus complement [17,18], or with antibodies linked to toxins or bound to magnetic beads [15,19], as well as physical removal by lectin agglutination and E-rosetting [20] or counterflow elutriation [21]. However, the beneficial effect of T cell depletion on preventing severe GvH reactions had been counterbalanced by the increased incidence of both graft rejection and leukemic relapse in recipients of T cell depleted marrow allografts [17,18].

Clinical manifestations of GvH reactions

Both posttransfusion and posttransplantation GvHD are characterized by abnormalities in three target organs: the skin, the liver, and the gastrointestinal tract [22-25]. The earliest symptoms, fever and rash, appear 3 to 30 days following transfusion and are followed by profuse watery diarrhea, marked jaundice, and pancytopenia. Since symptoms of fever, rash, hepatitis, and diarrhea are relatively nonspecific, it may be difficult to support the diagnosis of posttransfusion GvHD on clinical grounds alone. Confirmatory studies may include cytogenetic analysis of donor and recipient tissues, especially in cases of sex disparity, and HLA typing of donor and recipient lymphocytes [26-29]. In addition, histologic confirmation can be achieved by skin biopsy, which typically shows hyperkeratosis, lymphocytic infiltration, and vacuolar degeneration [30], and by bone marrow biopsy, which often reveals a histiocytic infiltrate with erythrophagocytosis [31].

In contrast to the clinical recognition of posttransplantation GvHD, which is easily identified whether the symptoms are mild or severe, cases of posttransfusion GvHD have been recognized only when the patient was severely affected, and the outcome has been fatal in 90% of cases. In accord with experience gained in the posttransplantation setting, attempts at treating established, severe posttransfusion GvHD with immunosuppressive agents have been uniformly unsuccessful [22-24]. Thus, similar to the posttransplantation setting, attention has focused on prevention of the disorder and determination of high risk groups.

Posttranfusion GvHD: patient risk groups

Premature and full term neonates have a small but well-documented risk of GvHD following blood transfusion. The disorder has been reported in seven infants who received either exchange transfusions or intrauterine as well as exchange transfusions [32-35], and in one infant who received only platelets of maternal origin [36] (Table 1). The outcome was uniformly fatal. Since it is likely that only fatal cases were recognized and confirmed by autopsy or HLA studies, the actual risk of posttransfusion GvHD in this population is unknown, and may be considerably higher than the small number of reported cases would suggest.

Children with congenital immune deficiency syndromes involving severe impairment in cellular immunity appear to be at considerable risk of posttransfusion GvH reactions. Eleven cases have been fully documented (Table 2) and include three patients whose transfusions consisted only of fresh nonfrozen plasma, containing less than 10^7 lymphocytes per unit [37-39]. In addition, engraftment of intrauterine-derived maternal lymphocytes is common

Table 1. Clinical features of neonates with posttransfusion GvHD.

Diagnosis	Age	Product transfused*	Ref.
1. Prematurity	33-wk gestation	ExTx (x2)	31
2. Prematurity	28-wk gestation	600 ml WB ExTx	32
3. HDN**	32-wk gestation	IU Tx (600 ml PRBC) ExTx (1000 ml WB)	33
4. HDN	Term	ExTx (1500 ml WB)	
5. HDN	33-wk gestation	IU Tx (x3); ExTx (x6)	34
6. HDN	36-wk gestation	IU Tx (230 ml PRBC) ExTx (x5)	35
7. HDN	36-wk gestation	IU Tx (220 ml PRBC) ExTx (x2)	35
8. NAIT***	Term	Maternal platelets	36

* ExTx = exchange transfusion; IU Tx = intrauterine transfusion; WB = whole blood; PRBC = packed red blood cells.
** HDN = hemolytic disease of the newborn.
*** NAIT = neonatal alloimmune thrombocytopenia.

Table 2. Posttransfusion GvHD in patients with congenital immunodeficiency syndromes.

Diagnosis	Age	Product transfused*	Ref.
1. Wiskott-Aldrich syndrome	32 mo	fresh plasma	37
2. SCID**	11 yr	fresh plasma	38
3. SCID	5 mo	fresh plasma	39
4. SCID	3 mo	50 ml WB	39
5. SCID	3 mo	WB, 2U	41
6. SCID	3.5 mo	5000 ml WB (ExTx)	42
7. SCID	4 mo	WB, 1U; PRBC, 2U	43
8. SCID	5 mo	WB, 1U	44
9. SCID	8 mo	750 ml BC	42
10. SCID	11 mo	125 ml WB	25
11. SCID	18 mo	200 ml PRBC	45

* 'U' indicates a one unit transfusion; ExTx = exchange transfusion; WB = whole blood; BC = buffy coat cells; PRBC = packed red blood cells.
** SCID = severe combined immunodeficiency disease.

in this disorder, and is occasionally associated with the development of GvHD [40]. Since the fevers, recurrent infection, and chronic diarrhea that characterize GvHD may mimic the symptoms of primary immunodeficiency, many cases of posttransfusion GvHD in this population of severely ill children have probably gone unrecognized, and the true risk is unknown.

Patients with acquired immunodeficiency syndrom (AIDS) commonly manifest profound lymphopenia and markedly altered T cell number and function [46]. However, despite disturbances in immunoregulation severe enough to result in lifethreatening opportunistic infections, patients with AIDS do not appear to be at risk of posttransfusion GvHD. There have been no documented cases of GvHD following transfusion in such patients, and no evidence of GvHD identified during autopsy of nearly 100 patients with AIDS at the N.I.H. (E. Lack, personal communication).

Patients with acute leukemia, Hodgkin's disease, and non-Hodgkin's lymphoma have been reported to develop GvHD following transfusion of either red cells, platelets, or granulocytes (Table 3). The GvH reactions occurred during periods of maximal immunosuppression induced by chemotherapy and/or radiation therapy. The outcome was uniformly fatal in the patients with lymphoma, although as many as a third of the patients with leukemia recovered. Estimations of the risk of posttransfusion GvHD in this population are extremely difficult to determine, and have ranged from 0.01% to 1.0% [52,53].

Only two patients with solid tumors, a two year child with neuroblastoma and a 59 year old female with glioblastoma have been reported to develop

Table 3. Posttransfusion GvHD in patients with acute leukemia and lymphoma.

Diagnosis	Age	Products transfused*	Ref.
1. AML**	6 yr	PRCB's, 2U; gran, 2U; platelets, 4U	47
2. AML	19 yr	washed RBC's, 4U; platelets, 1 pack	48
3. AML	38 yr	washed RBC's, 12 U; plts 14U, gran, 12 U	48
4. AML	50 yr	granulocytes, 10U	49
5. AML	45 yr	PRBC's, 2U; gran, 3U; platelets, 2 packs	50
6. AML	60 yr	PRBC's, 4U; gran, 2U; platelets, 5 packs	50
7. ALL	7.5 yr	granulocytes, 2U	23
8. ALL	10 yr	granulocytes	26
9. ALL	5 yr	whole blood, 5U	26
10. NHL	6 yr	150 ml buffy coat	22
11. NHL	30 yr	granulocytes, 5U	27
12. NHL	34 yr	granulocytes	30
13. HD, III_A	18 yr	PRBC, 2U	28
14. HD, III_A	6 yr	granulocytes, 3U	29
15. HD, II_B	24 yr	WB, 2U; plts, 2U	51
16. HD, III_A	30 yr	platelets, 4U	52

* WB = whole blood; PRBC = packed red blood cells; plts = platelet concentrates; gran = granulocyte concentrates.

** ALL = acute lymphocytic leukemia; AML = acute myelocytic leukemia; NHL = non-Hodgkin's lymphoma; HD = Hodgkin's disease.

Table 4. Lymphocyte contamination in blood products.*

Component	Lymphocytes per unit
Whole blood	$1.0\text{-}2.0\text{x}10^9$
Washed red cells	$1.0\text{-}2.0\text{x}10^8$
Filtered red cells	$1.0\text{x}10^7$
Frozen, deglycerolized red cells	$5.0\text{x}10^7$
Platelet pack (one unit)	$4.0\text{x}10^7$
Platelet pheresis pack	$3.0\text{x}10^8$
Granulocyte concentrate	$1.0\text{x}10^{10}$
Single donor plasma	$1.5\text{x}10^5$
Fresh frozen plasma	0
Cryoprecipitate	0

* Data derived from N.I.H. Department of Transfusion Medicine.

posttransfusion GvHD [24,29]. The disorder was fatal in both cases. It is notable that GvH reactions have not occurred in patients with the more common solid tumors treated with multimodality immunosuppressive therapy, such as breast, ovarian, and testicular carcinoma.

Recipients of autologous stored marrow undergo a preparative regimen of ablative chemotherapy and total body irradiation similar to that given to recipients of allogeneic marrow grafts [54]. Posttransfusion GvHD has not yet been reported in this setting. However, since most autologous marrow recipients are treated on protocols involving transfusion of irradiated blood products only, the actual risk in this group cannot be determined at present.

Lymphocyte contamination in blood products

GvHD has been attributed to the passenger lymphocytes contained in units of whole blood and packed cells, washed red cells, platelet and granulocyte concentrates, and even single units of nonfrozen plasma. In the case of plasma only $8\text{x}10^4$ lymphocytes per kg were estimated to have been transfused [39]. Since the lymphocyte content of various blood products ranges for $1.5\text{x}10^5$ cells per unit of nonfrozen plasma to $5.0\text{x}10^9$ cells in a granulocyte concentrate, any of the blood products listed in table 4 may potentially be capable of initiating a lethal GvH reaction in a susceptible host.

GvHD has not been reported to follow transfusions of frozen deglycerolized red cells. However, while deglycerolization may remove up to 95% of the original lymphocytes in a unit of red cells, the remaining white cells are predominantly mononuclear and exhibit intact functional activity in vitro [55]. Newer depth-type blood filters, made from cotton wool, polyester, or cellulose acetate, are capable of removing greater than 99% of the leukocytes in a red cell unit. No cases of posttransfusion GvHD have been reported in recipient of such filtered units, but experience with these filters is limited.

Transfusions of frozen, cryopreserved blood components, such as plasma and cryoprecipitate, have not been associated with GvH reactions. Since a cryoprotective agent is not used during the preparation of these components, the final product does not contain functional cells and would not be expected to elicit a GvH reaction.

Standard blood bank techniques to reduce the lymphocyte content in blood components may thus lower the number of mononuclear cells, but do not eliminate them entirely. In contrast, ionizing radiation has been shown to completely inhibit lymphocyte mitotic potential [56]. Prophylactic irradiation of blood products prior to transfusion is presently the safest way to prevent posttransfusion GvHD. The remaining discussion will focus on identifying an optimum dose of radiation that will prevent lymphocyte engraftment while preserving intact red cell, platelet and granulocyte function.

Effects of irradiation on circulating blood cells

In order to initiate a GvH reaction, donor lymphocytes must both recognize the MHC antigens of the recipient as foreign, and respond to this stimulus by proliferating and producing cytotoxic factors. Small circulating lymphocytes are extremely radiosensitive. The mean dose of radiation associated with loss of reproductive capacity in these cells is less than 2 Gy. [57]. Lymphocyte proliferation in response to tissue alloantigen, as measured in a mixed lymphocyte culture (MLC), can be completely abolished by exposure to 5 Gy [56,58], although a higher dose of radiation, approaching 50 Gy, is necessary to completely inhibit blast transformation in response to mitogens [59,60]. Blast transformation only reflects the ability of cells to recognize and react to a stimulus and can occur without cell division. Since MLC reactivity directly reflects the mitotic potential of lymphocytes, irradiation of cells with a dose sufficient to abolish MLC reactivity (5 Gy) should eliminate the ability of such cells to induce a GvH reaction following transfusion. A certain nonuniformity in dose distribution is inherent in the actual irradiation of irregularly shaped blood products, and a three to four fold margin of safety is usually allowed. We would thus consider 12-20 Gy as the minimal radiation dose to use in the prophylactic irradiation of blood products. There have been no reports of posttransfusion GvHD in susceptible patients receiving blood products irradiated with at least 15 Gy [8].

In contrast to lymphocytes, mature erythrocytes are not mitotically active and are among the most radioresistant of circulating blood cells. Following exposure to 100 Gy, the in vivo survival of ^{51}chromium-labeled autologous red cells was not significantly different from that of nonirradiated controls [59]. Similarly, red cell units stored for 21 days and then exposed to up to 200 Gy of gamma radiation exhibited the same ATP, 2,3-DPG, and free hemoglobin levels as nonirradiated units [59]. However, packed red cell units exposed to 40 Gy and then stored for 35 days in CPDA-1 were recently shown to have slightly lower ATP and 2,3-DPG levels and higher free hemoglobin levels when compared with concurrently stored nonirradiated units [61]. The in vivo significance of these changes in stored irradiated cells remains to be demonstrated.

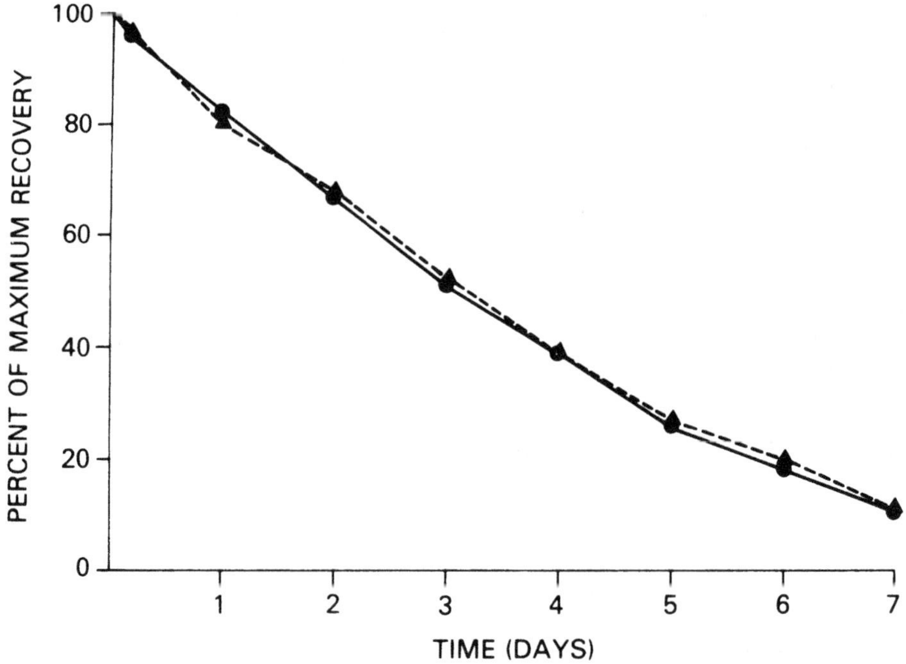

Figure 1. In a pair-controlled manner, platelet concentrates were collected from six donors on two occasions each and stored for 5 days at 22°C. One of each of the paired collections was irradiated with 30 Gy prior to storage. The in vivo survival of autologous ^{111}Indium-labeled platelets that had been irradiated prior to storage (▲ ---▲) did not differ from that of platelets stored in the nonirradiated state (●——●). Each point represents the mean of six values (Kodis C, Read EJ, Leitman SF).

Platelets, which are also mitotically inactive, appear to be similarly resistant to damage by ionizing radiation. Several small studies have suggested that in vivo ^{51}Cr-labeled platelet survival is unchanged after exposure to doses of radiation ranging from 50 to 750 Gy [59,62]. Platelets stored for 5 days and then treated with 50 Gy were shown to have normal shape, size, LDH and beta-thromboglobulin release, to generate normal amounts of thromboxane B_2, to exhibit normal responses to hypotonic stress, and to undergo equivalent degrees of synergistic aggregation to ADP plus collagen when compared to nonirradiated similarly stored platelet packs [63]. A recent pair-controlled study analyzed the effects of irradiation prior to storage on subsequent survival of indium-labeled autologous platelets [64]. Exposure to 30 Gy followed by 5 days of storage at 22°C was associated with normal in vivo recovery and survival (Fig. 1). Thus no additional storage lesion appeared to result from prolonged storage of platelets in the irradiated state.

Unlike erythrocytes and platelets, mature granulocytes contain an intact nucleus and, when stimulated, may engage in biochemical activities that lead to free radical formation. It is not surprising to find that the function of these cells may be significantly impaired by moderate doses of radiation. A dose-related decline in granulocyte locomotion has been demonstrated over exposures that ranged from 5 to 1200 Gy, although bactericidal capacity was affected only after exposure to 400 Gy [58]. Other investigators have similarly found that exposure to less than 50 Gy did not appear to alter endotoxin-stimulated nitroblue tetrazolium (NBT) reduction, bactericial capacity, or chemotaxis [65,66]. The effect of ionizing radiation on superoxide production in granulocytes has been difficult to characterize, however. In one study, a twenty percent reduction in phorbol ester-stimulated superoxide production was noted after exposure of granulocytes to 50 Gy [59]. Others have demonstrated a highly variable reduction (5 to 72%, mean 41%) in the number of phorbol ester-stimulated NBT-positive granulocytes following exposure to 25 Gy [67]. The results of these studies suggest that irradiation of granulocytes prior to transfusion may lead to defects in oxidative metabolism, but that these effects are highly variable.

Techniques of blood product irradiation

Cesium-137, a gamma emitter with a half-life of 30 years, is the most commonly used radioactive source for delivering a fixed dose of radiation to blood components. The cesium source is generally purchased as part of a free-standing blood irradiator containing a rotating platform for placement of the blood product, and double lead shields to encase the radioactive material. The current price of such a device ranges from $40,000 to $50,000 [68]. Depending on the strength of the cesium source, which ranges from 600 to 2400 curies in most commercially available devices, the dose rate at which a blood product is irradiated will range from 5 to 20 Gy per minute. The total dose delivered depends on the length of time the blood pack is exposed to the source, such that delivery of 15 to 50 Gy can be accomplished in 1 to 5 minutes if an 1800 curie source is used. Dosimetry checks are usually performed on a yearly basis, and the time of exposure adjusted to account for radioactive decay in the source.

Blood product irradiation may also be accomplished using conventional cobalt-60 sources or linear accelerators located in radiation therapy departments. In this case, the radiation is delivered using two standard anteroposterior fields. Lymphocyte proliferative ability can also be completely eliminated by exposure to ultraviolet light, which is significantly less expensive to employ than gamma radiation [69]. However, standard polyvinylchloride blood storage plastics do not allow penetration by ultraviolet light in the UV-B range (290-320 nm), the wavelength at which the desired cellular inhibitory effects are seen. Although routine blood product irradiation via UV exposure is thus impractical at present, synthesis of newer blood storage plastics or collection devices may make it possible to overcome this obstacle.

Since many smaller transfusion services do not have access to in-house irradiators, consideration has been given to maintaining an inventory of irradiated components, wherein radiation was delivered at another institution, usually a regional blood collection center. Such a practice raises two questions:

(1) Can irradiated units be stored as long as nonirradiated untis? (2) Can irradiated blood products be safely given to recipients not necessarily requiring such a special product?

To answer the storage question first, it is necessary to recall that the molecular interaction of ionizing radiation with cellular DNA is extremely rapid. The damage done by gamma radiation is nearly instantaneous; it will not increase during prolonged storage of an irradiated unit. This has been confirmed in vitro for red cell units irradiated and stored for 35 days [61] and in vivo for platelet concentrates irradiated and stored for 5 days [64]. Both the metabolic activity of red cells and the in vivo survival of platelets were not significantly impaired following prolonged storage in the irradiated state. These considerations do not apply to granulocytes, which should be transfused as soon as possible after collection.

In terms of the carcinogenic potential of an irradiated unit, at the very high dose rates used in irradiating blood packs, usually 10 Gy per minute or greater, there is no opportunity for repair of sublethal damage to DNA. All exposed cells will subsequently die an intramitotic or intermitotic death [57]. There is no potential for sustained proliferation of cells whose nucleic acid has been damaged by such high unfractionated doses of radiation. In addition, once a blood pack has been exposed to radiation and removed from the radiation source, it is not 'radioactive'. It does not pose the potential for radiation exposure to staff members manipulating it or to transfusion recipients. In view of these considerations, it appears that irradiated blood products may be safely transfused to patients who do not necessarily require irradiated blood. Due to the adverse effects of irradiation on granulocyte function, however, this practice should be limited to red cells and platelets. Irradiated blood products should be clearly labeled as such.

Summary and conclusions

Blood product irradiation is currently the most efficient and dependable way to prevent posttransfusion graft-versus-host disease. Doses of less than 30-40 Gy appear not to interfere with red cell or platelet function, however doses of greater than 20 Gy can significantly impair granulocyte metabolism. In contrast, lymphocyte mitotic activity can be completely inhibited by exposure to as little as 5 Gy. In balancing the considerations of minimal damage to non-mononuclear cells with the need for complete inhibition of lymphocyte proliferative capacity, we have selected 15-20 Gy as an optimum dose for the prophylactic irradiation of blood products.

Preliminary data suggest that red cells and platelets may be stored following irradiation for the full shelf-life of the original product. Adoption of such usage in transfusion practice would greatly aid inventory maintenance for transfusion services lacking on-site facilities for blood irradiation. There is no evidence that irradiated blood products pose either a carcinogenic or a radiation hazard to transfusion recipients.

Indications for blood product irradiation are given in table 5. Patients at highest risk of developing GvHD following transfusion include children with

Table 5. Indications for blood product irradiation.

Absolute indications	Relative indications	No definite indications
Congenital immune defeciency syndromes	Intrauterine transfusions	Non-premature neonates
Allogeneic and autologous bone marrow transplants	Neonatal exchange transfusions	Solid tumors
	Lymphoma	Acquired immunodeficiency syndrome (AIDS)
	Acute leukemia	

severe congenital immunodeficiency syndromes involving T lymphocytes and recipients of autologous and allogeneic bone marrow transplants. All cellular products given to such patients should be irradiated. It does not appear necessary to irradiate non-cellular frozen blood products such as fresh frozen plasma or cryoprecipitate.

At considerably less risk are patients receiving immunosuppressive therapy for hematologic malignancies, in whom no definite statement can be made about the likelihood of a GvH reaction following transfusion. At the height of sustained and severe therapy-induced cytopenias, the safest product for such patients is probably irradiated blood.

The risk assessment of posttransfusion GvH reactions in infants receiving intrauterine and/or exchange transfusions is extremely difficult. Although routine irradiation of blood products given to all premature infants or full-term neonates is not indicated, it appears reasonable to irradiate blood intended for intrauterine transfusion or for exchange transfusion following intrauterine transfusion.

Prophylactic irradiation of blood products is not necessary for patients with solid tumors receiving standard chemotherapy. Similarly, patients with AIDS do not appear to be at risk of posttransfusion GvHD and routine use of irradiated blood is not recommended in this setting. Until a fuller understanding of the disorder is achieved, irradiation of blood products should be limited only to those clinical settings in which disease risk has been definitively demonstrated.

Acknowledgements

The expert assistance of Ms. Trisha Stein in the preparation of this manuscript, and of Dr. Dennis Klinman and Dr. Elaine Sloand in reviewing the manuscript, are gratefully appreciated.

References

1. Billingham RE, Brent L. A simple method for inducing tolerance of skin homografts in mice. Transplant Bull 1957;4:67-71.
2. Simonsen M. The impact on the developing embryo and newborn animal of adult homologous cells. Acta Pathol Microbiol Scand 1957;40:480-500.
3. Korngold P, Sprent J. Lethal graft-versus-host disease after bone marrow transplantation across minor histocompatibility barriers in mice. J Exp Med 1978;148:1687-98.
4. Rolink AG, Gleichman E. Allosuppressor- and allohelper- T cells in acute and chronic graft-vs.-host disease. III. Different Lyt subsets induce different pathological syndromes. J Exp Med 1983;158:546-58.
5. Yunis EJ, Good RA, Smith J, Stutman O. Protection of lethally irradiated mice by spleen cells from neonatally thymectomized mice. Proc Natl Acad Sci USA 1974;71:2544-8.
6. Vallera DA, Soderling CC, Carlson GJ, Kersey JH. Bone marrow transplantation across major histocompatibility barriers in mice. Effect of elimination of T cells from donor grafts by treatment with monoclonal Thy-1.2 plus complement. Transplantation 1981;31:218-22.
7. Korngold R, Sprent J. Features of T cells causing H-2-restricted lethal graft-vs.-host disease across minor histocompatibility barriers. J Exp Med 1982;155: 872-83.
8. Thomas ED, Storb R, Clift RA, et al. Bone marrow transplantation. N Engl J Med 1975;292:832-43.
9. Storb R. Pathophysiology and prevention of graft-versus-host disease. In: McCullough J, Sandler SG (eds). Advances in immunobiology: Blood cell antigens and bone marrow transplantation. New York: Alan R. Liss 1984:337-66.
10. Deeg HJ, Storg R. Graft-versus-host disease: pathophysiological and clinical aspects. Ann Rev Med 1984;35:11-24.
11. Rose WC, Rodey GE, Rimm AR, Truitt RI, Bortin M. Mitigation of graft-versus-host disease in mice by treatment of donors with bacterial endotoxin. Exp Haematol 1976;4:90-6.
12. Ramsay NKC, Kersey JH, Robinson LL, et al. A randomized study of the prevention of graft-versus-host disease. N Engl J Med 1982;306:392-7.
13. Deeg HJ, Storb R, Thomas ED, et al. Cyclosporine as prophylaxis for graft-versus-host disease: a randomized study in patients undergoing marrow transplantation for acute nonlymphoblastic leukemia. Blood 1985;65:1325-34.
14. Storb R, Deeg HJ, Whitehead J, et al. Methotrexate and cyclosporine compared with cyclosporine alone for prophylaxis of acute graft-versus-host disease after marrow transplantation for leukemia. N Engl J Med 1986;314:729-35.
15. Prentice HG, Janossy G, Price-Jones L, et al. Depletion of T lymphocytes in donor marrow prevents significant graft-versus-host disease in matched allogeneic leukemic marrow transplant recipients. Lancet 1984;i:472-5.
16. Waldmann H, Hale G, Cividalli G, et al. Elimination of graft-versus-host disease by in vitro depletion of alloreactive lymphocytes with a monoclonal rat anti-human antibody. Lancet 1984;ii:483-5.
17. Mitsuyasu RT, Champlin RE, Gale RP. Treatment of donor bone marrow with monoclonal anti-T-cell antibody and complement for the prevention of graft-versus-host disease. An Intern Med 1986;105:20-6.
18. Martin PJ, Hansen JA, Buckner CD, et al. Effects of in vitro depletion of T cells in HLA-identical allogeneic marrow grafts. Blood 1985;66:664-72.

19. Filipovich AH, Vallera DA, Youle RJ, et al. Ex vivo treatment of donor bone marrow with anti-T-cell immunotoxins for prevention of graft-versus-host disease. Lancet 1984;i:469-71.
20. Reisner Y, Kapoor N, Kirkpatrick D, et al. Transplantation for severe combined immunodeficiency with HLA-A,B,D, DR incompatible parental marrow cells fractionated by soybean agglutinin and sheep red blood cells. Blood 1983;61: 341-48.
21. Noga SJ, Donnenberg AD, Schwartz CL, Strauss LC, Civin CI, Santos GW. Development of a simplified counterflow centrifugation elutriation procedure for deletion of lymphocytes from human bone marrow. Transplantation 1986;41:220-9.
22. Betzhold J, Hong R. Fatal graft-versus-host disease after a small leukocyte transfusion in a patient with lymphoma and varicella. Pediatrics 1978;62:63-6.
23. Rosen PC, Huestis DW, Corrigan JJ. Acute leukemia and granulocyte transfusion: Fatal graft-versus-host reaction following transfusion of cells obtained from normal donors. J Pediatr 1978;93:268-70.
24. Woods WG, Lubin BH. Fatal graft-versus-host disease following a blood transfusion in a child with neuroblastoma. Pediatrics 1981;67:217-21.
25. Hathaway WE, Fulginiti VA, Pierce CW, et al. Graft-versus-host reaction following a single blood transfusion. JAMA 1967;201:139-44.
26. Siimes MA, Koskimies S. Chronic graft-versus-host disease after blood transfusions confirmed by incompatible HLA antigens in bone marrow. Lancet 1982; i:42-3.
27. Wieden PL, Zuckerman N, Hansen JA. Fatal graft-versus-host disease in a patient with lymphoblastic leukemia following normal granulocyte transfusions. Blood 1981;57:328-32.
28. Dinsmore RE, Straus DJ, Pollack MS, et al. Fatal graft-versus-host disease following blood transfusion in Hodgkin's disease documented by HLA typing. Blood 1980;55:831-4.
29. Schmidmeier W, Feil W, Gebhart W, et al. Fatal graft-versus-host reaction following granulocyte transfusion. Blut 1982;45:115-9.
30. De Dobbeleer GD, Ledoux-Corbusier MH, Achten GA Graft-versus-host reaction. An ultrastructural study. Arch Dermatol 1975;111:1597-602.
31. Seemayer TA, Bolande RP. Thymic involution mimicking thymic dysplasia. A consequence of transfusion-induced graft-versus-host disease in a premature infant. Arch Pathol Lab Med 1980;104:141-4.
32. Hathaway WE, Brangle RW, Nelson TL, Roeckel IE. Aplastic anemia and alymphocytosis in an infant with hypogammaglobulinemia: Graft-versus-host reaction? J Pediatr 1966;68:713-22.
33. Bohm N, Kleine W, Enzel U. Graft-versus-host disease in two newborns after repeated blood transfusions because of rhesus incompatibility. Beitr Path Vol 1977;160:381-400.
34. Naiman JL, Punnett HH, Lischner HW, Destine ML, Arey JB. Possible graft-versus-host reaction after intrauterine transfusion for Rh erythroblastosis fetalis. N Engl J Med 1969;281:697-701.
35. Parkman R, Mosier D, Umansky I, Cochran W, Carpenter CB, Rosen FS. Graft-versus-host disease after intrauterine and exchange transfusions for hemolytic disease of the newborn. N Engl J Med 1974;290:359-63.
36. Martin B, Robin H, Williams R, Ornela W. Neonatal graft-versus-host disease following transfusion of maternal platelets. Transfusion 1983;23:417a.
37. Douglas SD, Fudenberg HH. Graft-versus-host reaction in Wiskott-Aldrich syndrome: Antemortem diagnosis of human GvH in an immunologic deficiency disease. Vox Sang 1969;16:172-8.

38. Rubinstein A, Radl J, Cottier H, Rossi E, Gugler E. Unusual combined immunodeficiency syndrome exhibiting kappa-IgD paraproteinemia, residual gut-immunity and graft-versus-host reaction after plasma infusion. Acta Pediatr Scand 1973;62:365-72.
39. Park BH, Good RA, Gate J, Burke B. Fatal graft-versus-host reaction following transfusion of allogeneic blood and plasma in infants with combined immunodeficiency disease. Transplant Proc 1974;6:385-7.
40. Pollack MS, Kirkpatrick D, Kapoor N, Dupont B, O'Reilly R. Identification by HLA typing of intrauterine-derived maternal T cells in four patients with severe combined immunodeficiency. N Engl J Med 1982;307:662-6.
41. Jacobs JC, Blanc WA, de Capoa A, et al. Complement deficiency and chromosomal breaks in a case of Swiss-type agammaglobulinemia. Lancet 1986;i:499-503.
42. Hathaway WE, Githens JH, Blackburn WR, Fulginiti V, Kempe CH. Aplastic anemia, histiocytosis and erythrodermia in immunologically deficient children. N Engl J Med 1965;273:953-8.
43. Niethammer D, Goldmann SF, Flad HD, et al. Graft-versus-host reaction after blood transfusion in a patient with cellular immunodeficiency: The role of histocompatibility testing. Eur J Pediatr 1979;132:43-8.
44. Gatti RA, Platt N, Pomerance HH, et al. Hereditary lymphopenic agammaglobulinemia associated with a distinctive form of short-limbed dwarfism and ectodermal dysplasia. J Pediatr 1969;75:675-84.
45. Robertson WR, Berry CL, Macaulay JC, Soothill JF. Partial immunodeficiency and graft-versus-host disease. Arch Dis Child 1971;46:571-4.
46. Fauci AS, Macher AM, Longo DL, et al. Acquired immunodeficiency syndrome: Epidemiologic, clinical, immunologic, and therapeutic considerations. Ann Intern Med 1984;100:92-106.
47. Cohen D, Weinstein H, Mihm M, Yankee R. Nonfatal graft-versus-host disease occurring after transfusion with leukocytes and platelets obtained from normal donors. Blood 1979;53:1053-7.
48. Schmitz N, Kayser W, Gassmann W, et al. Two cases of graft-versus-host disease following transfusion of nonirradiated blood products. Blut 1982;44:83-8.
49. Ford JM, Cullen MH, Lucey JJ, Tobias JS, Lister TA. Fatal graft-versus-host disease following transfusion of granulocytes from normal donors. Lancet 1976; ii:1167-9.
50. Lowenthal RM, Menon C, Challis DR. Graft-versus-host disease in consecutive patients with acute myeloid leukemia treated with blood cells from normal donors. Aust NZ J Med 1981;11:179-83.
51. Groff P, Torhorst J, Speck B, et al. Die Graft-versus-Host Krankheit, eine wenig bekannte Komplikation der Bluttransfusion. Schweiz Med Wschr 1976;106:634-9.
52. Von Fliedner V, Higby DJ, Kim U. Graft-versus-host reaction following blood transfusion. Am J Med 1982;72:951-61.
53. Schiffer CA, Aisner J, Dutcher JA, Wiernik PH. Sustained post-transfusion granulocyte increments following transfusion of leukocytes obtained from donors with chronic myelogenous leukemia. Am J Hematol 1983;15:65-74.
54. Yeager AM, Kaizer H, Santos GW, et al. Autologous bone marrow transplantation in patients with acute nonlymphocytic leukemia, using ex vivo marrow treatment with 4-hydroperoxycyclophosphamide. N Engl J Med 1986;315:141-7.
55. Crowley JP, Skrabut EM, Valeri CR. Immunocompetent lymphocytes in previously frozen washed red cells. Vox Sang 1974;26:513-7.

56. Sprent J, Anderson RE, Miller JF. Radiosensitivity of T and B lymphocytes. II. Effect of irradiation on response of T cells to alloantigens. Eur J Immunol 1974;4:204-10.
57. Hall EJ. Radiobiology for the radiologist. Hagerstown: Harper & Row 1978.
58. Valerius NH, Johansen KS, Nielsen OS, Platz P, Rosenkvist J, Sorensen H. Effect of in vitro x-irradiation on lymphocyte and granulocyte function. Scand J Hematol 1981;27:9-18.
59. Button LN, de Wolf WC, Newburger PE, Jacobson MS, Kevy SV. The effects of irradiation on blood components. Transfusion 1981;21:419-26.
60. Coifman RE, Good RA, Meuwissen HJ. The function of irradiated blood elements. I. Limitations on the response to phytohemagglutinin as an indicator of immunocompetence in irradiated lymphocytes. Proc Soc Exp Biol Med 1971; 137:155-60.
61. Moore GL, Ledford ME. Effects of 4000 rad irradiation on the in vitro storage properties of packed red cells. Transfusion 1985;25:583-5.
62. Greenberg ML, Chanana AD, Cronkite EP, Schiffer LM, Stryckmans PA. Extracorporeal irradiation of blood in man, radiation resistance of circulating platelets. Radiat Res 1968;35:147-54.
63. Moroff G, George VM, Siegl AM, Luban NLC. The influence of irradiation on stored platelets. Transfusion 1986;26:453-6.
64. Kodis C, Read EJ, Leitman SF, Carter CS, Klein HG. Effect of pre-storage irradiation on posttransfusion platelet survival. Transfusion 1986;26:568a.
65. Holley TR, van Epps DE, Harvey RL. Effect of high doses of radiation on human neutrophil chemotaxis, phagocytosis, and morphology. Am J Pathol 1974;75:61-8.
66. Patrone F, Dallegri F, Brema F, Sacchetti C. Effects of irradiation and storage on granulocytes harvested by continuous-flow centrifugation. Exp Hematol 1979;7:131-6.
67. Buescher ES, Holland PV, Gallin JI. Radiation-induced defective oxygen metabolism in leukocytes prepared for transfusion as assessed by nitroblue tetazolium reduction. Clin Res 1983;31:309a.
68. Atomic Energy of Canada Limited. Gammacell 1000 – Blood Irradiator. Kanata, Ontario 1984;1-4.
69. Kahn RA, Duffy BF, Rodey GG. Ultraviolet irradiation of platelet concentrates abrogates lymphocyte activation without affecting platelet function in vitro. Transfusion 1985;25:547-50.

PERSPECTIVES FOR LYMPHOKINE THERAPY: FROM GENETIC ENGINEERING TO IMMUNOLOGIC ENGINEERING*

R.T. Schooley

Introduction

In the three years since interferon therapy was last discussed at this symposium [1], there have been major advances in both our basic understanding of cellular immune mechanisms, and in our ability to produce large quantities of human lymphokines by recombinant and non-recombinant DNA techniques. These advances have greatly expanded our horizons in the development of innovative therapeutic modalities using interferons and other biologic response modifiers. In parallel with these basic and applied advances in our knowledge of cellular immunology, a broader array of antiviral chemotherapeutic agents has been developed [2-6]. These developments, coupled with early observations about pharmacokinetics and toxicities of interferons, have resulted in a change in the primary focus of lymphokine therapy. Rather than being limited to the area of antiviral therapy, there is now a much wider view of the prospects for the therapeutic application of lymphokines. A final development over the past three years has been the spread of human immunodeficiency virus (HIV), and an increasing sense of urgency in developing effective therapies for this devastating pathogen [6,7]. In that cellular immunodeficiency is the basic mechanism by which HIV induces morbidity, the potential use of lymphokines in immune restoration has become an area of very intense investiation [8-10].

At the in vitro level, a large number of lymphokines have been described and characterized to various degrees, but up to this point only three (interferon alpha, interferon gamma, and interleukin-2 have been produced in large quantities and used in large scale human trials. These human trials have focused on a wide array of diseases, including cancer, viral diseases, congenital and acquired immunodeficiencies, and neurology disorders. Although on could expend a great deal of effort recounting in detail the results of these clinical trials, it might be more productive to concentrate on a more restricted group of topics in order to outline future directions for the clinical utility of lymphokines rather than to simply catalogue the large number of clinical trials which have been carried out over the past several years. Thus, the focus of this manuscript will be on the potential utility of interferons and interleukins

* Supported in part by a grant from the National Cancer Institute (CA-37461).

in the therapy of neoplasia, and of the possible role of immunomodulatory agents in the treatment of the acquired immune deficiency syndrome (AIDS). Given the central role of blood banks in several aspects of lymphokine therapy (Table 1), it is very appropriate that this topic be one of the features of this symposium.

Table 1. Roles of blood banks in adoptive immunotherapy.

1. Collection of large numbers of peripheral blood mononuclear cells
   a. preparation of lymphokines
   b. starting materials for in vitro manupulations of autologous cells
2. Administration of cellular products following in vitro manipulation
3. Quality control of blood components

Basic mechanisms

The cellular immune response is comprised of a complex network of cellular effectors, and soluble mediators which function primarily to coordinate the cellular immune response. The initial phase in the induction of a cellular immune response requires processing of antigen by cells of the monocyte/macrophage lineage. When such processed antigen is presented to lymphocytes of the helper/inducer (primarily T4 expressing) surface phenotype in the presence of both the compatible HLA class II molecules and interleukin-1, these cells are induced to produce interleukin-2 (IL-2) and to express receptors for IL-2. In addition, IL-2 operates in a positive feedback loop by the induction of additional IL-2 receptors. Such activated T4 cells proliferate, and participate in the activation of natural killer (NK) cells, cytotoxic-T cells, lymphokine activated killer (LAK) cells, and B-cells through the elaboration of interleukin-2. IL-2 driven T-cells also produce interferon gamma which plays a further role in the activation of NK cells and HLA restricted cytotoxic T-cells. In addition, interferon gamma enhances the expression of HLA class II molecules on the surface of activated monocyte/macrophage which then in turn further enhances the cellular immune response. Defects in one or several of these steps can have profound effects on the coordination and intensity of the cellular immune response. In the case of antineoplastic therapy, interferons (alpha and gamma) have additional direct antitumor effects which may be operative above and beyond the immunomodulatory effects which are primarily exhibited by interferon gamma.

Toxicities and pharmacokinetics of interferons and interleukin-2

Interferon alpha for clinical trials has been produced by both non-recombinant and recombinant DNA techniques [11-14]. The initial clinical trials were made possible by preparations which were produced by Kari Cantell utilizing pooled buffy coat preparations from Finish Red Cross blood donors. After a series of purification steps, a material was produced which contained 1-2x10^4 U interferon alpha/mg of protein. Lymphoblastoid interferon, as this form of interferon is termed, achieved peak levels 4-6 hours after intramuscular or subcutaneous injection and exhibits a serum half-life of 4-8 hours. Interferon alpha diffuses poorly into the central nervous system and other extravascular sites. With the recent advances in molecular biology, it has become apparent that there are at least 14 different species of interferon alpha. These forms of interferon alpha vary both in molecular structure and in activity against specific viruses, but pharmacokinetics in these species which have been most extensively studied are similar to lymphoblastoid interferon. Although recombinant DNA techniques have allowed for the development of much more highly purified interferon preparations, interferon toxicity has co-purified with biologic activity.

The toxicity of interferon alpha is dependent on several factors: (1) dose, (2) routine of administration, (3) length of administration, and (4) the host (Table 2). Interferon toxicity can be divided into both systemic and organ system-specific effects. Systemic toxicity is dose-related with most adults exhibiting fever, chills, malaise, myalgias and headache in doses of 1x10^6 U or greater (Table 3). In one study, however, these effects appeared to be more

Table 2. Factors affecting systemic toxicity of interferon.

1. Dose
2. Route of administration
3. Length of administration
4. Host immune status

Table 3. Toxicities of parenterally administered interferons.

Systemic	
Chills	Fever
Headache	Malaise
Myalgias	Nausea
Diaphoresis	Syncope
Organ system specific	
Bone marrow suppression	Cardiovascular
Nephrotoxicity	Peripheral neuropathy

pronounced after subcutaneous or intramuscular injection, compared to a slow intravenous injection [15]. This study suggested that the magnitude of these effects may relate as much to the peak serum interferon level as to the total dose. With chronic administration tachyphylaxis develops to many of these effects so that during the second or third week of daily administration, systemic side effects are much less severe. Finally, it has been our impression that immunocompromised patients (e.g. organ allograft recipients and those with AIDS) tolerate the systemic effects of interferon better than those who are immunocompetent. In addition, organ sytem-specific interferon toxicity is also observed. These toxicities include reversible bone marrow suppression, nephrotoxicity, and cardiac toxicity [16]. Interferon gamma has also been produced by recombinant DNA techniques. Such interferon has been administered to patients with cancer and with AIDS. Preliminary data suggest that pharmacokinetics and toxicities are similar to those exhibited by interferon alpha.

Interleukin-2 was initially prepared for clinical administration by the fractionation of supernatant fluid from human peripheral blood lymphocytes cultured in the presence of lectins. Since these earlier trials, production of IL-2 by recombinant DNA techniques has been achieved. Although this material is not glycosylated, the biologic activities appear to be identical to material produced by mammalian cells [17].

Pharmacokinetic studies have been performed with both non-recombinant and recombinant IL-2. The serum half-life following intravenous administration of recombinant IL-2 is quite short, being in the range of 6-7 minutes [18-19]. Despite the short serum half-life of IL-2 itself, the biological effects may be much longer, given the fact that the effects of IL-2 on the host are mediated indirectly by effector cells. Once these effector cells are stimulated by IL-2, their effects may last for a much longer period of time.

Interleukin-2 is one of the better-tolerated lymphokines. The most serious toxicity at high doses is fluid retention, which appears to be due to increased capillary permeability [20]. This effect can result in peripheral edema, pulmonary edema, or both. In addition, patients may exhibit fever, chills, malaise or gastrointestinal disturbances. In certain patients, IL-2 administration appears to induce a graft-versus-host-like reaction with fever, a maculopapular eruption, diarrhea, and pleural and pericardial inflammation.

Therapy of cancer with interferons and interleukin-2

Strategies for the immunotherapy of neoplasia have been in existence for many years (Table 4). It was not until the advent of molecular biological techniques in the early 1980s which made possible the inexpensive production of large quantities of interferons for clinical use, that such therapies became a practical reality.

The initial interest in interferons focused on the direct antitumor effects of these biological response modifiers. Early trials with non-recombinant interferon-alpha, particularly in such situations as osteogenic sarcoma prophylaxis and adjuvant therapy of non-Hodgkin's lymphoma, were sufficiently

Table 4. Interleukin-2: Stages in the development of effective clinical applications.

1. Initial description
2. Biochemical and functional characterization
3. Molecular cloning and development of techniques for large scale in vitro production
4. Clincial trials:
   a. Parenteral IL-2
   b. Adoptive immunotherapy:
      i. lymphokine activated killer cells + IL-2
      ii. task specific effectors (e.g. TIL cells) ± IL-2

interesting to induce major efforts on the part of the American Cancer Society and of the National Cancer Institute to make sufficient interferon available for widespread clinical trials. Over the past five years, there have been many clinical trials with interferons. Most have been accomplished with interferon produced by recombinant DNA techniques. Although there are several exceptions, the initial enthusiasm for interferon alpha as a major form of therapy for a wide variety of tumors was waned. There are, however, at least three tumors in which recombinant interferon alpha has shown clear-cut benefit: hairy cell leukemia, renal cell carcinoma, and Kaposi's sarcoma [21-24]. Recombinant interferon alpha has recently been licensed in the USA for the former two indications. In other neoplastic diseases, interferon therapy has exhibited much less clear-cut benefit. Although clinical trials with interferons in cancer will clearly proceed, most investigators expect a much more limited role for interferons as single agents in the therapy of most forms of cancer than was hoped by some as recently as three years ago.

The potential role of IL-2 in the therapy of neoplastic disease is currently of both great theoretical and practical interest. Cellular effectors with cytotoxic capabilities against autologous and syngeneic tumors have been demonstrated in a wide variety of in vitro and animal systems. Depending on the specificity and lineage of these cellular effectors they have been designated as natural killer (NK), lymphokine activated killer (LAK), and cytotoxic T-lymphocytes. The pivotal role of Il-2 in both the initial induction of these cells and in the stimulation of proliferation of these cells is well recognized. Initial clinical trials with IL-2 served mainly to confirm the fact that it is relatively non-toxic following parenteral administration. Direct antitumor effects of this dosing strategy were, however, rarely demonstrable.

A large number of well-executed animal studies have formed the basis for a much more innovative approach to the use of IL-2 in the therapy of neoplasia [25-33]. These animal studies have demonstrated that IL-2 can be used very effectively in vitro to selectively expand subsets of cells with specific functional capabilities. In the first generation of these studies, IL-2 has been used to stimulate the proliferation of a subset of cells, termed lymphokine activated killer (LAK) cells [20,29-33]. These cells of non-B, non-T lineage are present in the bone marrow, spleen, lymph nodes and peripheral blood. In human studies which have been carried out primarily at the National Cancer Institute, 5×10^9 to 5×10^{10} peripheral blood mononuclear cells were harvested from the peripheral blood of patients with a variety of tumors, by continuous flow cell separator. These cells were then cultured in vitro in the presence of high concentrations of IL-2 for 3-4 days, washed, and reinfused into the patient in conjunction with high doses of IL-2 (Table 5). In the initial studies, which consisted of 25 patients with solid melanoma exhibited a complete response which has lasted for at least 10 months (Table 6). The major toxicity exhibited by this approach was fluid retention which could be attributed to the high dose of IL-2 which was required for the continued activity of the infused cells in vivo.

Recently a much more tumor-specific approach has been investigated in the murine system. In these studies, tumor biopsies were obtained, minced, and established in culture in the presence of IL-2 [34]. After a week, the tumor cells regress and lymphocytes remain. With further in vitro cultivation

Table 5. Adoptive immunotherapy using lymphokine activated killer cells.

5×10^9 – 5×10^{10} peripheral blood mononuclear cells collected by continuous flow cell separation

Ficoll hypaque separation

3-4 day in vitro cultivation with 1000 U rIL-2/ml

administration of 10^8 cells with rIL-2

Table 6. Lymphokine-activated killer cells: Interim results.

1. 25 patients treated with several types of tumors including:
   a. melanoma
   b. colon or rectal cancer
   c. osteogenic and other sarcomas
   d. renal cell cancer
   e. esophageal cancer
2. Regression: 11 of 25 patients
   Complete regression: 1 patient
3. Toxicity:
   a. fever, chills
   b. fluid retention

with IL-2, the number of tumor-infiltrating lymphocytes (TIL) can be expanded 100-fold. These cells are much more active in vitro against the tumor from which they arise than are LAK cells derived from peripheral sites. In the presence of immunosuppressive therapy with cyclophosphamide, TIL cells coupled with IL-2 are highly effective in both the reduction of established micrometastases and in reducing hepatic metastases, in the MCA-105 sarcoma and MC-38 colon adenocarcinoma systems respectively. In addition to the clear-cut therapeutic activity of this approach, there is a need for much less parenteral IL-2. This should significantly reduce the toxicity of this approach. These techniques are in the process of being applied to humans. TIL with anti-tumor activity have been generated from human tumors. Clinical results have not yet been reported.

Thus, from the standpoint of anti-neoplastic therapy, it is clear that lymphokines will play an increasingly important role. Over the post decade we have witnessed an increasingly refined approach to cancer therapy in which efforts have progressed from simple parenteral administration of relatively impure preparations, to the in vitro application of highly purified materials produced by recombinant DNA techniques in the in vitro induction and expansion of specific subsets of narrowly directed effector cells.

Lymphokines in the therapy of AIDS

As has been noted above, the central feature of the acquired immune deficiency syndrome is the immunoincompetence induced by the etiologic retrovirus, HIV ([8,10]. Although the lytic interaction between HIV and lymphocytes of the T4 surface phenotype has been perceived as the major mechanism for HIV induced immunoincompetence, it is also clear that other cells including monocytes and cells of the central nervous system are also susceptible to infection by HIV [35-39]. In addition, humoral mediators of the immunoincompetence induced by HIV have also been demonstrated.

Interest in immune reconstitution in patients with HIV infection stems from two underlying tenets. The first is that since immunoincompetence is the major means by which HIV induces morbidity, immune reconstitution will prevent the indirect clinical expression of HIV in the form of opportunistic infections and neoplasms. The second is that it is quite likely that part of the reason for the differences in the clinical expression of HIV from patient to patient may relate to HIV specific immune function. Lymphokine therapy of patients with HIV infection might be expected, therefore, to be directed at manipulation of either global or HIV-specific immune function. Two other objectives of therapy with lymphokines might relate to either the direct effects of these agents on a complication of AIDS (e.g. Kaposi's sarcoma) or on the virus itself (e.g. interferons).

Studies by our group and by others have demonstrated the activity of interferon alpha against HIV in vitro [40]. Using recombinant Roche interferon-alpha A we have noted marked inhibition of HIV replication in either H9 cells or peripheral blood mononuclear cells at therapeutically achievable concentrations of interferon. Interferon gamma is less active against HIV in lymphocyte target cells, but appears to be more active than interferon alpha against HIV with monocyte target cells. Thus, at least in vitro, the activity of interferons against HIV is target cell specific.

Clinical trials of interferons in AIDS patients have included trials of interferon alpha or gamma against Kaposi's sarcoma [24], and a double-blinded placebo-controlled study of recombinant interferon alpha A in patients with AIDS-related complex or AIDS. The studies of interferon alpha against Kaposi's sarcoma have demonstrated partial remissions in a subgroup of patients. Patients most likely to respond are those who have not had an opportunistic infection and those who do not have endogenous levels of circulating acid labile interferon alpha. Although not yet formally reported, interferon gamma did not exhibit beneficial results in patients with Kaposi's sarcoma.

A multicenter trial of interferon alpha in patients with AIDS-related complex, or patients with AIDS who have recently recovered from *Pneumocystis carinii* pneumonia has been recently completed. Although the data analysis is not yet complete, it does not appear that Roche interferon alpha A in doses of 3 or 9×10^6 U three times weekly has a significant effect on patient survival (Friedland, G, personal communication). We are currently performing a study designed to determine whether the same interferon preparation has a demonstrable antiviral effect in vivo (Schooley, RT, Hirsch, MS, ongoing studies). Although we have, as yet, studied only a small number of patients, we have not demonstrated that these doses of recombinant interferon alpha A decrease the ability to isolate HIV from the peripheral blood.

Interleukin-2 has also received attention as a possible therapeutic adjunct in patients with HIV infection. Defects in both IL-2 elaboration in response to mitogens, and in IL-2 responsiveness have been demonstrated in patients with HIV infection [8-9,41-44]. We and Quinnan et al., have demonstrated in the EBV and CMV systems respectively, the ability of IL-2 to reconstitute cytotoxic effector cell function against autologous virally-infected cells [45-48].

The parenteral administration of IL-2 to patients with AIDS has, however, been disappointing to date. Extensive studies at the NIH by Clifford Lane have demonstrated the feasibility of long-term parenteral administration of IL-2 in this patient population. Although modest transient improvement in several immunologic parameters have been noted in occasional patients, no clear-cut clinical benefits have been demonstrated.

Toxicities of parenteral IL-2 in this patient population have been considerable. In addition to the toxicities observed in the Rosenberg cancer trials, we have observed a graft-versus-host-like reaction in a patient participating in an escalating dose tolerance trial of recombinant IL-2 administered by intravenous infusion over 30 minutes at weekly intervals (Schooley RT, Hirsch MS, unpublished observations). This individual developed exfoliative dermatitis, fever, diarrhea, and pleural and pericardial effusions four days after receiving 10 million units of IL-2. This may be the result of the activation and expansion of a subset of cells with autoimmune properties [49].

Thus, despite a good theoretical basis for the application of lymphokine therapy in patients with HIV infections, clinical benefits have to date been extremely modest in that they have been limited to a subgroup of patients with Kaposi's sarcoma treated with interferon alpha.

Is there likely to be a role for lymphokine therapy in patients with AIDS? Two approaches which have been utilized in the application of anticancer therapy appear to warrant further investigation in HIV infection. The first of these relates to combination chemotherapy; the second to in vitro manipulation of specific effector cell subpopulations.

Recently the multicenter placebo controlled trial of the reverse transcriptase inhibitor, azidothymidine (AZT) in patients with AIDS and ARC was terminated, because of excess mortality in the placebo group. Although the data analysis is currently not complete, several benefits were observed in the group of patients receiving azidothymidine (Table 7). Because of these benefits, it was deemed prudent to terminate the study in order to offer the drug to all participants. Although it is not yet clear whether these studies which were performed in severe ARC patients and AIDS patients who have recently recovered from *Pneumocystis carinii* pneumonia can be extrapolated to other subgroups of HIV-infected individuals, and what, if any, long-term toxicity will be exhibited by AZT, it is clear that effective antiviral therapy results in both improved survival, and in improved in vitro assessments of immunologic function.

Table 7. Benefits of azidothymidine therapy.

Decreased mortality
Fewer recurrent or new opportunistic infection
Improved delayed hypersensitivity testing
Increased number of T4 cells
Increased performance status
Weight gain

We have studied in vitro interactions of antiviral drugs such as azidothymidine and phosphonoformate (PFA) with recombinant interferon alpha, and have noted additional or synergistic effects with both interferon alpha and AZT and interferon alpha and PFA [50]. Thus, it seems reasonable to advocate the cautious exploration of the clinical utility of such combinations in selected subgroups of patients.

The other potential role of lymphokines in the therapy of HIV infection relates to the potential use of these agents in the manipulation of HIV specific immune responsiveness. Although antibodies which neutralize HIV have been studied extensively in the pursuit of vaccines for HIV, little is yet known about the cellular immune response to HIV. In ongoing collaborative studies with dr. Bernard Moss of the National Institute of Allergy and Infectious Diseases, we have demonstrated the existance of HIV-specific cytotoxic T-lymphocytes in two patients with AIDS-related complex. In these studies we have observed significant cytotoxic activity in a ^{51}Cr release assay using autologous targets infected with vaccines/HIV-env recombinant virus. We are currently extending these studies to determine the potential role of this response in determining the natural history of HIV infection, to determine the range of epitopes at which their response is directed, and to explore whether this response might be expanded in vitro using lymphokines such as IL-2. If this response proves to be important, it is conceivable that adoptive immunotherapy might play a role in the therapy of HIV infection, as it is beginning to be applied to patients with neoplastic disease.

References

1. Schooley RT, Hirsch MS, Rubin RH, Cantell K. The role of interferons in viral infections in immune compromised patients. In: Smit Sibinga CTh, Das PC, Opelz G (eds). Transplantation and blood transfusion. 1984:83-9.
2. Hirsch MS, Schooley RT. Treatment of herpesvirus infection. N Engl J Med 1983;309:963-70, 1034-9.
3. Dolin R. Antiviral therapy and chemoprophylaxis. Science 1985;227:1296-303.
4. Felsenstein D, D'Amico DJ, Hirsch MS, et al. Treatment of cytomegalovirus retinitis with 9-[2-hydroxy-1-(hydroxymethyl)ethoxymethyl]guanine (BWB759U). Ann Int Med 1985;103:377-80.
5. Hall CB, McBride JT, Walsh EE, et al. Aerosolized ribavirin treatment of infants with respiratory syncytical viral infection. N Engl J Med 1983;308:1443-8.
6. Hirsch MS, Kaplan JC. Prospects for therapy of infection with human lymphotropic virus type III. Ann Int Med 1975;103:750-5.
7. Curran J. AIDS trends: Projections from limited data. Science 1985;230:1018-21.
8. Bowden DL, Hane HC, Fauci AS. Immunopathogenesis of the acquired immune deficiency syndrom. Ann Int Med 1985;103:704-9.
9. Quinnan GC, Siegal JP, Epstein JS, Manischewitz JF, Barnes S, Wells MA. Mechanisms of T-cell functional deficiency in the acquired immune deficiency syndrom. Ann Int Med 1985;103:710-4.
10. Lane HC, Fauci AS. Immunologic reconstitution and the acquired immune deficiency syndrom. Ann Int Med 1985;103:714-8.
11. Cantell K, Hirvonen S, Kauppinean H-L, Myllyla G. Production of interferon in human leukocytes from normal donors with the use of Sendai virus. Methods Enzymol 1981;78:29-38.
12. Cantell K, Hirvonen S, Kostinea V. Partial purification of human leukocyte interferon on a large scale. Methods Enzymol 1981;18:499-505.
13. Maeda S, McCandliss R, Gross M, et al. Construction and indentification of bacterial plasmids containing nucleotide sequence for human leukocyte interferon. Proc Natl Acad Sci USA 1980;77:7010-3.
14. Staehelin T, Hobbs DS, Kung HF, Lai CY, Pestka S. Purification and characterization of recombinant human leukocyte interferon (IFLrA) with monoclonal antibodies. J Biol Chem 1981;256:9750-4.
15. Wills RJ, Dennis S, Spiegel HE, Gibson DM, Nadler PI. Interferon kinetics and adverse reactions after intravenous, intramuscular, and subcutaneous injection. Clin Pharmacol Ther 1984;35:722-7.
16. Averbuch SD, Austin HA, Sherwin SA, Antonovych T, Bunn PA, Longo DL. Acute interstitial nephritis with the nephrotic syndrom following recombinant leukocyte a interferon therapy for mycosis fungoides. N Engl J Med 1984;310:32-5.
17. Burton DT, Richardson LB, Taylor RJ. Biological activity of recombinant human interleukin-2 produced in Escherichia coli. Science 1984;223:1410-1.

18. Bindon C, Czerniecki M, Ruell P, et al. Clearance rates and systemic effects of intravenously administered interleukin-2 (IL-2) containing preparations in human subjects. Br J Cancer 1983;47:123-33.
19. Donohue JH, Rosenberg SA. The fate of interleukin-2 after in vivo administration. J Immunol 1983;130:2203-8.
20. Rosenberg SA, Lotze MT, Muul LM, , et al. Observations on the systemic administration of autologous lymphokine-activated killer cells and recombinant interleukin-2 to patients with metastatic cancer. N Engl J Med 1985;313:1485-92.
21. Quesada JR, Reuben J, Manning JT, Hersh EM, Gutterman JU. Alpha interferon for induction of remission in hairy-cell leukemia. N Engl J Med 1984;310: 15-8.
22. Golumb HM. Interferons: present and future use in cancer therapy (editorial). J Clin Oncol 1986;4:123-5.
23. Quesada JR, Swanson DA, Trindade A, Gutterman JU. Renal cell carcinoma: anti tumor effects of leukocyte interferon. Cancer Res 1973;43:940-7.
24. Krown SE, Real FX, Cunningham-Rundles S, et al. Preliminary observations on the effect of recombinant leukocyte A interferon in homosexual men with Kaposi's sarcoma. N Engl J Med 1983;308:1071-6.
25. Borberg H, Oettgen HF, Choudry K, Beattie EJ Jr. Inhibition of established transplants of chemically induced sarcomas in syngeneic mice by lymphocytes from immunized donors. Int J Cancer 1972;10:539-47.
26. Cheever MA, Greenberg PD, Fefer A. Specificity of adoptive chemoimmunotherapy of established syngeneic tumors. J Immunol 1980;125:711-4.
27. Fernandez-Cruz E, Halliburton B, Feldman JD. In vivo elimination by specific effector cells of an established syngeneic rat Moloney virus-induced sarcoma. J Immunol 1979;123:1772-7.
28. Mazumder A, Rosenberg SA. Successful immunotherapy of natural killer-resistant established pulmonary melanoma metastases by the intravenous adoptive transfer of syngeneic lymphocytes activated in vitro by interleukin-2. J Exp Med 1984;159:495-507.
29. Mule JJ, Shu S, Schwartz SL, Rosenberg SA. Adoptive immunotherapy of established pulmonary metastases with LAK cells and recombinant interleukin-2. Science 1984;225:1487-9.
30. Mule JJ, Shu S, Rosenberg SA. The anti-tumor efficacy of lymphokine-activated killer cells and recombinant interleukin-2 in vivo. J Immunol 1985;135:656-2.
31. Grimm EA, Mazumder A, Zhang HZ, Rosenberg SA. Lymphokine-activated killer cell phenomenon: lysis of natural killer-resistant fresh solid tumor cells by interleukin-2 activated autologous human peripheral blood lymphocytes. J Exp Med 1982;155:1823-41.
32. Rosenstein M, Yron I, Kaufmann Y, Rosenberg SA. Lymphokine-activated killer cells: lysis of fresh syngeneic natural killer-resistant murine tumor cells by lymphocytes cultured in interleukin-2. Cancer Res 1984;44:1946-53.
33. Grimm EA, Ramsey KM, Mazumder A, Wilson DJ, Djeu JY, Rosenberg SA. Lymphokine-activated killer cell phenomenon. II. Precursor phenotype is serologically distinct from peripheral T lymphocytes, memory cytotoxic thymus-derived lymphocytes, and natural killer cells. J Exp Med 1983;157:884-97.
34. Rosenberg SA, Spiess P, Lafreniere R. A new approach to the adoptive immunotherapy of cancer with tumor-infiltrating lymphocytes. Science 1986; 233:1318-21.
35. Klatzmann D, Barre-Sinoussi F, Nugeyre MT, et al. Selective tropism of lymphoadenopathy associated virus (LAV) for helper-inducer T lymphocytes. Science 1984;225:59-62.

36. Ho DD, Rota TR, Hirsch MS. Infection of monocyte/macrophages by human T lymphotropic virus type III. J Clin Invest 1986;77:1712-5.
37. Shaw GM, Harper ME, Hahn BH, et al. HTLV-III infection in brains of children and adults with AIDS encephalopathy. Science 1985;227:177-82.
38. Ho DD, Rota TR, Schooley RT, Kaplan JC, et al. Isolation of HTLV-III from cerebrospinal fluid and neural tissues of patients with neurologic syndromes related to the acquired immunodeficiency syndrome. N Engl J Med 1985;313: 1493-7.
39. Gabuzda DH, Ho DD, de la Monte SM, Hirsch MS, Rota TR, Sobel RA. Immunohistochemical identification of HTLV-III antigen in brains of patients with AIDS. Ann of Neurol 1986;20:289-95.
40. Ho DD, Hartshorn KL, Rota TR, Andrews CA, Kaplan JC, Hirsch MS. Recombinant human interferon alpha A suppresses HTLV-III replication in vitro. Lancet 1985;i:602-3.
41. Prince HE, Kermani-Arab V, Fahey JL. Depressed interleukin-2 receptor expression in acquired immune deficiency and lymphadenopathy syndromes. J Immunol 1984;133:1313-6.
42. Donnelly RP, Tsang KY, Galbraith GMP, Wallace JI. Inhibition of interleukin-2-induced T cell proliferation by sera from patients with the acquired immune defiency syndrome. J Clin Immunol 1986;6:92-101.
43. Murray HW, Rubin BY, Masur H, Roberts RB. Impaired production of lymphokines and immune (gamma) interferon in the acquired immuno deficiency syndrome. N Engl J Med 1984;310:883-9.
44. Murray HW, Welte K, Jacobs JL, Rubin BY, Mertelsmann R, Roberts RB. Production of and in vitro response to interleukin-2 in the acquired immunodeficiency syndrome. J Clin Invest 1985;76:1959-64.
45. Rook AH, Hooks JJ, Quinnan GV, et al. Interleukin-2 enhances the natural killer cell activity of acquired immuno deficiency syndrome patients through a gamma interferon-independent mechanism. J Immunol 1985;134:1503-7.
46. Rook AH, Masur H, Lane HC, et al. Interleukin-2 enhances the depressed natural killer and cytomegalovirus specific cytotoxic activity of lymphocytes from patients with the acquired immune deficiency syndrome. J Clin Invest 1983;72:398-403.
47. Blumberg RS, Paradis T, Byington R, Henle W, Hirsch MS, Schooley RT. Effects of human T lymphotropic virus type III (HTLV-III) on the cellular immune response to Epstein Barr virus in homosexual men. Characterization of the cytotoxic response and lymphokine production. (Submitted for publication 1986).
48. Lifson JD, Mark DF, Benike CJ, Koths K, Engleman EG. Human recombinant interleukin-2 partly reconstitutes deficiency in vitro immune responses of lymphocytes from patients with AIDS. Lancet 1984;i:698-702.
49. Sondel PM, Hank JA, Kohler PC, Chen BP, Minkoff DZ, Molenda JA. Destruction of autologous human lymphocytes by interleukin-2-activated cytotoxic cells. J Immunol 1986;137:502-11.
50. Hartshorn KL, Sandstrom EG, Neumeyer D, et al. Synergistic inhibition of human T-cell lymphotropic virus type III replication in vitro by phosphonoformate and recombinant alpha A interferon. Antimicrob Ag Chemother 1986; 30:189-91.

DISCUSSION

M.R. Halie and S.B. Moore

S.B. Moore (Rochester): Dr. Leitman, since severity and mortality of the graft-versus-host disease is obviously quite different in patients who have received bone marrow transplantation and within the group of patients who receive a blood product do you think that perhaps what we now call graft-versus-host disease is really several immunologically and perhaps clinically distinct entities, which tend to manifest themselves in a similar fashion. Are we looking at a highly heterogeneous mixture?

S.F. Leitman (Bethesda): That is a difficult question. I think that posttransfusion graft-versus-host reactions are much more common than we appreciate. Grade I and II reactions can be quite mild. They are immediately recognized in the posttransplant setting, because they are watched for so closely. But they may not be recognized as a consequence of transfusion in a sick patient. A little rash, diarrhea, jaundice, and fever can be attributed to multiple other processes. I think that one can probably, with the appropriate degree of suspicion, see the same spectrum of grade I to grade IV posttransfusion GvHD as one sees in the posttransplantation setting.

H.R. de Vries (Enschede): Prof. The, is there any relation between the detection of early and late CMV antigens to the infectivity of blood transfusion. And if so could you elaborate on the best tests to screen blood for transfusion.

T.H. The (Groningen): With regard to your question about selection of blood donors with the direct test on circulating blood leukocytes, I have to emphasize that the positive cells are only detectable in acute CMV cases. In normal healthy blood donors this test is to my feeling less usable. For screening blood donors a sensitive CMV ELISA method is the most practical test available.

S.B. Moore: Prof. The, the antibody to the immediate early antigen of CMV appears to be perhaps one of the more important antibodies developed from the selfprotection standpoint of the individual. Would you speculate on the possibility of using this antibody to determine the epitope characteristics and from the epitope characteristics to derive a vaccine. This then would be a non-infectious vaccine, but would in fact contain the antigen which would induce the protecting immune response.

T.H. The: The immediate early antigen I was dealing with is an intracellular antigen located in the nucleus. So, this antigen has a significance as a marker to recognize CMV infected cells. These cells are in fact fixed in vitro, so the antigens in the nucleus can be reached. With regard to immunosurveillance of the host against virus and specially the virus in its latent stage one would look more at the cell surface instead of inside the cell. Immediate early antigens are probably also expressed at the cell surface but these are not yet detectable by monoclonal antibodies.

H.R. de Vries: Dr. de Wolf, in your excellent paper you drew the conclusion that 17 days or even older units of blood are free of mononucleated cells. In my opinion that does not mean that they are free of antigens. It sounded like a suggestion that you could make blood non-immunogenic by simply storing it for three or more weeks and that it could be compared in that fashion with filtered blood, which is almost entirely leukocyte free.

J.Th.M. de Wolf (Groningen): In 1978 Bachelor had a publication in Nature*, concerning rats transfused with membrane fragments bearing HLA antigens. They followed the animals for 50 days and no immunization occurred. Only if viable cells were transfused alloimmunization occurred. In blood stored for 17 days HLA bearing lymphocytes have almost disappeared.

H.R. de Vries: Would you suggest that to store blood for three weeks or more will be as good as to deplete it completely of leukocytes as we do now for instance by using cellulose acetate or cotton wool filters or by washing the cells or freezing and thawing? Do you suggest that, as a method it is equivalent to depleting red blood cells from leukocytes?

J.Th.M. de Wolf: I think that the leukocytes present in platelet suspensions are more important for alloimmunization than fragments of leukocytes in blood stored for three weeks, because they are stored at room temperature and therefore are viable cells. The last three years we have used red blood cells stored for two or three weeks and then filtered. However, our percentage of alloimmunization and the requirement of HLA-matched platelets is not higher than elsewhere.

C.Th. Smit Sibinga (Groningen): There is indeed some evidence that when cells ex vivo age they become less immunogenic. An intriguing point mentioned is that these cells show less mitotic or progenitor activity and therefore lead to less expression of GvHD or might even not be causative for that. That is something we need to sort out further.

Prof. The, could you give us some further clues of how to prevent CMV infections. Because to my knowledge it is know that when blood of CMV positive individuals apparently infected with the virus, is stored at 4°C, the virus rather rapidly looses infectivity. Is that true?

T.H. The: Yes, but I hesitate whether this is absolute.

* Bachelor JR. Nature 1978;273;54-7.

C.Th. Smit Sibinga: So, if we do not agree upon the absoluteness of the loss of infectivity, the vitality of the virus, it means that we should try to either eliminate white cells from blood products or try to come to the use of CMV negative blood. Your screening method is sensitive and picks up a very early phenomenon. What we usually do in blood donor screening is using an overall test, which is less sensitive and does not pick up an early infection. What do you think we should do?

T.H. The: It may happen that certain seemingly healthy blood donors might have a primary CMV infection. That might be detected with the direct test on their blood leukocytes even before the appearance of circulating antibodies, but in practice this would be a minority. I think it is not very practical to look at the donor cells. The sensitive CMV ELISA test is better to look for CMV seropositivity and CMV latency, but I agree that acute cases before onset of clinical symptoms could be missed.

S.J. Slichter (Seattle): As there is a large amount of data suggesting that CMV may be predominantly transmitted within white cells, it may be that leukocyte-poor blood products will have two potential benefits. One is the previously discussed decrease in platelet alloimmunization, and the second may be a reduction in CMV transmission. The virologists associated with the Bone Marrow Transplant Unit in Seattle are currently conducting a study evaluating CMV transmission in bone marrow transplant candidates with leukocyte-poor blood products compared to standard transfusion products. This study is being conducted in a special group of marrow transplant patients who have a high risk of CMV seroconversion with transfusion of CMV-positive blood products but little risk for development of active infection. This study is being performed because of the very large requirements for CMV-negative blood products to bone marrow transplant patients that must be provided by our Blood Center. In CMV-negative transplant patients who also have a CMV-negative bone marrow donor, it has clearly been shown that CMV-negative blood products result in a substantial reduction in CMV infection. However, because the CMV-positive rate in our donor population is in the range of 50%, providing consistently CMV-negative blood products to a transplant programme, which does over 400 bone marrow transplants a year, is a logistical problem. Therefore, the leukocyte-poor transfusion trial is being conducted to determine if this may be a way to provide safe blood products even from CMV-positive donors. The data is too preliminary to have any results, but at least, for the first several patients, there has been no evidence of CMV seroconversion from leukocyte-poor blood products. However, one remaining question to be addressed both for CMV transmission as well as platelet alloimmunization is the potential effect of leukocyte disintegration during blood storage on these problems. There is conflicting data in the literature concerning whether antigens have to be present on intact cells in order to be recognized as foreign, or whether membrane fragments are themselves immunogenic. Furthermore, as the white cell breaks down and the CMV virus is released into the plasma, does this make the virus more or less susceptible to clearance following transfusion into a recipient?

C.Th. Smit Sibinga: Dr. Schooley, could you give some more information on the recent clinical trial using adoptive immunotherapy?

R.T. Schooley (Boston): The FDA just released their guidelines. They have not yet decided what to do about patients whose fate is very complex, because of the time constrains. This study had both AIDS and ARC patients present. There were more deaths among the AIDS patients, but there was a trend towards increased survival in the ARC patients as well. The study was set up to be terminated as soon as there was an overall difference or difference in either subgroup. So it was terminated before statistically significant differences were seen amongst the ARC patients. If I were an ARC patient, I likely, on an emotional basis would want the drug. The development of the drug sofar has been very rapid; it was just given to the first patient last summer. The biggest drawback has been until recently the availability of the starting material. Burroughs Wellcome has enough drug they tell me to be able to treat 30,000 new patients per year, which is a large number of patients. But if you look at the number of ARC patients even only in the United States, that would not come close to providing drug for ARC patients. But in the United States now the easiest subgroup of patients to get drugs for, are the patients with AIDS who had no pneumocystis. Clinical trials will continue. I think we will know a lot more about this in the next three or four months. It is a very exciting position to finally have something to offer, but I think we are still a long way from having something to offer every patient.

III. PRODUCTION ASPECTS

PRACTICAL ASPECTS OF PLATELET CONCENTRATE PRODUCTION AND STORAGE*

S.J. Slichter

Introduction

Major advances in platelet concentrate production and storage have ensured the ready availability of this transfusion product. The storage procedures required to achieve a quality product are determined by monitoring selected in vitro measurements together with the incremental response, survival, and function of the platelets following their transfusion into either normal volunteers or aplastic thrombocytopenic recipients.

Over time, a standardized approach for evaluating new platelet storage procedures has been developed. Such an approach uses a limited number of in vitro tests that have been documented to correlate with poststorage in vivo platelet viability measurements. If the preliminary in vitro test results are acceptable, poststorage radiolabeled platelet recovery and survival measurements are performed in normal volunteers. Finally, transfusion studies in selected stable thrombocytopenic patients provide conclusive evidence of platelet viability and function in clinical practice.

Methods

1 Methods of measuring poststorage platelet viability and function
1.1 In vitro measurements
1.1.1 pH

Several studies have documented a progressive fall in pH during storage of platelet concentrates at 22°C. The pH changes are primarily a consequence of lactate accumulation through glycolysis with some contribution from accumulated CO_2 [1,2]. Generally, the fall in pH with room temperature storage has been directly correlated with increasing platelet concentration [1-3] and maybe further increased by residual white blood cells [4,5]. However, pH is not affected by contaminating red cells [3]. If pH falls to less than 6.0, platelet viability is markedly compromised; i.e., recoveries $<15\%$ and survivals of <2.5 days compared to recoveries of $>30\%$ and survivals of >7.9 days at

* Supported by NHLBI Grant HL 33375. A portion of this work was also conducted through the Clincal Research Center, University of Washington which is supported by NIH Grant RR-37.

higher pH [6-8]. Platelet concentration can be appropriately reduced by increasing the residual plasma volume which maintains pH by buffering the acid load. Carbon-dioxide loss is enhanced by continuous gentle agitation during storage. Under some circumstances, it may be necessary to further facilitate gas transport (O_2 in and CO_2 out) by decreasing the thickness of the bag wall or increasing the surface-to-volume ratio by storing the concentrates in larger bags [1]. The latter changes in the storage bag are usually only required if the platelet concentration cannot be appropriately reduced.

Higher pH values between 7.2 and 7.8 may occur if concentrates are stored in large, thin bags which permit excessive CO_2 loss, or even in regular bags, if the platelet count is very low. These concentrates show a direct inverse relationship between increasing pH and decreasing posttransfusion recovery [1]. Thus, extremes of pH are positively correlated with reduced posttransfused platelet viability. However, in the range of 6.0-7.2, the pH does not reflect differences in platelet viability of individual units [1].

1.1.2 Morphology

1.1.2.1 Disc-to-sphere transformation (shape change)

Normally, platelets circulate in the blood stream as discs. As the pH falls during storage at 22°C, there is a progressive change in the percentage of platelets in disc form compared to those which have become sphered. At pH values between 6.8 and 7.2, platelets maintain a normal disc configuration even after 3 days of storage. When the poststorage pH is between 6.0 and 6.4, 40-70% of platelets are sphered; at pH values <6.0 or >7.2, platelets are all sphered with spiny projections, correlating with major losses in platelet viability [1].

A morphologic index, rather than the percentage of cells in disc form, has also been shown to predict viability after 22°C storage [9]. The number of discs identified in a 100 cell count was multiplied by 4, spheres by 2, platelets with dendrites by 1, and balloon forms by 0. The calculated answers were added together and a perfect score was 400. The morphology score was found to directly predict both posttransfusion platelet recovery and survival with correlation coefficients of 0.67 and 0.82, respectively.

As a more quantitative way to measure disc-to-sphere transformation, or more accurately 'shape change', samples of platelet concentrates before and after storage were added to an aggregometer and stirred at two different speeds [10]. The amount of light transmitted through the PRP was found to be dependent on stirring rate with disc-shaped cells, but was independent of rate for spherical cells. As shown in Figure 1, if after 3 days of platelet concentrate storage at 22°C, pH values were between 6.8 and 7.1, the ratio of light transmission of the two stirring rates was comparable to that of fresh platelets. At intermediate poststorage pH values of 6.1-6.5, there was a significant change in the ratio which was reversed after pH adjustment to 7.0. This reversibility in shape may correlate with in vivo data showing maintenance of platelet viability in this pH range. Conceivably, a similar restoration of disc shape occurs in vivo as the cells are brought to physiologic pH following transfusion. In contrast, platelet concentrates with poststorage pH values of

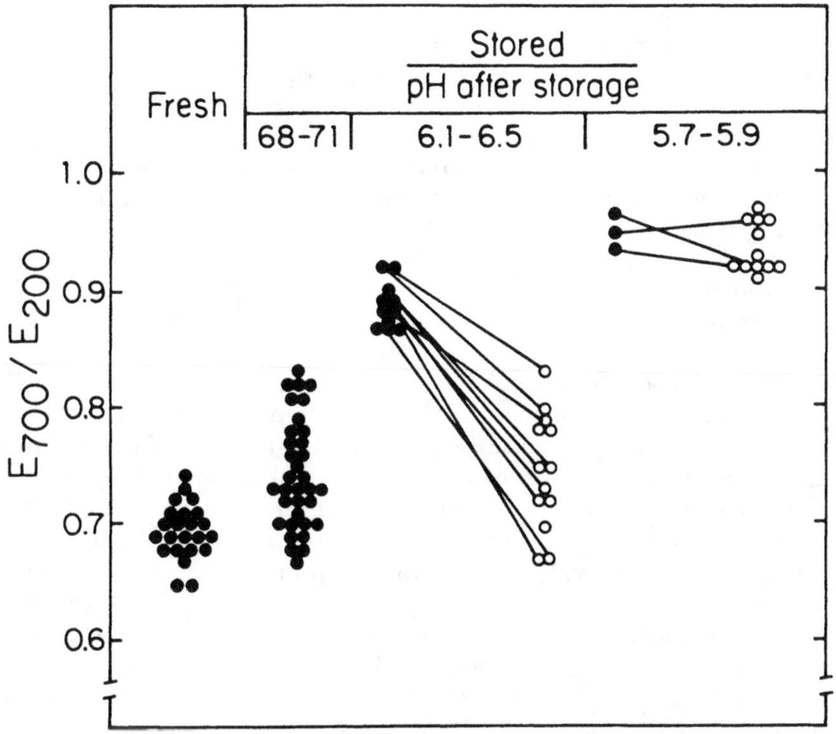

Figure 1. Shape change. Effect of 3 days of storage of platelet concentrates (PC) at 22°C on E_{700}/E_{200}. In those cases where the final pH of the PC was below 6.6, the diluted platelet suspensions were divided into two parts. The pH of one part was adjusted to that of the final pH of the PC after storage with 1 N HCl, and the pH of the other was adjusted to 7.0 with 1 N NaOH. E_{700} is the extinction or optical density at a stirring rate of 700 rpm in a Payton aggregometer, and E_{200} is the extinction at 200 rpm. Light transmission is dependent on stirring rate for disc-shaped platelets, but is independent of rate for spherical cells. At pH values between 6.1 and 6.5, sphering is reversible as evidenced by changes in E_{700}/E_{200} with pH adjustment. ● = pH not corrected; ○ = pH corrected to 7.0. From Holme and Murphy [10].

less than 6.0 showed no change in light transmission with stirring at different rates, reflecting the spherical transformation known to occur below this pH level. Furthermore, the change in shape was not reversible with in vitro pH adjustment to 7.0. This result is compatible with the confirmed in vivo loss of viability of these platelets.

1.1.2.2 Size range

One additional morphologic measurement which has been correlated with in vivo platelet recovery and survival is the size range. Poststorage platelets were measured by a Coulter channel analyzer arbitrarily set to record the number of platelets in seven different windows. Increased platelet size was considered to reflect disc-to-sphere transformation, while decreased size was thought to represent the effect of a release reaction. An increase in the size range of stored platelets correlated with decreased in vivo platelet recovery with a correlation coefficient of 0.83, and, with percent discs, the value was 0.67 [11]. There was no relationship with in vivo platelet survival.

Although there have been a variety of other in vitro tests evaluated, the tests discussed are among the most reliable and simplest to perform. A comprehensive review of the relationship between in vitro tests and in vivo transfusion data is available [12].

1.2 In vivo measurements

1.2.1 Normal volunteers

Evaluation of platelet efficacy involves determining the recovery, survival, and function of transfused platelets in thrombocytopenic recipients. However, variables related to the patient's disease [13,14], or therapy [15] often limit the interpretation of posttransfusion results. A useful alternative approach has been to measure the recovery and survival of fresh or stored ^{51}Cr or ^{111}Indium-labeled autologous platelets in normal volunteers. Normal variations in recovery and survival measurements among individuals may obscure minor differences between storage parameters unless paired studies are done in the same volunteer [11]. The validity of using radiolabeled platelet viability measurements in normal volunteers has been documented by confirmatory platelet transfusion studies in selected, clinically stable thrombocytopenic patients [16].

1.2.2 Thrombocytopenic patients

Although preliminary studies on the effect of storage conditions on platelet viability are best performed in normal volunteers, major changes in platelet storage techniques still require confirmatory studies in thrombocytopenic patients. However, finding appropriate thrombocytopenic recipients to reliably determine posttransfusion platelet viability and function is difficult but extremely important. Such patients should not have hypersplenism, viral or bacterial infections, extensive malignant disease, or other conditions known to be associated with platelet consumption, or be taking medications known to interfere with platelet function. If the posttransfusion data suggest that the storage procedure has compromised either platelet viability or function, a repeat transfusion of fresh platelet concentrates will determine if the product or the recipient is producing the abnormality.

1.2.2.1 Platelet viability

Posttransfusion platelet survival is determined by measuring pretransfusion and multiple posttransfusion platelet counts, or by determining the disappearance rate after transfusion of radio-labeled platelets.

Platelet recovery is calculated by:

$$\text{platelet recovery (\%)} = \frac{\text{1 hr posttransfusion plt ct} - \text{baseline plt ct}}{\text{plt ct of concentrate} \times \text{volume injected}}$$

1.2.2.2. Platelet function

There is a direct inverse relationship between bleeding time and platelet count in aplastic thrombocytopenic patients [17,18] (see Fig. 2). This bleeding time/platelet count relationship forms the basis for determining the function of stored platelets; i.e., whether there has been an appropriate improvement in the bleeding time for the posttransfusion platelet count achieved [17]. The best differential between baseline and posttransfusion data is achieved if only patients with severe thrombocytopenia and correspondingly long bleeding times are studied; i.e., a baseline platelet count of $<20{,}000/\mu l$ and a bleeding time of >30 minutes. Posttransfusion platelet aggregation studies, as another approach to determining platelet function, are rarely performed because platelet increments are usually not sufficient to obtain reliable results.

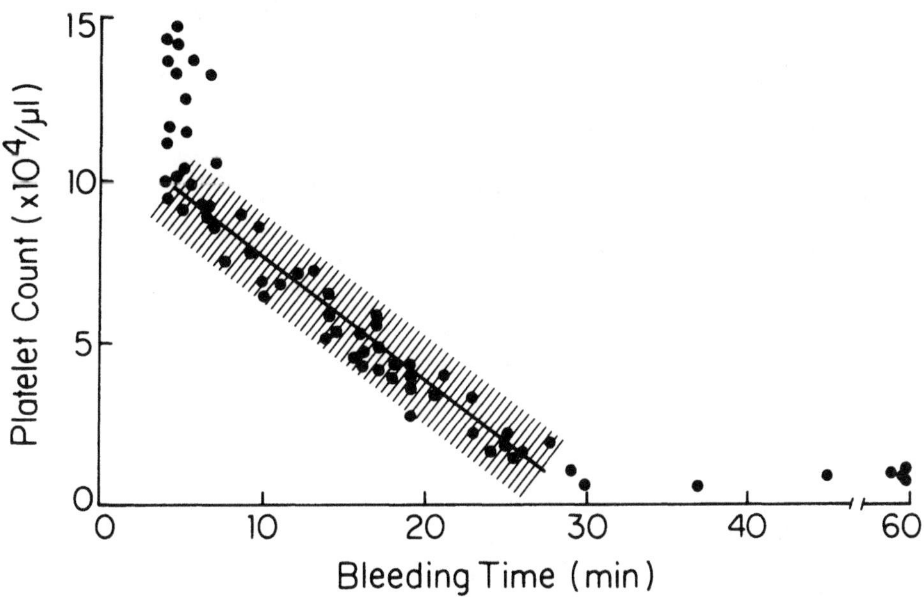

Figure 2. The relationship between bleeding time and platelet count was determined in 70 individuals with marrow failure and platelet counts of less than 150,000/μl. In individuals with platelet counts of greater than 100,000/υl, the bleeding time averaged 4½ ± 1½ minutes. In patients with platelet counts between 10 and 100,000/μl, there was a direct inverse relationship between bleeding time and platelet count that could be predicted by the equation,

$$\text{bleeding time (min)} = 30.5 - \left(\frac{\text{platelet count} \times 10^9/\text{l}}{3.85}\right)$$

At platelet counts less than 10,000/μl, bleeding time was greater than 30 minutes [17]. From Harker and Slichter [17].

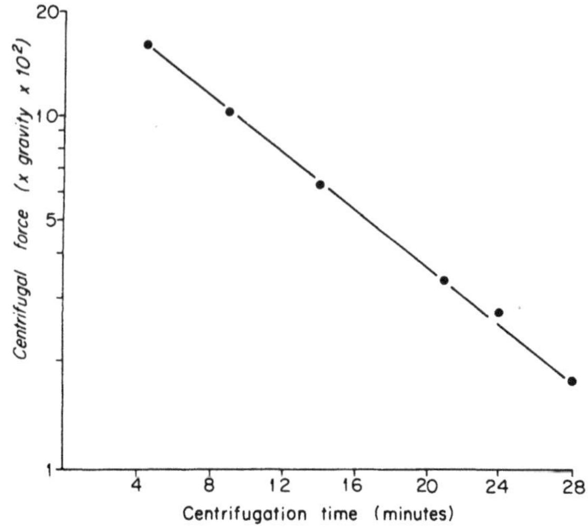

Figure 3. Six centrifugal forces between 175 and 1600 g were evaluated for the centrifugation time required to achieve the maximum platelet yield from the whole blood into the platelet-rich plasma (PRP). The optimum time to achieve maximum platelet yield for each **g** force is inversely proportional to the logarithm of the force applied. From Slichter and Harker [19].

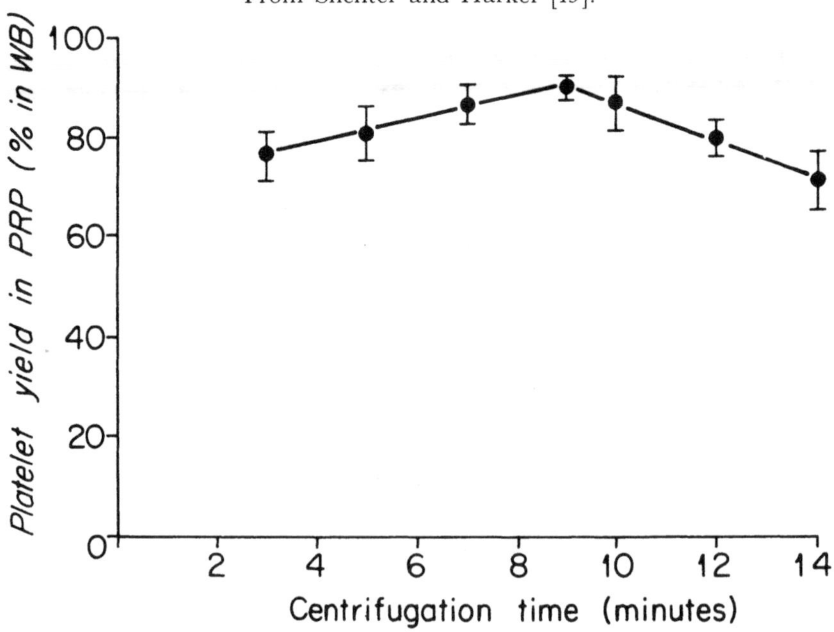

Figure 4. For each **g** force tested, too short a centrifugation time did not allow adequate separation of PRP from other cells, resulting in poor yield while too long a centrifugation time sedimented the platelets into the buffy coat, reducing platelet yield. In this example, a centrifugal force of 1000 **g** was used with an optimum centrifugation time of 9 minutes to yield 89±1% of the whole blood platelet into the PRP. From Slichter and Harker [19].

Results

1 Techniques of optimum platelet concentrate preparation and storage
1.1 Platelet concentrate production

The yield of platelets in a platelet concentrate varies with the time and force of centrifugation used to separate the platelet-rich plasma (PRP) from whole blood and, subsequently, the sedimentation of platelets from the PRP. Centrifugation conditions should yield the maximum number of platelets in the shortest time while perserving platelet viability and function.

Using an RC-3 Sorvall centrifuge with horizontal head, extensive studies have been performed to obtain maximum platelet yield [19]. For each centrifugation force tested for PRP preparation, an optimum time for centrifugation was found (Fig. 3). Too short a centrifugation time for the **g** force did not allow adequate separation of PRP from other cells, while too long a centrifugation sedimented the platelets into the buffy coat (Fig. 4). The maximum platelet harvest of 89±1% of the whole blood platelets was determined using a **g** force of 1000 for 9 minutes (Fig. 5).

The data in Figure 5 show that, as long as the optimum centrifugation time is used for each **g** force (Fig. 3), the differences between the platelet yield in

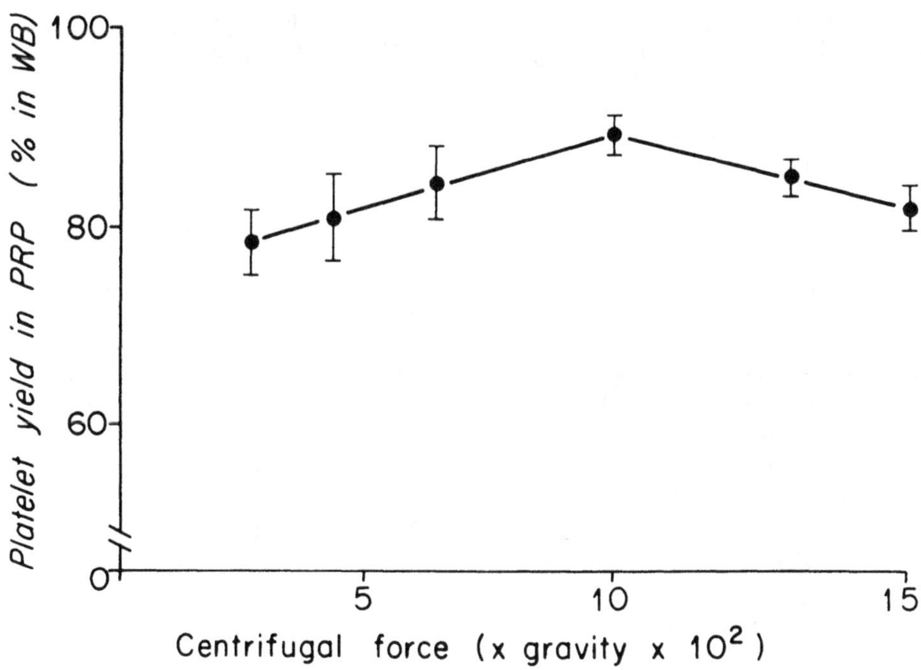

Figure 5. Plotting the optimum platelet yield in the PRP for each centrifugal force evaluated indicates a optimum platelet yield at 1000 **g**. From Slichter and Harker [19].

PRP over a wide range of **g** forces is not great: 79-89% of the platelets in whole blood are separated into the PRP. This finding may explain why different strategies of optimum platelet harvesting have resulted in a number of different recommendations for PRP preparation [19-21]. Furthermore, to achieve reliable data, a large number of units must be examined, because of differences in blood sedimentation characteristics of individual donors.

Another factor that may need to be considered in the PRP preparation process is the number of contaminating white cells. This is a variable that has not been systematically addressed, but high white counts in the platelet concentrate appear to contribute to a pH fall during storage, leading to loss of platelet viability [4,22] (see below). It may also contribute to platelet alloimmunization [22,24]. Prolonged centrifugation at low **g** forces gives the greatest reduction in white cell contamination (Table 1).

Table 1. PRP centrifugation conditions determine WBC contamination of platelet concentrate.

	PRP preparations			**WBC contamination platelet concentrate**
Investigator	**# units**	**time (min)**	**force (g)**	**WBC's $\times 10^8$/unit***
Herzig [24]	252	3	1500	8.36** (4.8-22.5)
Moroff [22]	66	3.5	2665	1.41 ± 1.27
Slichter	12	5	1500	0.95 ± 0.69
Gottschall [4]	290	6	1032	0.92 ± 1.1
Slichter	12	9	1000	0.70 ± 0.57

* Average ± S.D.
** Median with range in parenthesis.

The objective of platelet sedimentation from PRP is to obtained all of the platelets without using a **g** force so high that it damages cells. The higher the **g** force used, the shorter is the centrifugation time required (Fig. 6). However, at the highest **g** force tested of 4000 **g** for 10 minutes, a decrease in platelet survival was found even when the platelets were transfused without storage [19]. This injury is potentiated after platelet storage for 3 days [6].

After centrifugation, it is important to leave an appropriate volume of platelet-poor plasma (PRP) with the platelet concentrate to facilitate storage (see below). This can best be achieved by placing the transfer pack on a shelf above the expressor. This system leaves the desired residual volume and prevents gravity syphoning of plasma beyond that required.

Resuspension of platelets is a critical step in the preparation process. After centrifugation, immediate attempts at resuspension result in platelet aggregation, completing the aggregation process initiated by platelet packing during centrifugation. If the platelets are left for 1½-2 hours at room temperature, spontaneous disaggregation occurs [25], and the platelet pack can be gently kneaded to facilitate resuspension, or placed on a rotator.

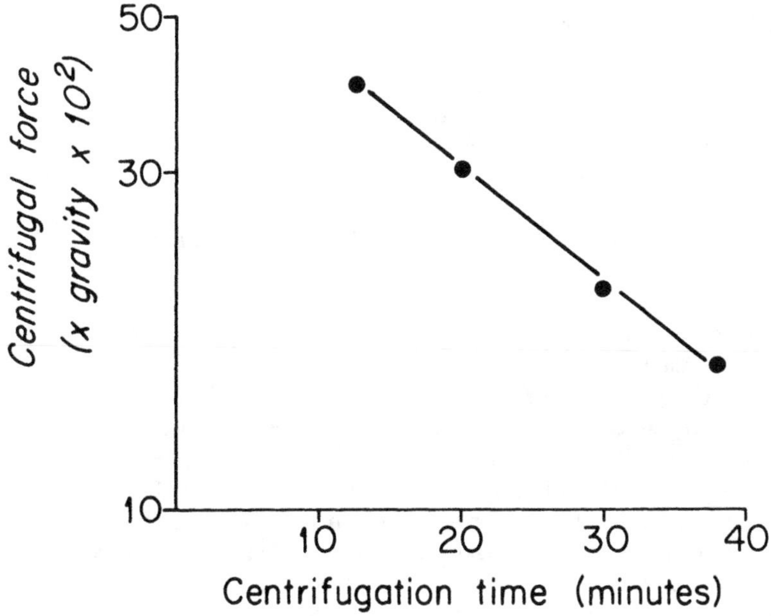

Figure 6. The minimum time required to sediment 95% of the platelets from the PRP into a PC was found to be inversely proportional to the centrifugal force applied. From Slichter and Harker [19].

Most patients require platelets from more than one donor, necessitating pooling of platelet concentrates. This procedure should be done before issuing the platelets from the central facility to ensure that all of the platelets are transferred to the pooling bag. Furthermore, as some storage procedures require large residual plasma volumes (up to 70 ml/unit), an additional centrifugation after pooling may be necessary to reduce the volume of plasma adminstered. Centrifuging up to 8 pooled concentrates at 1745 **g** for 15 minutes recovers over 95% of the platelets and does not reduce posttransfusion platelet recovery and survival, even if the platelets have been stored for 3 days before pooling (personal observations).

1.2 Platelet concentrate storage

There are several variables that directly effect poststorage platelet viability and function (see below). However, it has been well-established that CPD anticoagulant solutions with or without adenine do not produce platelet injury storage [26-28] and that 22°C is the optimum storage temperature [29]. Thus, these latter parameters will not be discussed further.

1.2.1 Agitation

Platelets require constant gentle agitation during room temperature storage to maintain viability [7,19]. In fact, even the type of agitation used – whether a horizontal to-and-fro movement at 40-70 cycles per minute (Eberbach, Ann Arbor, MI), and end-over-end type of tumbler agitation (Helmer Laboratories), elliptical rotation (Fenwal), or a 'ferris wheel' rotation at 5 cycles/minute – had different effects on platelet viability [11,30]. Equally good transfusion results were obtained with either the horizontal or the tumbler agitator, while the other two agitation methods (elliptical and ferris wheel) produced substantially inferior results.

1.2.2 Platelet count, white cell count, residual plasma volume and gas exchange through the storage bag

Several interrelated variables affect platelet viability during storage. There is a direct inverse relationship between platelet count and pH change during storage [6,26,30]. To explain this pH change, the relationships between pH, platelet count, lactate production, oxygen tension, and PCO_2 levels have been evaluated [1,2,30,31]. The higher the platelet concentration, the lower the poststorage PO_2 level (Fig. 7), and lactic acid and PCO_2 levels are reciprocally elevated. Low poststorage pH's are exacerbated if the platelets are not agitated during storage and are lessened if: (1) platelets are stored in either more permeable bags or those with a large surface area to improve gas transport, or (2) the platelet concentration is reduced by increasing the residual plasma volume.

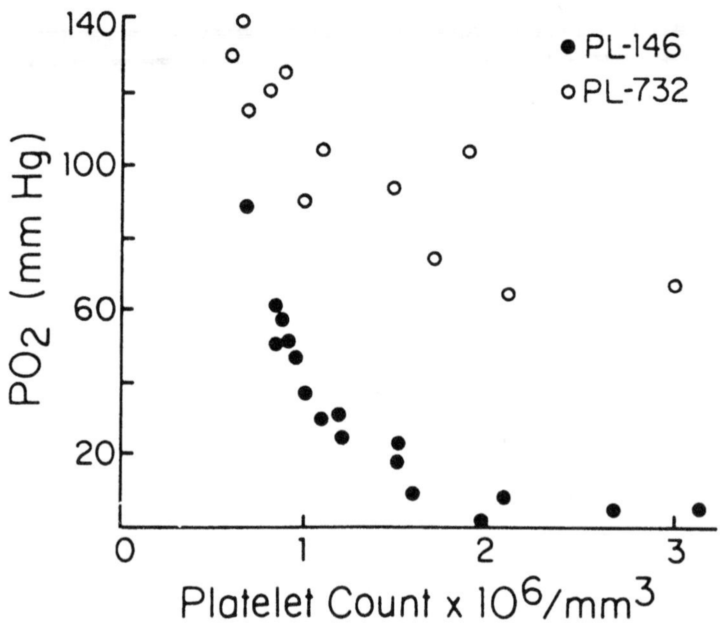

Figure 7. Platelet concentrates were stored in 50 ml of plasma for 24 hours. In PL-146 plastic bags (Fenwal), poststorage PO_2 was markedly reduced in PC with high platelet counts, suggesting oxygen transport across the plastic bag was inadequate to replenish the oxygen consumed. PO_2 was higher in PL-732 plastic bags (Fenwal), consistent with its increased permeability to oxygen. From Murphy et al. [30].

Oxygen is utilized by platelets to support aerobic metabolism during 22°C storage. If the number of stored platelets produces a requirement for oxygen that cannot be met by gas exchange through the bag's plastic walls, platelet metabolism changes from aerobic to anaerobic, and the increase in glycolysis produces excessive lactic acid. If there is not sufficient plasma present to buffer the lactic acid, the pH falls. In addition, pH varies with production of CO_2 and its transfer across the bag; i.e., high PCO_2 levels further contribute to low pH's.

When using the standard PL-146 (Fenwal) and CL-3000 (Cutter) 3-day storage bags, the best method of preventing the pH fall associated with high platelet yields is to increase the residual plasma volume. The plasma volume required is determined by the storage time; i.e., for 1-day storage a residual plasma volume of 20 ml is sufficient; for 2 days, 50 ml; and for 3 days, 70 ml [6]. A platelet concentration of less than $1.7 \times 10^{12}/l$ is necessary to maintain pH above 6.0 after 3 days of 22°C storage. However, even when optimum plasma-platelet ratios were used so that the pH did not fall below 6.0, platelets showed substantial losses in viability if storage in these bags was extended beyond 3 days [6,29].

Fortunately, a new generation of bags has been developed that permits platelet storage for up to 7 days. These bags were designed to facilitate gas transport by using either a more permeable polyolefin plastic (Fenwal PL-732) [30] or a thinner bag (Cutter CLX™) [32].

Using the CLX™ plastic bag with a 50 ml residual plasma volume, 149 of 167 (89%) of platelet concentrates stored for 5 days maintained a post-storage pH greater than 6.0. Those with low pH had platelet concentrations of greater than $2.0 \times 10^{12}/l$, indicating that this is the maximum allowable platelet concentration for 5-day storage. For those concentrates with a pH of greater than 6.0 at the end of the storage interval, there was no difference between recovery and survival data using radio-labeled measurements in normal volunteers after 3 or 5 days of storage [32].

After 7 days of storage CLX™ bags with a 50 ml volume, 15/20 units (75%) had a pH below 6.0. For those 15 units with a pH greater than 6.0, posttransfusion recovery was above 40%, and half-time survivals were reduced to 2.8 days as compared to 3.3 days for 5-day-stored platelets. Transfusion studies in four patients showed improved bleeding time measurements in all but one, whose maximum posttransfusion platelet count was only 39,000/μl.

After 5 days of storage in PL-732 plastic bags containing 30-60 ml of plasma, 93 of 101 platelet concentrates had a pH between 6.7 and 7.4. One had a pH of 6.1, and 7 had pH's of greater than 7.5. Thus, 8% of the stored concentrates had unacceptable pH values. ^{51}Chromium-labeled platelet viability studies in normal volunteers showed there was no difference in platelet recovery or survival after 5 days, compared to 1 day of storage at room temperature [30]. These viability results were confirmed in patient transfusion studies. Even with this improved container, acceptable platelet recoveries depend on residual plasma volume as demonstrated in Figure 8. After 7 days of storage with 50 ml of residual plasma, recoveries were significantly less than at 5 days with the same volume. One of the 8 units has a pH of less than 6.0 for 7 days, but even those with a pH greater than 6.0 had reduced recoveries.

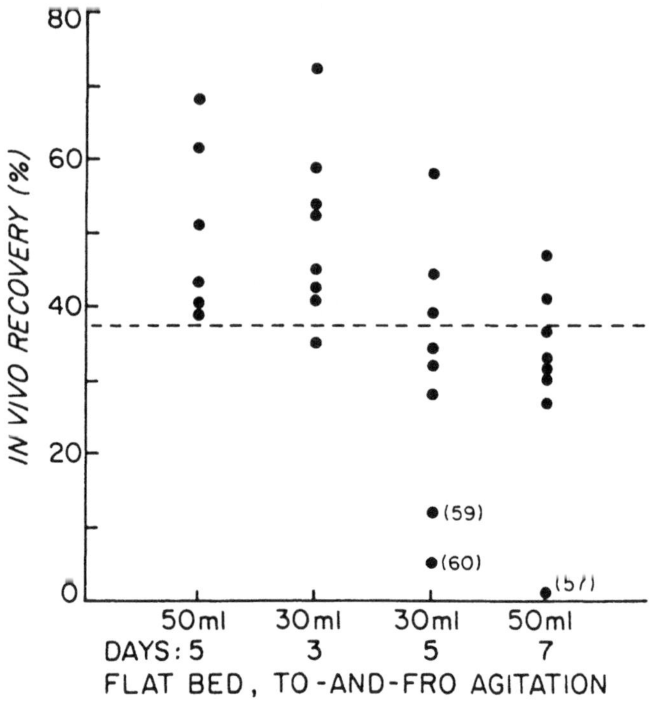

Figure 8. In vivo recovery using ^{51}Cr-labeled autologous platelets in normal volunteers after 3-7 day storage intervals in either 30 or 50 ml of residual plasma in PL-732 plastic with flatbed agitation. The symbols represent individual studies and the numbers in parentheses represent the final poststorage pH. The horizontal line represents the lower limit of the results when 50 ml of plasma were stored with the platelet concentrate for 5 days. Use of 30 ml of residual plasma for 5 days or only 50 ml for 7-day storage resulted in reduced platelet recoveries. From Murphy et al [30].

Recently, the Food and Drug Administration (USA) has shortened the accepted platelet storage time in the new bags from 7 to 5 days. This change was based on concerns about bacterial contamination following extended storage and a progressive loss in platelet viability over the storage interval.

Discussion

The value of any proposed change in the conditions of platelet preparation and storage requires a systematic approach. Platelet preparation procedures are designed to optimize platelet yield into a platelet concentrate without compromising platelet viability or function. Critical steps in this process are the sedimentation force used to prepare the platelet concentrate and resuspension of the concentrated platelets.

If a procedure results in a poststorage pH below 6.0, there are sufficient transfusion data to document that this change will be harmful, and the procedure should be abandoned. Less information exists on the detrimental effects of a high pH, but the available studies suggest that pH values greater than 7.4 are sometimes associated with decreased platelet recovery.

If poststorage pH is satisfactory, an evaluation of platelet morphology is indicated to determine if platelets have undergone disc-to-sphere transformation. However, disc-to-sphere transformation begins during 22°C storage at pH's less than 6.8 and progresses to complete platelet sphering at pH's less than 6.0. Since acceptable poststorage recoveries and survivals have been shown for platelets at pH's between 6.8 and 6.0, partial disc-to-sphere transformation cannot by itself be taken as evidence for loss of platelet viability. This may be related to a reversal to disc form following transfusion.

If the in vitro determinations give acceptable results, poststorage chromium or indium-radio-labeled platelet recovery and survival measurements in normal volunteers should be performed. Finally, if a significant change in the storage procedure has been introduced, serial measurements of posttransfusion platelet counts and corresponding improvements in bleeding times in stable thrombocytopenic patients will confirm the effectiveness of the storage procedure in maintaining platelet viability and function.

Platelets should be continuously agitated during 22°C storage either by a horizontal to-and-fro motion (Eberbach rotator) or an end-over-end process (Helmer Laboratories). With the newer platelet storage bags (Fenwal PL-732 or Cutter CLX™), platelet concentrations of between 2 and $3 \times 10^{12}/l$ in 50 ml of residual plasma are well-preserved for at least 5 days of storage. Because of the excellent gas transport provided by these new storage containers, it is important for blood centers to closely monitor poststorage pH values for unacceptably high results greater than 7.4. Such results may occur in poor-yield platelet concentrates with large residual plasma volumes; either reducing the residual plasma volume or improving platelet yield will solve the problem (Table 2).

Table 2. Correction of poststorage pH's.

	Resolution[1]			
Problem	**Residual plasma volume**	**Platelet yield**	**WBC contamination**	**Gas transport**
Poststorage pH < 6.0	Increase	–	Reduce[2]	Improve[3]
Poststorage pH > 7.4	Decrease	Improve	–	Reduce[4]

1. One or more of these procedural changes should resolve the problem.
2. Use PRP centrifugation time and force that reduces WBC contamination (see Table 1).
3. Use more permeable storage bag or a storage bag with a larger surface area. In addition, bags should be stored individually on open wire racks with small bag labels to facilitate gas transport.
4. Use less permeable storage bag or storage bag with a smaller surface area.

References

1. Murphy S, Gardner FH. Platelet storage at 22°C: Role of gas transport across plastic containers in maintenance of viability. Blood 1975;46:209-18.
2. Rock G, Figuerdo A. Metabolic changes during platelet storage. Transfusion 1976;16:571-9.
3. Filip DJ, Aster RH. Relative hemostatic effectiveness of human platelets stored at 4°C and 22°C. J Lab Clin Med 1978;91:618-24.
4. Gottschall TL, Johnston VL, Rzad L, Anderson AJ, Aster RH. Importance of white blood cells in platelet storage. Vox Sang 1984;47:101-7.
5. Beutler E, Kuhl W. Platelet glycolysis in platelet storage. IV. The effect of supplemental glucose and adenine. Transfusion 1980;20:97-100.
6. Slichter SJ, Harker LA. Preparation and storage of platelet concentrates. II. Storage variables influencing platelet viability and function. Br J Haematol 1976;34:403-19.
7. Murphy S, Sayer SN, Gardner FH. Storage of platelet concentrates at 22°C. Blood 1970;35:549-57.
8. Becker GA, Tuccelli M, Kunicki T, Chalos MK, Aster RH. Studies on platelet concentrates stored at 22°C and 4°C. Transfusion 1973;13:61-8.
9. Kunicki TJ, Tuccelli M, Becker GA, Aster RH. A study of variables affecting the quality of platelets stored at 'room temperature'. Transfusion 1975;15:414-21.
10. Holme S, Murphy S. Quantitative measurement of platelet shape by light transmission studies; application to storage of platelets for transfusion. J Lab Clin Med 1978;92:53-64.
11. Holme S, Vaidja K, Murphy S. Platelet storage at 22°C: Effect of type of agitation on morphology, viability and function in vitro. Blood 1978;52:425-35.
12. Slichter SJ. In vitro measurements of platelet concentrates stored at 4 and 22°C: Correlation with post-transfusion viability and function. Vox Sang 1981;40:72-86.
13. Harker LA, Slichter SJ. Platelet and fibrinogen consumption in man. N Engl J Med 1972;287:999-1005.
14. Freireich EJ, Kliman A, Gaydos LA, Mantel N, Frei E. Response to repeated transfusions from the same donor. Ann Intern Med 1963;59:277-87.
15. Brown CH, Bradshaw MW, Natelson EA, Afriey CP, Williams TW. Defective platelet function following the administration of penicillin compounds. Blood 1976;47:949-56.
16. Slichter SJ. Post-storage platelet viability in thrombocytopenic recipients is reliably measured by radiochromium labelled platelet recovery and survival measurements in normal volunteers. Transfusion 1986;26:8-13.
17. Harker LA, Slichter SJ. Bleeding time as a screening test for evaluating platelet function. N Engl J Med 1972;287:155-9.
18. Kahn RA, Merryman HT. Storage of platelet concentrates. Transfusion 1976;16:13-6.
19. Slichter SJ, Harker LA. Preparation and storage of platelet concentrates. I. Factors influencing the harvest of viable platelets from whole blood. Br J Haematol 1976;34:393-402.
20. Reiss RF, Katz HA. Optimizing recovery of platelets and platelet-rich plasma by the simplex strategy. Transfusion 1976;16:370-4.
21. Racz Z, Thek M. Buffy coat or platelet-rich plasma? Comparison of two platelet processing techniques. Vox Sang 1984;47:108-13.
22. Moroff G, Friedman A, Robkin-Kline L. Factors influencing changes in pH during storage of platelet concentrates at 20-24°C. Vox Sang 1982;42:33-45.

23. Eernisse JG, Brand A. Prevention of platelet refractoriness due to HLA antibodies by administration of leukocyte-poor blood components. Exp Haematol 1981;9:77-83.
24. Herzig RH, Herzig GP, Bull MI, et al. Correction of poor platelet transfusion responses with leukocyte poor HLA-platelet concentrates. Blood 1975;46:743-50.
25. Mourad N. A simple method for obtaining platelet concentrates free of aggregates. Transfusion 1968;8:48.
26. Scott EP, Slichter SJ. Viability and function of platelet concentrates stored in CPD-adenine (CPDA-1). Transfusion 1980;20:489-97.
27. Bolin RB, Cheney BA, Simpliciano OA, Peck CC. In vitro evaluation of platelets stored in CPD-adenine formulations. Transfusion 1980;20:409-18.
28. Bolin RB, Cheney BA, Smith V, Gildengorin V, Shegekawa R. An in vivo comparison of CPD and CPDA-2 preserved platelet concentrates after an 8 hour preprocess hold of whole blood. Transfusion 1982;22:491-5.
29. Murphy S, Gardner FH. Effect of storage temperature on maintenance of platelet viability – deleterious effect of refrigerated storage. N Engl J Med 1969;280:1094-8.
30. Murphy S, Kahn RA, Holme S, et al. Improved storage of platelets for transfusion in a new container. Blood 1982;60:194-200.
31. Murphy S. The storage of platelets for transfusion at 22°C. In: Baldini MG, Ebbe S (eds). Platelets: Production, function, transfusion and storage. New York: Grune and Stratton 1974:373.
32. Simon TL, Nelson EJ, Carmen R, Murphy S. Extension of platelet storage. Transfusion 1983;23:207-12.

SURGE PLATELETAPHERESIS

M.K. Elias, H. Pol, M. Weggemans, A. Maas, P.C. Das, C.Th. Smit Sibinga

Introduction

Minimizing alloimmunization of multitransfused platelets recipients is increasingly becoming a challenge. The use of non-selected single donor platelets or HLA-matched platelets reduces the rate of alloimmunization to only 50% and 30% respectively.

The use of leukocyte-poor platelets seems to gain increasing support. Indepenent studies [1-5] report a similar low incidence of alloimmunization in recipients of leukocyte-poor blood components. This incidence was reduced to 0% when using platelets which are both leukocyte-poor and matched [3].

There are 3 possibilities to deplete platelet concentrates of contaminating leukocytes:

1. An extra centrifugation step of 300 **g** for 10 minutes completely removed the leukocytes from standard platelet concentrates [6]. However, this results in loss of at least 30% of the thrombocytes.
2. Filtration through a cotton wool column [7] recovers almost all the platelets, but the final leukocyte contamination varies according to the initial pre-filtration leukocyte count in the platelet concentrate.
3. The third possibility is the surge technique; this is a plateletapheresis method which combines centrifugal separation with elutriation. The elutriation method allows a cell separation based on the balance between cell sedimentation speed and plasma speed in the opposite direction. As sedimentation speed is principally a function of cell surface, elutriation can be considered as a small cell collection technique. It therefore increases the resolution of platelets from leukocytes producing a high-yield product equal to 7-8 standard platelet concentrates, with a minimal possible leukocyte contamination (Table 1). However, this contamination still seems to be of considerable amount as regards alloimmunization.

At present, there is a lack of consensus on the minimal dose of leukocytes per transfusion which is capable of inducing sensitization. Some investigators report to the absence of a dose response relationship [8]. Others suggested that the critical level for febrile reactions to occur is 0.25×10^9 leukocytes per transfusion [9]. A recent study [10] reported that platelets with fewer than 5 million lymphocytes per transfusion do not seem to stimulate a response to major histocompatibility antigens, while a contaminating dose of 15 million leukocytes appears to be highly immunogenic. Accordingly, we attempted to deplete the leukocyte-poor surge platelets even further by filtration through cotton wool.

Table 1. The platelet yield and the leukocyte contamination obtained with various preparation techniques.*

Method	**Mean platelets** $\times 10^{11}$	**Leukocyte contamination** $\times 10^{8}$	**Donor equivalent**
Standard	0.55	4-10	1
Manual thrombapheresis (multiple bag)	1.8 – 3.6	6 – 8	2 – 6
Machine thrombapheresis	3.2 – 6.4	54 – 67	6 – 8
Surge	3.4 – 5.8	0.7 – 6.7	6 – 8

* The absolute content of one donor equivalent of standard PC is 0.55×10^{11} thrombocytes with a contamination of 4×10^{8} leukocytes in a 50 ml volume prepared from a donation of 450 ml blood.

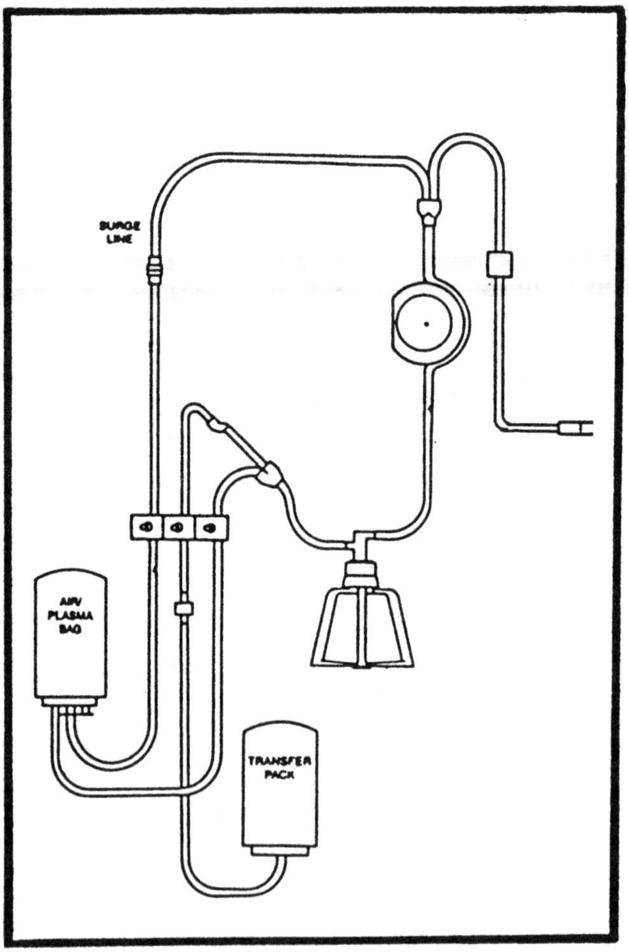

Figure 1. The surge technique (Haemonetics V50-1).

Methods used

The surge technique (Fig. 1)

The Haemonetics V50 hemapheresis machine with a platelet elutriation programme was used. Blood is pumped into the bowl at 60-70 ml/min. When the buffy coat is 1.1 cm from the exit port, the blood pump is stopped automatically and the surge pump activated to eject part of the plasma collected in the air/plasma bag, into the spinning bowl.

This fast stream of plasma, called 'surge', elutes the platelets from the buffy coat leaving white and red cells behind. The surge technique evoluted rapidly in three generations: the manual, the semiautomated and the autosurge.

In the early surge trials [11] a line was drawn 1.05 cm from the bowl rim to serve as an indicator to start the surge pump by pressing a button. Again, collection of platelets was terminated by noting a clearing in the turbidity of plasma when platelets have passed through the exit port. This manual and visual control of the surge collection was not very accurate. The surge was further semiautomated by supplying optical sensors at the shoulder of the bowl and on the effluent line allowing more accurate timing for the start and termination of collection.

Prior to each procedure three parameters must be adjusted according to the composition of the donor's blood in an attempt to modify the collection procedure for that donor. These parameters are: the VO, the CDV and the P/WC factor:

a. Volume offset (VO) determines the surge starting point, which is the point where the surge of plasma exiting from the air/plasma bag towards the bowl begins. This starting point can be delayed for donors with low hematocrit to give more time for the buffy coat to reach the shoulder of the bowl. It is possible to recognize whether the VO should be increased or decreased based on the sequence of events observed during the first pass (Fig. 2).
   - If the VO is too low the surge begins too early. The graph in this situation would be elongated on the time axis. The product would have a high volume, low platelet concentration because the buffy coat (BC) did not have enough time to be well formed. This results in a poor total yield and very low or no contaminating white and red cells.
   - if on the other hand the VO is too high, the surge starts too late. The graph in this situation would be compressed on the time axis with the cell population overlapping each other to a greater extend. This is the packing phenomenon. The product would be low in volume, with a high platelet concentration but still poor in total yield and with increased white and red blood cells.

   There is an inverse relationship between VO and donor hematocrit. The higher the hematocrit, the lower the VO and vice versa. This relationship is not directly linear because of the presence of other factors such as donor precount, thickness of the platelet band, plasma viscosity, packing characteristics and indiviual machine operating range. Therefore, observation of the first pass is essential to predict what the VO for a particular donor

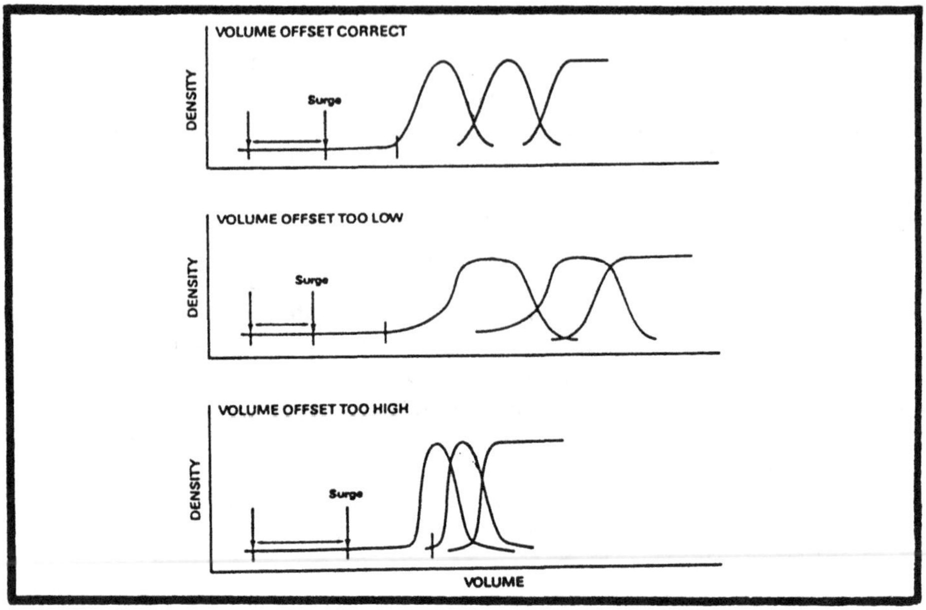

Figure 2. The situations which may be encountered with different VO adjustments (adapted from publications of Haemonetics).

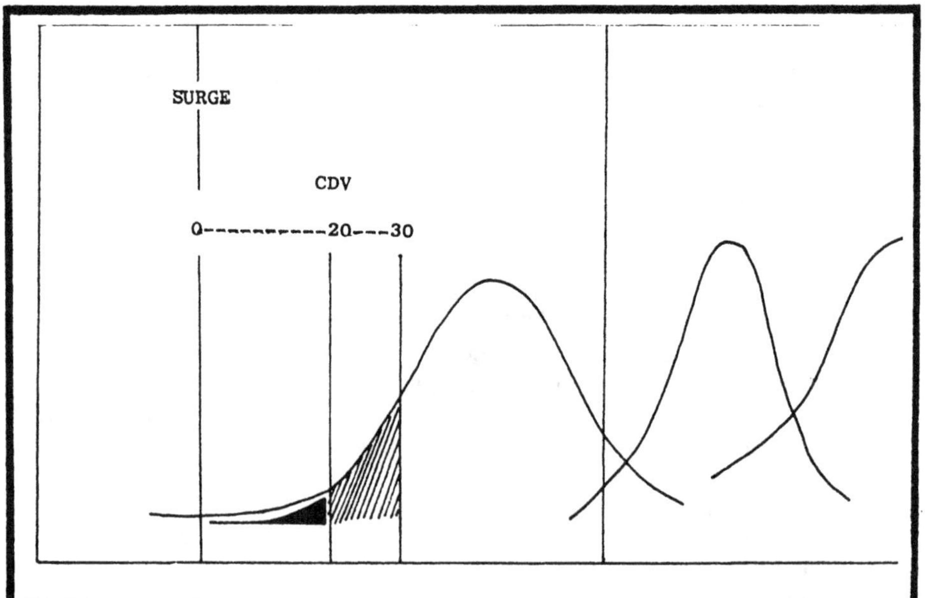

Figure 3. Determination of the product volume by adjusting the CDV parameter.

should be. In a previous study [12] we developed a range of VO adjustments according to different hematocrits. The platelet yield obtained using an adjusted VO was significantly higher than that obatined using the surge protocol with standard VO parameter.

b. The second parameter to be adjusted is the collection delay volume (CDV). This determines the collection starting point (Fig. 3). Prior to the start of the surge there is a long period where the separated PPP enters the air/plasma bag. After activation of the surge pump the concentration of platelets in the effluent line remains low for a further 20 ml (the preset value of the CVD) after which collection begins. The concentration of platelets then steadily increases within the next 20 ml. The peak is detected, then steadily decreases within the next 20 ml before the concentration of white cells increases. When the CDV parameter is adjusted in an appropriate way, the volume and therefore the concentration of the final product could be altered to meet specific needs; for example a high volume for storage or a low volume for radio-active labeling etc.

c. The third surge control parameter is the platelet/white cell factor (Fig. 4). This determines the end point of the surge. It is measured as the number of seconds during which the surge continues after the platelet peak has been detected by the line sensor. The preset value is 3 seconds. Increase of the P/WC factor yields more platelets, but carries the risk of increasing white cell contamination in the product.

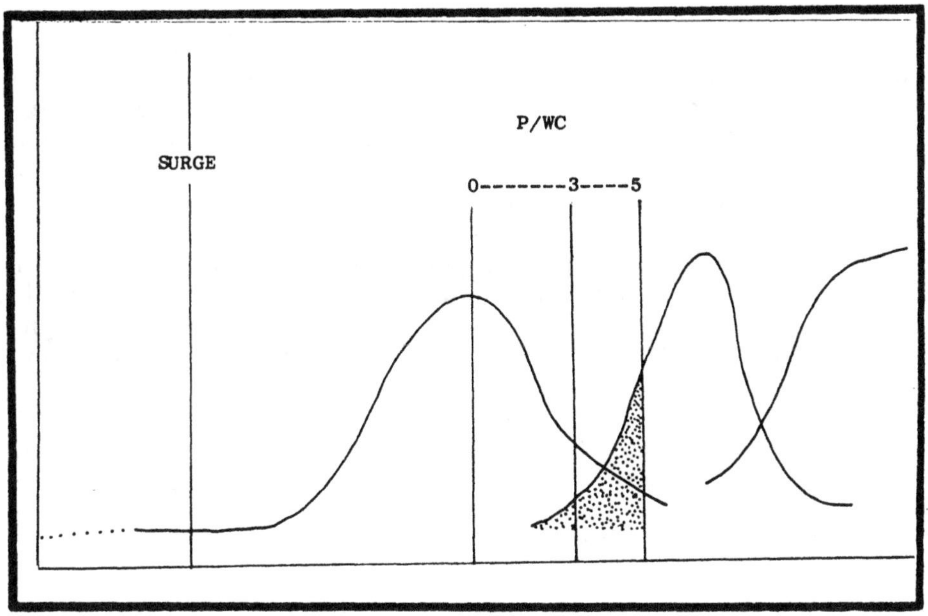

Figure 4. Determination of the end of collection through adjusting the P/WC parameter.

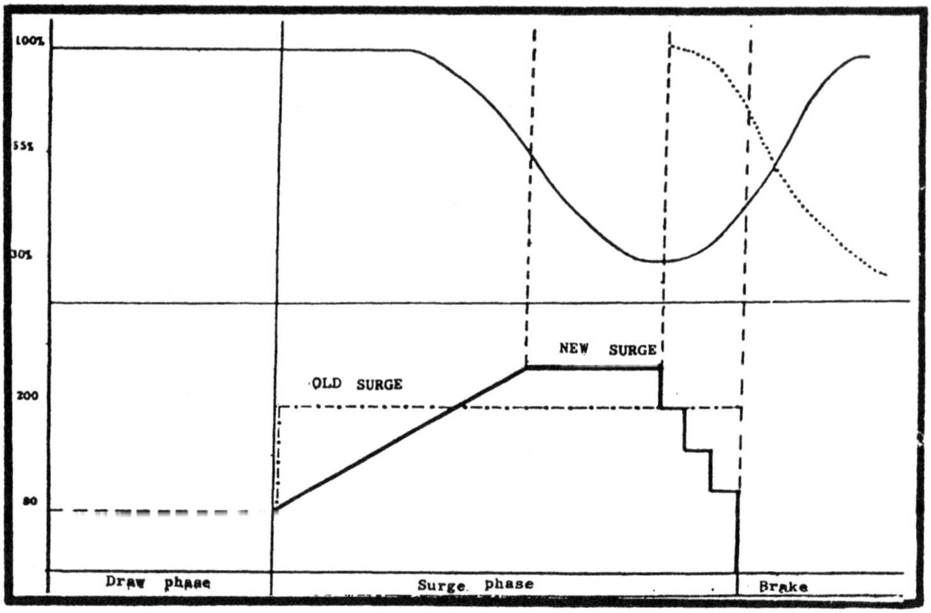

Figure 5. Comparison between the old surge and the autosurge. The reference value of the donor's plasma is taken as 100%.

The interaction of these three control parameters VO, CDV and P/WC factor especially in the light of the donor's hematologic profile modifies the surge technique to obtain the best product possible from each individual donor. However, a major disadvantage of the surge technique is the difficulty to find the correct BC position through adjusting the VO prior to each procedure. Since elutriation is dependent on a good BC position, the resolution between platelets and leukocytes is imcomplete unless this position is found. Also the interruption of the surge after predetermined volume (P/WC factor) may be too early or too late, according to the thickness of the platelet band. This makes the surge procedure a semiautomated platelet collection programme which lacks standardization.

Another disadvantage is that part of the platelets already processed is remixed with white and red cells during the sudden start and sudden brake of the surge. To circumvent these problems a fully automated platelet elutriation programme has been developed called 'autosurge' (Fig. 5). In this programme the surge always starts at the same BC position detected by the bowl optics irrespective of the donor hematocrit. Elutriation starts with a surge speed of 80 rpm and increases its speed every second by 5 ml per minute. When the platelet concentration in the effluent line increases and the line sensor voltage drops to 65% of the reference value, the surge acceleration stops meaning that the surge incremental limit (SIL) is reached. This optimal

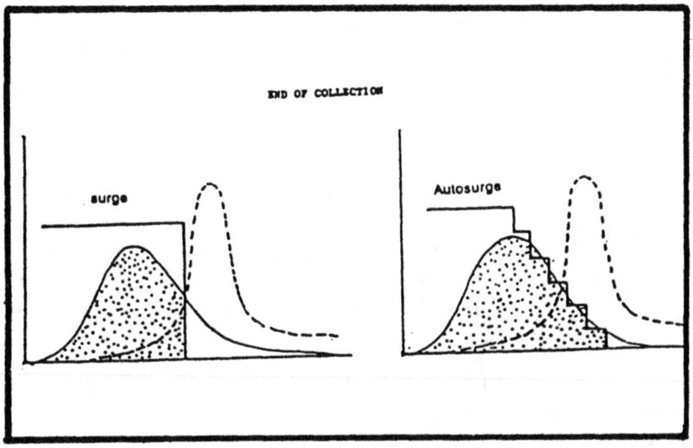

Figure 6. Comparison between the end of collection in the old surge and the autosurge.

elutriation speed (range 170-230 ml/min) is then kept constant until the platelet peak is detected. If the line sensor detects a small platelet peak, the machine automatically reduces the SIL for the next cycle to prevent contamination. This gradual surge acceleration allows automatic adaptation to each cycle and each donor. It also generates less turbulence in the BC and thus minimizes remixing of platelets with white cells.

Another modification in the autosurge (Fig. 6) is that the end of collection is not suddenly terminated as in the traditional surge. Once the platelet peak has been detected, the surge pump slows down at a rate predetermined by the contamination factor until it reaches the baseline speed. the preset value is 30ml/min every second. This gradual decrease of the surge speed allows collection of the last platelets. The CDV in this programme is equal to 20ml for the first cycle meaning that the line sensor is disabled during the first 20 ml of surge. The line sensor signal is read every 2 ml. When it reaches 70% of the reference plasma value the CDV is recorded by the machine (V). The CDV for the next cycle is then automatically calculated as $^3/_5 \times V$. This new platelet elutriation programme has some major donor related disadvantages namely overshooting of the surge acceleration in case of thin platelet band and in case of initial turbid or lipemic plasma. This jeopardizes the principles of the technique and leads to unpredictable white cell contamination.

Surge filtration

The Imugard IG500 cotton wool filter (Terumo Corporation, Japan) was used as described [7] except that the first 50 ml of platelet-poor plasma were discarded; the filter volume is approximately 80 ml. The capacity of the Imugard IG500 filter in retaining the leukocytes has been evaluated by filtration of other products with increasing leukocyte contamination gradients such as pools of standard platelet concentrates and pools of buffy coats. Care was taken to keep the volume of these products equal to that of the surge platelet concentrates (±300 ml). the filtrates where thoroughly shaken and the first few ml's in the tubing were discarded before taking a sample for in vitro tests. The platelet concentrates were allowed to run over the filter by gravity.

Laboratory tests

Manual counting by the Bürker chamber technique was done before and after filtration. Pellets from the filtrates which were 10× concentrated, were counted to confirm the presence or absence of leukocytes. The reliability of the automatic counters was also considered by comparing the results obtained by the Sysmex PL110 and the Coulter S plus counters with those obtained by the Bürker chamber technique. The absence of leukocytes was confirmed by Coulter histograms, cytospin preparations using antilymphocyte monoclonal antibodies and by blood smears.

As the platelets prepared by surge technique and filtration are subjected to two different handling techniques, we investigated the extend to which their function and integrity have been affected. The recovery from hypotonic shock was determined, the increase in lactic dehydrogenase percentage leakage and β-thromboglobulin percentage release were calculated. The two latter tests are known to correlate inversely with platelet survival [13]. The morphology score was performed according to Kunicki [14] before and after filtration. The ultrastructure of the surge platelets before and after filtration was examined by electron microscopy. The filter was tested for possible pyrogen release by the Limulus assay test. Random samples were cultured after filtration to assess the sterility since both elutriation and filtration are in principle open systems.

Results

Table 2 shows the results of 540 surge procedures carried out with the semi-automated as well as the autosurge protocols. Mean volume was 354 ml with a mean platelet yield of 3.7×10^{11} and a leukocyte contamination of 2.5×10^{8}, mostly lymphocytes. The unsuccessful surge procedures, in which the buffy coat was not detected, were excluded from the statistical analysis. The standard deviations of the leukocyte contamination in the platelet concentrates were almost approaching the means. In the autosurge protocol, when the donor platelet precounts are exceeding 200×10^{9}/l. No significant difference in

Table 2. Comparison of results (Haemonetics V50). n = 540

	Volume	Platelets $\times 10^{11}$	Leukocytes $\times 10^{8}$	PL/WC ratio	n
1984 semiautomated	401 (74)	4.3 (1.0)	2.0 (1.1)	2150	370
1985 autosurge	315 (58)	3.3 (1.0)	2.5 (2.2)	1320	110
1986 autosurge	346 (41)	3.5 (0.9)	2.9 (2.0)	1200	60
mean	354	3.7	2.5	1557	540

Standard deviation in parentesis.

platelet yield was found with different SIL settings. At low precount, however the SIL needed to be adjusted to a lower setting. It is therefore advisable to reject donors with low platelet precounts, although this is not always practically feasible. The volume of the platelet products obtained by the autosurge correlated inversely with the donor hematocrit and this explains the correlation between the total platelet yield and the donor hematocrit.

Table 3 shows the results of filtration of platelet concentrates with different initial leukocyte contaminations.

Table 3. Comparative filtration study.

	% platelet recovery	Absolute leukocyte count $\times 10^8$					
		Bürker		Sysmex		Coulter	
		before	after	before	after	before	after
Surge (n=28)	95	3.4	0.0	3.9	0.1	2.0	0.1
Pools of 6 standard PC (n=10)	75	12.4	0.0	10.1	0.33	9.9	0.5
Pools of 6 BC (n=3)	57	105.4	16.3	93.0	11.8	90.5	12.4

Platelet recovery – The mean platelet recovery of the surge PC's is 95% with a range of 89-100%, while the mean platelet percentage recovery of the standard pooled PC's is 75% and only 57% of the buffy coat platelets are recovered.

Residual leukocytes – Although no residual leukocytes could be detected by the Bürker's chamber counting technique after filtration of either the surge PC's or the pooled PC's, yet in the automatic counting technique a considerable amount of contamination ($30\text{-}50 \times 10^6$) of the pooled PC was detected when the prefiltration leukocyte counts are in the range of 10×10^8. The readings were nil or within the blanc level for the surge PC's. This observation suggests that the filter is not equally effective in depleting both products and that confirmatory methods are needed when low leukocyte counts are dealt with.

Confirmatory tests – No leukocytes were detected in the blood smears or the cytospin preparations after filtration of the surge PC. No lymphocyte histogram could be plotted by the Coulter S plus after filtration.

Table 4 summarizes the results of filtration of the surge platelets. The pH remained optimal after filtration excluding the possibility of acid release by the filter. The Limulus test was negative excluding a possible pyrogen release by the filter. No significant change was found in the hypotonic shock response before and after filtration. The increase in LDH percentage leakage and BTG percentage release after filtration was not significant. However, the latter was found to be increased after the surge procedure suggesting centrifugation induced platelet activation. The morphology score after either elutriation or filtration was above 200.

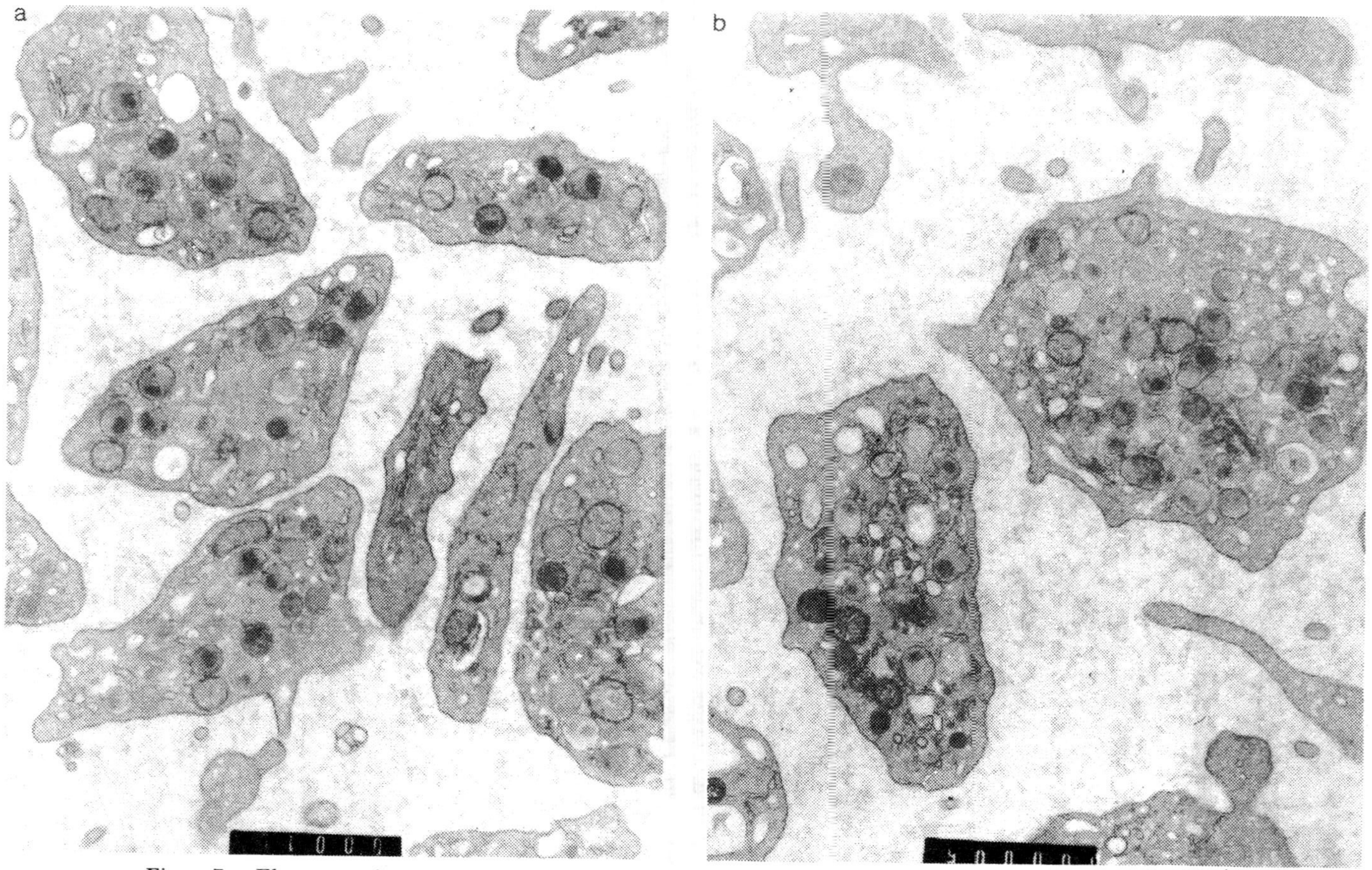

Figure 7. Electron micrographs of the surge platelets before (left) and after (right) filtration through Imugard cotton wool filter (magnification 15,000×).

Table 4. Surge-filtration study.

Platelet recovery	Residual leukocytes (Bürkers)	Mean pH	Mean HSR %	Increase LDH % leakage	Increase B-TG % release	Morph. score change
89-100%	0.0	6.94	71.3	0.7	0.5	14

The morphological features of the surge platelets before and after filtration are shown in Figure 7. The discoid configuration was preserved after the surge elutriation while after filtration the platelets acquired a more rounded configuration with the appearance of short stubby pseudopods. However, the ultrastructure of the platelets remained intact with normally distributed dense and α-granules and with moderate number and size of vacuoles. The platelet membrane displayed an electron density consistent with preseved cell membrane integrity.

Conclusion

We concluded that surge filtration seems to be a suitable technique to almost completely deplete platelets of contaminating leukocytes without compromising platelet yield. Preconnecting the filter with the surge software in one closed system could overcome the sterility problem for future clinical application and allows extended storage of the surge platelets.

Acknowledgements

We are most grateful to Mr. Eddy Ligeon from the Central Clinical Chemical Laboratory, Mr. Robert Bloem from the Paediatric Haematology Laboratory and Miss Nel Blom and Miss Marja van Luyn from the Haematology Research Laboratory of the University Hospital Groningen for the morphometric analysis of the electron micrographs.

Special thanks for the contribution of the voluntary blood donors, the Apheresis section, the Blood Processing department, the Laboratory team at the Red Cross Blood Bank Groningen-Drenthe and Miss Maya ten Cate for typing this manuscript.

References

1. Eernisse JG, Brand A. Prevention of platelet refractoriness due to HLA antibodies by administration of leukocyte-poor blood components. Exp Haematol 1981;9:77-83.
2. Herzig H, Herzig GP, Bull MI, et al. Correction of poor platelet transfusion response with leukocyte-poor HLA-matched platelet concentrates. Blood 1975;46:743-50.

3. Murphy MF, Metcalfe P, Thomas H, et al. Use of leukocyte-poor blood components and HLA-matched platelet donors to prevent HLA alloimmunisation. Brit J Haematol 1986;62:529-34.
4. Robinson EAE. Single donor granulocytes and platelets. Clin in Haematol 1984; 13(1):185-216.
5. Schiffer CA, Dutcher JP, Aisner J, Hogge D, Wiernik PH, Reilly JP. A randomized trial of leukocyte-depleted platelet transfusion to modify alloimmunization in patients with leukaemia. Blood 1983;62:815-20.
6. Cott ME, Oh JH, Vroon DH. Isolation of leukocyte-free platelets from standard platelet concentrates by centrifugation. Transfusion 1986;26:272-3.
7. Sirchia G, Parravicini P, Rebulla P, Bertolini F, Morelati F, Marconi M. Preparation of leukocyte-free platelets for transfusion by filtration through cotton wool. Vox Sang 1983;44:115-20.
8. Dutcher JP, Schiffer CA, Aisner J, Wiernik PH. Alloimmunization following platelet transfusion: The absence of a dose-response relationship. Blood 1981;57: 395-8.
9. Perkins HA, Payne R, Ferguson J, Wood M. Non-haemolytic transfusion reactions. Qualitative effects of blood components with emphasis on iso-antigenic incompatibility of leukocytes. Vox Sang 1966;11:578-600.
10. Fisher M, Chapman JR, Ting A, Morris PJ. Alloimmunisation to HLA antigen following transfusion with leukocyte-poor and purified platelet suspensions. Vox Sang 1985;49:331-5.
11. Hogge DE, Schiffer CA. Collection of platelets depleted of red and white cells with the 'surge pump' adaptation of a blood cell separator. Transfusion 1983;23: 177-81.
12. Elias M, Oenema B, Scholten JT, Das PC, Smit Sibinga CTh. Surge pump plateletapheresis: A method for effective depletion of white cells from machine-collected single donor platelets. Plasma Ther & Transf Technol 1985;6:381-6.
13. Snyder EL, Hezzey A, Katz AJ, Bock J. Occurrance of the release reaction during preparation and storage of platelet concentrates. Vox Sang 1981;41:172-7.
14. Kunicki TJ, Tucilli M, Becker GA, Aster RH. A study of the variables affecting the quality of platelets stored at room temperature. Transfusion 1975;15:414-21.

PLATELETS AND PROPYLENE GLYCOL: AN APPROACH TO FREEZING PLATELETS IN THE PRESENCE OF A NEW CYROPROTECTANT*

F.G. Arnaud, Ch.J. Hunt, D.E. Pegg

Introduction

Banking of cryopreserved platelets would make it possible to adjust the balance between supply and demand, and would facilitate the availability of typed [1,2] and autologous [3,4] platelets and random blood groups in cases of emergency [5]. The cryopreservation of platelets, at slow cooling rates, using conventional cryoprotectants (CPAs) remains unisatisfactory when assessed in vitro [6-8] although some have considered the results sufficiently good for clinical use [9,10]. Since the first attempts [11,12] platelet freezing has proved less satisfactory than that of many other cells, such as red blood cells [13]. This poor response might be explained by greater osmotic fragility of platelets [14] or by an inadequate concentration of CPA [15] due to the limitations imposed by toxic effects.

Recently, there have been reports of bacterial infection associated with long-term liquid storage of platelets leading to death of the recipient [16,17]. Although, it is an expensive technique, cryopreservation should be seriously considered as a means of platelet preservation.

CPAs are chemical compounds which must be water soluble, non toxic in the concentrations used [18], and if they belong to the group of permeating CPAs then the more permeable, the easier is their addition and dilution. Therefore, platelets should be given better protection during freezing in high concentrations of a permeable, non toxic CPA [15]. Propylene glycol (or propane-1,2-diol) (PG) has been proposed as a CPA for platelets because it is known to have low toxicity and to permeate the cell membrane rapidly. Some authors have favored PG [20-22] because of its ability to inhibit ice formation; it has a strong glass forming tendency and the amorphous state is remarkably stable [23]. However, the tolerance of platelets to PG should be investigated and the toxic limits should be found before cryopreservation is attempted. Moreover, toxicity cannot be assessed without first establishing the permeability of platelets to PG [15,24] so that methods of addition and removal can be used that avoid osmotic damage. Normal cell physiology is maintained only when cell volume is kept within a specific range [25] and it has been shown that platelets can tolerate volume variations between 60 and 130% of their initial volume [15].

* This work was funded by the Medical Research Council.

The purpose of this study was to measure the effect of several concentrations of PG at several temperatures and for various lengths of time. The details of the methods and the complete data will be described elsewhere; only the data from experiments at room temperature are included in this paper.

Methods

Preparation of the cells

Platelet concentrate (PC) was prepared from fresh blood by the standard method shown in Figure 1. First a gentle spin at 250 **g** for 20 min to produce the platelet rich plasma (PRP); then a hard spin 2000 **g** for 15 min to provide the platelet concentrate (PC) (Centrifuge MSE Mistral 6L from Fison Scientific Equipment, UK). After 20 min at 20°C the platelets were resuspended.

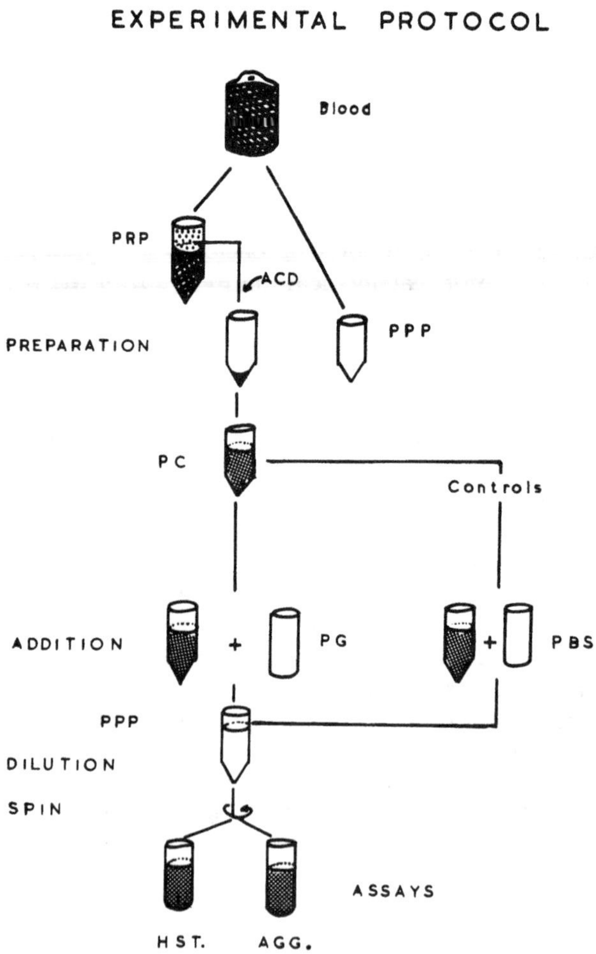

Figure 1. Protocol for the preparation of platelets from fresh blood.

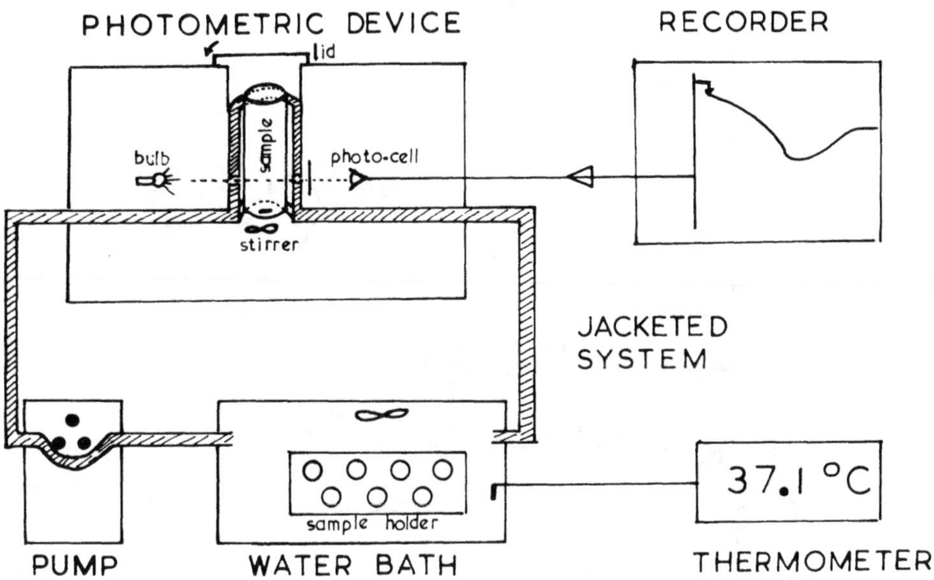

Figure 2. Photometric device to measure the changes in volume of platelets at various temperatures. The jacketed system allows the circulation of water around the sample cuvette from the water bath.

Method for measuring permeability to PG

Changes in cell volume [19,25] were measured following the addition of glycerol or propylene glycol (PG) (Glycerol Analar from BDH Ltd. Poole, UK; PG Purissimum from Fluka AG. 9470 Buchs, Switzerland); 0.5 ml of CPA solution (isotonic regarding the salt concentration) was added to 1 ml of PRP, producing a final concentration of 0.333 mol/l. The consequent change in platelet volume was monitored by a photometric device [25,26] (Fig. 2). Solutions of known osmolality were used to produce platelets of known volume, calculated by means of the Boyle van 't Hoff equation [27] (see appendix); these were used to calibrate the chart recorder in volume terms. The experimental curves from 6 individual experiments (Fig. 3a) were visually matched with curves (Fig. 3b) obtained by applying the equations of Kedem & Katchalsky [28]. This was done on a 380Z-D microcomputer (Research Machines Ltd. Oxford, UK) using a Pascal programme (see appendix). The shape of the curves is governed by the permeability parameters hydraulic conductivity (Lp), solute permeability (ω), and the reflexion coefficient (σ), and best fit values were obtained by curve fitting.

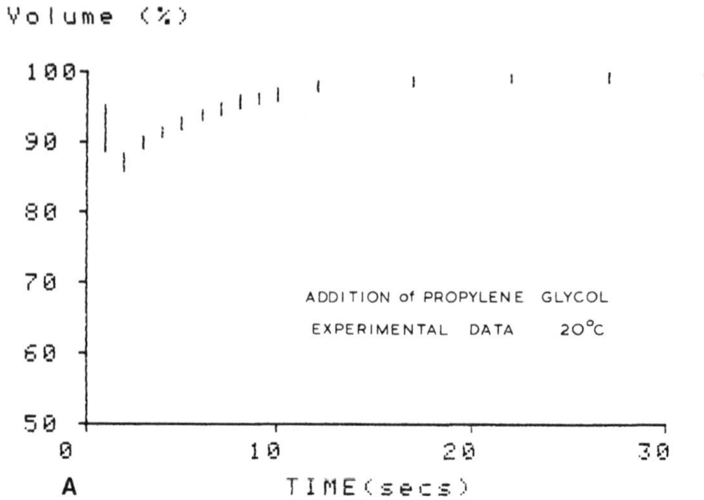

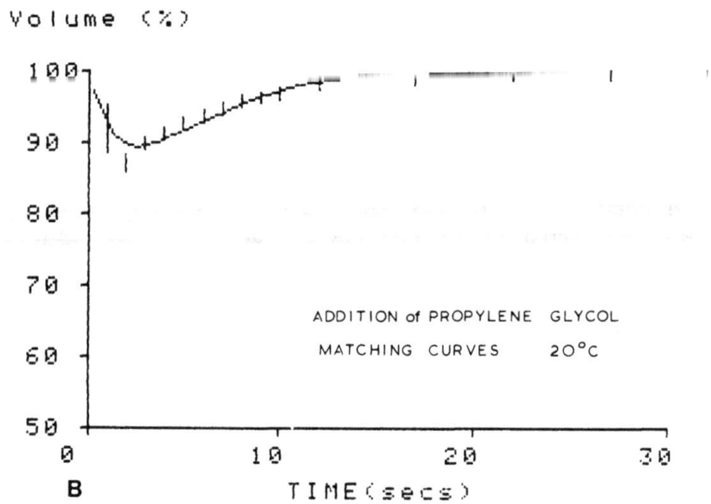

Figure 3. (A) Visual matching of the experimental data (||||) (mean of 6 experiments; the bars (|) indicate ± SEM).
(b) The computerized curves (———) were obtained from the equations of Kedem & Katchalsky.

Protocols of addition and dilution of PG

The permeability parameters were then used in the same Kedem & Katchalsky equations [28] to calculate the volume response to various step changes in concentration of PG. It was then possible to define steps such that the cell volume remained above 60% of initial volume during the addition and remained below 130% during dilution of PG.

Method of studying the toxicity of PG

Aliquots (10 ml) of platelet concentrate were equilibrated at 20°C (Fig. 1). The solutions of PG studied were also kept at this temperature and contained respectively 0, 0.5, 1, 2 and 2.5 mol/l of PG. All solutions were prepared in phosphate buffered saline, PBS, (Oxoid Ltd. Basingstoke, UK). Such solution was made up on a molar basis and contained salts equivalent to 9 g NaCl/l; thus they were all isotonic. PG was added stepwise to the suspension according to each protocol. The cell suspension was exposed to PG for 0, 15 min or 2 hours, then the dilution of the CPA was carried out by the appropriate stepwise dilution protocol. Finally PG was completely removed from the suspension by a 10 min spin at 2000 **g**, and the pellet was resuspended, either in platelet poor plasma (PPP) or PPP + ACD depending upon the test to be performed.

Assays

Hypotonic stress test:

When exposed to hypotonic conditions [29], platelets first swell due to the influx of water and then gradually return to their initial volume by efflux of water. In a spectrophotometer, the transmitted light increases due to dilution of the cells, and swelling also increases transmission (Fig 4). The final trans-

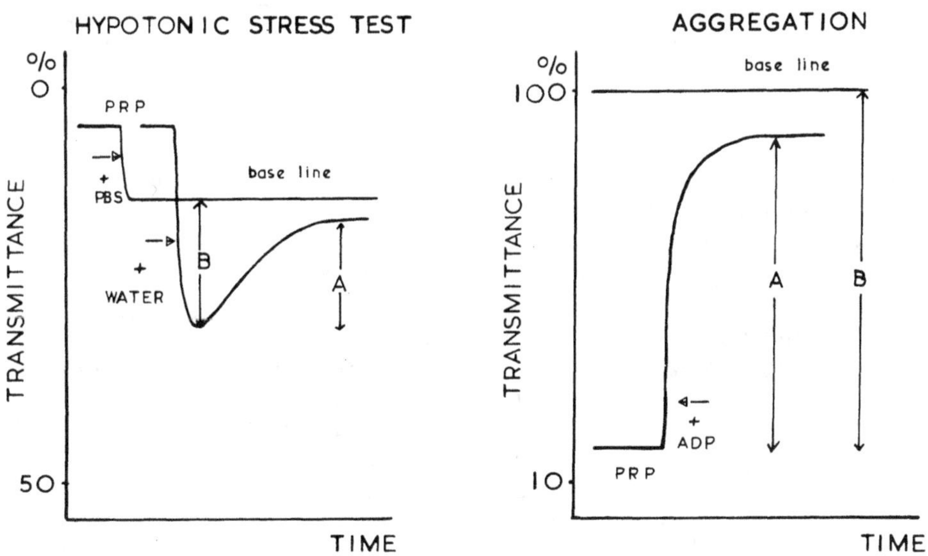

Figure 4. The assays. The hypotonic stress test (HST), 0.5 ml of water (or PBS for the baseline) was added to 1 ml of PRP, and recovery was calculated after 10 min as the ratio A/B. The aggregation test. Complete aggregation was induced by 1.5 μM ADP and recovery was calculated as the ratio A/B.

Table 1. Permeability parameters obtained from the best match between experimental and calculated curves (T=20°C).

Coefficients	Solute	
Hydraulic conductivity	PG	LP = $8x10^{-7}$ cm • s^{-1} • atm^{-1}
	Glycerol	LP = $8x10^{-7}$ cm • s^{-1} • atm^{-1}
Solute permeability	PG	ωRT = $1.1x10^{-5}$ cm • s^{-1}
	Glycerol	ωRT = $1x10^{-5}$ cm • s^{-1}
Reflexion coefficient	PG	σ = 0.4
	Glycerol	σ = 0.9

Table 2. Stepwise method of addition of PG at room temperature 20°C. The platelets were not allowed to shrink below 60% of their initial volume (T=20°C).

Time (sec)	Steps	PG concentration (mol/l)
0	1	0→ 1.4
15	2	1.4 → 2.15
30	3	2.15→ 2.6
45	4	2.6 → 2.9
60	5	2.9 → 3.1
75	6	3.1 → 3.21

Table 3. Stepwise method of dilution of PG at 20°C. The platelets were not allowed to swell above 130% of their original volume (T=20°C).

Time (sec)	Steps	PG concentration (mol/l)
0	1	2.5 → 2.4
30	2	2.4 → 2.2
60	3	2.2 → 2.0
90	4	2.0 → 1.75
120	5	1.75→ 1.45
150	6	1.45→ 1.05
180	7	1.05→ 0.6
210	8	0.6 → 0

mission if only dilution occurred was obtained by addition of isotonic PBS to the suspension and swelling was induced by adding water to PC. Transmittance was measured at 610 nm (SP spectrophotometer, Pye Unicam, UK) and the recovery was calculated as illustrated by Figure 4.

Platelet aggregation:

This was induced by 13 μmol/l ADP [30]. The suspension was continuously mixed and the optical transmission was recorded in a Malin aggregometer (Malin Electronics Ltd., UK). The increase in transmittance was recorded until total aggregation had occurred and recovery was calculated as illustrated by Figure 4. Platelet counts were performed with a Coulter counter (Model D from Coulter Electronics, Luton, UK).

Electron microscopy was used selectively in this study but not as a method of investigating function. The technique used was previously described [14]. The results were analyzed using Student's t-test.

Results and discussion

Permeability parameters

Permeability parameters deduced from the visual matching of experimental and theoretical curves are shown in Table 1. The data obtained for glycerol are in good agreement with those obtained by W.J. Armitage [19,24]. PG appears to be 110 fold more permeable at room temperature than glycerol. The reflexion coefficient is a representation of the semi permeability of the membrane for a specific solute [25]. The difference found between PG (0.4) and glycerol (0.9), although the molecules of PG and glycerol are of comparable size (radius=2.7Å) [31], suggests that these solutes cross the cell membrane by different mechanisms, or at least, not through the same fixed pores [32]. Using these coefficients protocols were designed, such that the step changes in CPA concentration allowed the platelets to contract and to expand within acceptable limits. The addition steps for PG at room temperature proved very convenient, and 2.5 mol/l PG could be reached in 3 steps of 15 seconds each (Table 2). Similarly, in the dilution protocol PG concentration could be reduced from 2.5 mol/l to 0.6 mol/l in 7 steps of 30 seconds each (Table 3).

Toxicity of PG

Using the previously described protocol, the effect of several concentrations of PG on platelet function has been ascertained (Fig. 5,6,8). No significant difference in numerical recovery (Fig. 5) was noted when each sample was tested immediately after a brief exposure, but the loss in platelets became significant after contact with 2 mol/l PG for 15 minutes or more. The information obtained from hypotonic stress test is presented in Figure 6. When PG was added to the platelet suspension and immediately diluted, simulating the conditions prior to freezing and after thawing, no differences were apparent with respect to the treated controls. However, the presence of 2.5 mol/l PG for 15 minutes or 2 mol/l for 2 hours did cause significant damage. Since the HST is an indication of membrane integrity [30], these results could be explained by alteration of the structure of the cell membrane.

EM of samples in contact with 2.5 mol/l PG for 10 minutes at 20°C appears similar to the controls: all organelles are present – microtubules, mitochondria and canalicular system (Fig. 7). However some cells had lost their discoid shape, and the canalicular system was highly developed, possibly because the platelets had been stored for 14 hours before being used. Treated and washed platelets responded very poorly to aggregation induced by ADP (Fig. 8). This is also ascribed to the time of storage, because controls aggregated poorly. Nevertheless, better aggregation was seen after the brief exposure of platelets to PG (time=0 on Fig. 8). Undeutsh et al [33] studied the effect of glycerol on platelet metabolism and reported an inhibitory action of glycerol on aggregation. They found it difficult to resuspend platelets after hard centrifugation, which caused a significant amount of aggregation. However, since their methods are different, it is difficult to compare this findings with our results. From our unpublished observations, aggregation appears to be

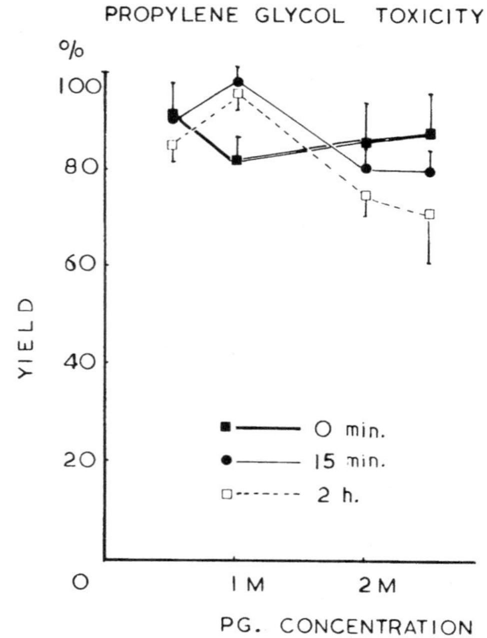

Figure 5. Numerical recovery of platelets after exposure to various concentrations of PG for 0, 15 min or 2 hours. N=5; error bars=SEM.

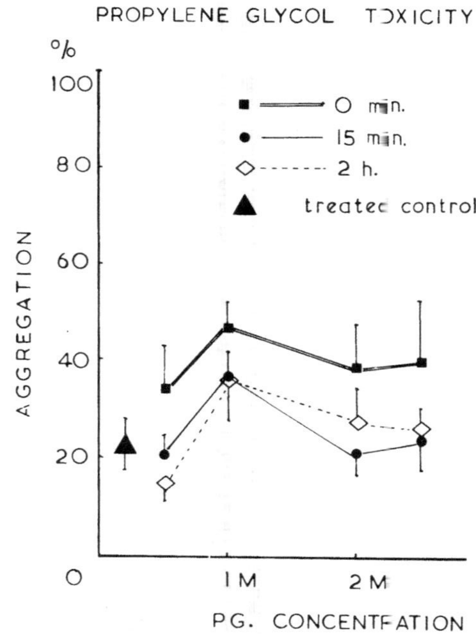

Figure 6. Recovery measured by the hypotonic stress test. Platelets were exposed to 0-2.5 mol/l PG for 0, 15 min or 2 hours. N=5; error bars=SEM.

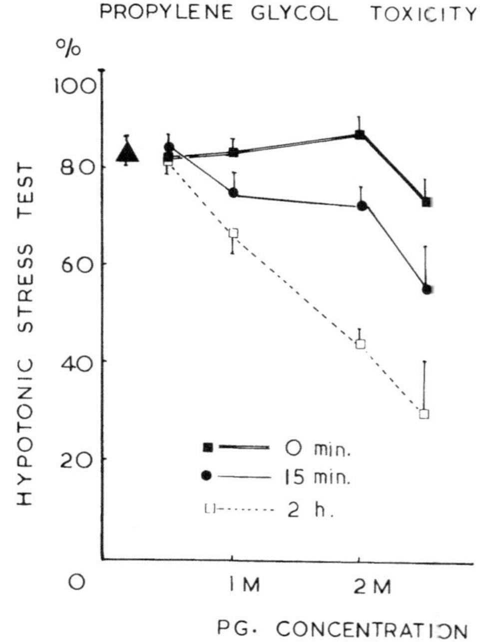

Figure 8. Recovery measured by aggregation. Platelets were exposed to PG (0-2.5 mol/l) for 0, 15 min or 2 hours. N=5; error bars=SEM.

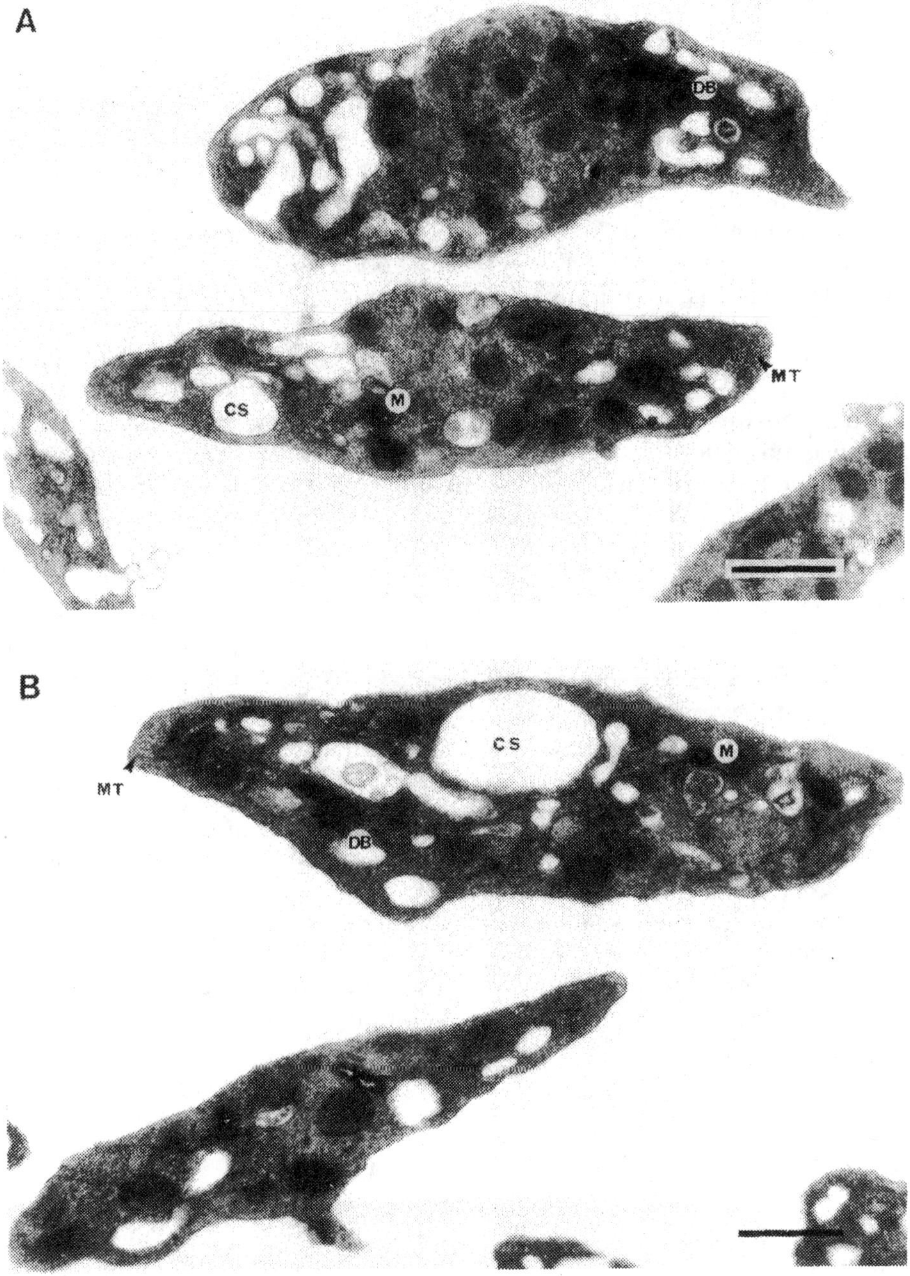

Figure 7. EM of platelets after 10 minutes in the presence of 2.5 mol/l PG at 20°C. The control (A) is a fresh platelet concentrate which underwent addition of PBS and subsequent dilution with PPP. Treated samples (B) appear similar to the control. Microtubule (MT), mitochodria (M), canalicular system (CS), dense bodies (DB) are present in both cells. Magnification (_____ scale = 0.5 μm).

stimulated by PG, and resuspension was easier after centrifugation and no aggregates were seen. It seems probable therefore, that PG affects platelet metabolism by a different mechanism than glycerol, but we have no evidence on this point.

Kim and Baldini [34] studied the effect of glycerol on platelets. They [34] and other authors [15] indicated that a gradual addition and removal of CPAs was beneficial for the function of platelets. It appears that glycerol and PG were of similar toxicity for platelets when low concentrations were used. They reported an HST response of 88% in 0.5% glycerol [34] and we obtained 82% in 0.5 mol/l PG. At 20°C glycerol requires 10 to 15 minutes to permeate the cell membrane [34,15, unpublished observations], and consequently glycerol, when it is used in high concentrations, exerts its toxicity during the incubation period. This would not happen with PG since its permeation is very rapid and virtually no incubation is necessary. This makes PG a solute safer at high concentration.

If platelets were tested within 15 minutes of the addition of PG (2.5 mol/l), there was no major decrease in viability. This suggests that platelet volume did respond in accordance with the model, but it should be stressed that it is not entirely proven that osmotic damage does not occur since we have not measured the relevant permeability coefficients at high concentrations of PG. Presumably the subsequent drop in viability was the result of toxicity of PG. Whatever the mechanism, it is shown that PG exerts its effects on platelets in a time-dependent manner, and consequently the quicker the cells are handled the higher the survival will be.

Conclusion

The results of the HST are sufficient proof that PG can be safely added at RT up to 2.5 mol/l, and we suggest that freezing should then be performed within 15 minutes. It would have been interesting to increase the concentration of PG to still higher levels where vitrification might conceivably happen, but the addition and dilution of the cryoprotectant will be then a long and tedious process. We therefore propose to start the study of platelet cryopreservation using 2.5 mol/l PG and to carry out the addition and dilution at 20°C.

Appendix

The Boyle van 't Hoff relationship

Platelets placed in solutions of different osmolalities of an impermeant solute such as NaCl are able to swell in hypotonic solutions or shrink in hypertonic solutions, thereby maintaining equality of chemical potential of water across the cell membrane. It is said that platelets behave as osmometers [31]. Consequently, there is a straight line relationship between the reciprocal of osmotic pressure and water volume. This is known as the Boyle van 't Hoff relationship.

The Boyle van 't Hoff equation calculated for platelets by W.J. Armitage [19] was:

$$V/V_0 = 0.87 \times \pi_0/\pi + 0.13 \qquad \text{(I)}$$

V/V_0: relative water volume
π_0/π: relative reciprocal osmolality
The physiological water content V_0 of the platelet occurs at the physiologic osmolality π_0.

The optical density of platelet suspensions of constant concentration is also linearly related to the reciprocal of osmolality; thus the chart of a recording of optical density can be calibrated in terms of cell water volume.

Kedem and Katchalsky equations

After addition of a permeable solute such as PG to a cell suspension, water will first flow out of the cell and then, accordingly to the ability of the solute to penetrate the membrane, the cell will increase in volume due to the penetration of solute and water. Cell volume will return to its initial value if the concentration of impermeant solutes is the same as initially. The shape of the volume curve is governed by the permeability parameters as follows:
Lp = hydraulic conductivity which controls the total volumetric flow.
ω = solute permeability which controls the solute flux through the plasma membrane.
σ = reflextion coefficient, which is an index of the semipermeability of the membrane.

The equations are:

$$Jv = Lp(\Delta P - A\pi_i - \sigma RT\Delta C_s \qquad \text{(II)}$$

$$Js = \omega RT\ \Delta C_s + Jv(1-\sigma)cs \qquad \text{(III)}$$

Jv = total volumetric flux
Js = solute flux
ΔP = hydrostatic pressure difference
$\Delta\pi_i$ = osmotic pressure difference due to impermeable solute
$\sigma RT\Delta C_s$ = osmotic pressure developed by permeable solute
ΔC_s = concentration difference of permeable solute
cs = mean concentration of permeable solute in the membrane.

These equations were solved simultaneously using the Euler method of numerical integration. A series of computerized curves (Fig. 3b) was then obtained by varying the 3 parameters Lp, ω, σ and imposing the following restrictions:

(a) Lp and σ values for glycerol should be similar to the values obtained by W.J. Armitage [19,24].
(b) Lp should be the same value for glycerol and PG.
(c) The surface area will remain constant and is equal to 2.6×10^{-7} cm^2 [19].
(d) The physiologic water volume is 6.6×10^{-12} cm^3 [19].

The experimental and theoretical curves were then visually matched as closely as possible.

Acknowledgements

We appreciate the collaboration of Adrian Hayes in the design and development of the photometric device. We would like to thank the Regional Blood transfusion and Immuno-Haematology Centre, Cambridge, which kindly provided the blood.

References

1. Hervé P, Masse M, Coffe C, Peters A. Cryopreserving HLA-typed platelets obtained on cell separators. Lancet 1977;ii:45.
2. Hester JP, McCredie P, Freireich EJ. Platelet replacement therapy. Prog Clin Biol Res 1978:281.
3. van Imhoff GW, Arnaud F, Postmus PE, Mulder NH, Das PC, Smit Sibinga CTh. Autologous cryopreserved platelets and prophylaxis of bleeding in autologous bone marrow transplantation. Blut 1983;47:203-9.
4. Schiffer CA, Aisner J, Wiernik PH. Frozen autologous platelet transfusion for patients with leukemia. N Engl J Med 1978;299:7-12.
5. Mollison PC. Blood transfusion in clinical medicine. London: Blackwell Scientific Publication 1983:157-90.
6. Dayian G, Rowe AW. Cryopreservation of human platelets for transfusion. A glycerol-glucose, moderate rate cooling procedure. Cryobiology 1976;13:1-8.
7. van Prooijen HC, van Heugten JG, Mommersteed ME, Akkerman JWN. Acquired secretion defect in platelets after cryopreservation in dimethyl sulfoxide. Transfusion 1986;26:358-63.
8. Law P, Meryman HT. Cryopreservation of platelets: current status. Plasm Ther Transfus Technol 1982;3:317-26.
9. Lazarus M, Kanieki-Green E, Warm S, Aikawa M, Herzig H. Therapeutic effectiveness of frozen platelet concentrates for transfusion. Blood 1981;57:243-9.
10. Hervé P, Potron G, Droule C, et al. Human platelets frozen with glycerol in liquid nitrogen. Biological and clinical aspects. Transfusion 1981;21:384-90.
11. Klein E, Toch R, Farber S, Freeman G, Florentino R. Hemostasis in thrombocytopenic bleeding following infusion of stored, frozen platelets. Blood 1956;11: 693-9.
12. Baldini M, Costea N, Dameshek W. The viability of stored human platelets. Blood 1960;16:1669-92.
13. Rowe AW, Lenny LL, Mannoni P. Cryopreservation of red cells and platelets. In: Ashwood-Smith MJ, Farrant J (eds). Low temperature preservation in medicine and biology. Pitman Medical Ltd. 1980:85-120.
14. Armitage WJ, Parman N, Hunt CJ. The effects of osmotic stress on human platelets. J Cell Physiol 1985;123:241-8.
15. Armitage WJ. Osmotic stress as a factor in the detrimental effect of glycerol on human platelets. Cryobiology (in press).
16. Heal JM, Singal S, Sardisco E, Mayer T. Bacterial proliferation in platelet concentrates. Transfusion 1986;26:388-9.
17. Braine HG, Kickler TS. Charache P, et al. Bacterial sepsis secondary to platelet transfusion: an adverse effect of extended storage. Transfusion 1986;26:391-4.
18. Nash T. Chemical constitution and physical properties of compounds able to protect living cells against damage due to freezing and thawing. In: Merymann HT (ed). Cryobiology. New York: Academic Press 1966:179-210.

19. Armitage WJ. Effect of solute concentration on intracellular water volume and hydraulic conductivity of human blood platelets. J Physiol (in press).
20. Boutron P, Arnaud F. Comparison of the cryoprotection of red blood cells by 1,2-propanediol and glycerol. Cryobiology 1984;21:348-58.
21. Renard JP, Bui-Xuan-Nguyen, Garnier V. Two-step freezing of two-cell rabbit embryos after partial dehydration at room temperature. J Reprod Fert 1984;71: 573-80.
22. Halasz NA, Collins GM. Studies in cryoprotection II: Propylene glycol and glycerol. Cryobiology 1984;21:144-7.
23. Boutron P, Kaufmann A. Stability of the amorphous state in the system water-1,2-propanediol. Cryobiology 1979;16:557-68.
24. Armitage WJ. Permeability of human blood platelets to glycerol. J Cell Phys 1986;128:121-6.
25. Dick DAT. Osmotic properties of living cells. Int Rev of Cytology 1959;8: 387-448.
26. Tedeschi H, Harris DL. Some observations on the photometric estimation of mitochondrial volume. Biochimica et Biophysica Acta 1958;28:392-402.
27. Nobel PS. The Boyle-van 't Hoff relation. J Theoret Biol 1969;23:375-9.
28. Kedem O, Katchalsky A. Thermodynamic analysis of permeability of biological membranes to non-electrolytes. Biochimica et Biophysica Acta 1958;27:229-46.
29. Valeri CR, Feingold H, Marchionni LD. The relation between response to hypotonic stress and the ^{51}Cr recovery in vivo of preserved platelets. Transfusion 1974;4:331-7.
30. Armitage WJ, Hunt CJ. The effect of glycerol on aggregation and ultrastructure of human platelets. Cryobiology 1982;19:110-7.
31. Stein WD. The movement of molecules across cell membranes. New York: Academic Press 1967:112.
32. Goldstein DA, Solomon AK. Determination of equivalent pore radius for human red cells by osmotic pressure measurement. J General Physiol 1960;44: 1-17.
33. Undeutsch K, Reuter H, Gross R. Investigation on the preservation of human platelets. I. The effect of glycerol on platelet metabolism and function. Thrombosis Res 1975;6:459-68.
34. Kim BK, Baldini MG. Glycerol stress and platelet integrity. Cryobiology 1986; 23:209-13.

BACTERIAL CONTAMINATION IN PLATELETS STORED AT AMBIENT TEMPERATURE

D.H. Buchholz

For many years blood products were stored at refrigerator temperatures in order to maintain cell quality and to prevent the growth of any bacteria introduced inadvertently into blood during the phlebotomy procedure. With the advent of integrally connected multiple plastic container systems, preparation of components such as plasma, red cells and platelets became feasible on a large scale. Platelet transfusion has played a major role in the supportive treatment of patients with thrombocytopenia and has permitted more aggressive attempts at the control/eradication of malignancy through the use of chemo- and radiotherapy.

In contrast to the 4°C storage conditions which appear optimal for red blood cells, platelets appear to benefit significantly if they are not stored under refrigerated conditions. Ambient temperature storage plus development of highly gas-permeable storage containers have permitted effective transfusion therapy after up to 7 days of 22°C storage. A theoretical risk of room temperature storage is the rapid proliferation of any microorganisms which may have been admitted along with blood at the time of collection. While controversial, several studies have indicated that bacteria can be recovered from room-temperature-stored platelets from one to seven percent of the time. Other studies have suggested that the recovery of bacteria from such platelets represents inadvertant contamination of the sample used for culture rather than true contamination of the platelet product.

Following an increase in reports of clinical/laboratory evidence of bacterial growth in platelets during 7 day storage, the United States Food and Drug Administration recently recommended that the maximum 22°C storage time be reduced from 7 to 5 days. The following historical review of studies dealing with bacterial recovery from platelets may be helpful in evaluating extended storage at ambient temperature conditions.

Murphy and Gardner [1], first demonstrated the beneficial effects of room temperature platelet storage in 1969. As part of their studies they cultured 137 units of platelet concentrate which had been stored for up to three days at 22°C. One-half ml samples of either platelet concentrate (PC) or platelet-rich plasma were inoculated into thioglycollate broth and maintained at 37°C for 72 hours. One non-hemolytic streptococcus was isolated.

The following year Silver et al. [2] studied 40 units of platelet concentrate prepared using ACD-A anticoagulant. A 1 ml sample of donor blood (segment) and a 2 ml sample of platelet-poor plasma from each unit were cultured. The PC had been stored at 30°C without resuspension; 10 different units were cultured in 10 ml of thioglycollate broth after 24, 48, 72 and 96 hours of storage, respectively. No bacterial growth was found.

In 1971 Buchholz et al. [3] reported that administration of platelet concentrate prepared immediately prior to transfusion from platelet-rich plasma stored at room temperature for 48 hours resulted in a shaking chill, hypotension and a fever to 41°C in a 20 year old outpatient with Hodgkins disease. *Enterobacter cloacae* was recovered from the recipient and later from platelet-poor plasma removed from one of the units which comprised the transfusion. Recovery of the recipient following antibiotic therapy was uneventful. Another platelet recipient experienced a shaking chill, fever (40.5°C), severe hypotension, and confusion following a transfusion of platelets stored for 24 hours at 22°C. Antibiotic therapy only slowly resolved symptoms. *E. cloacae* was recovered from the patient and the platelet pooling container.

As part of the evaluation of these patient septicemias, 258 platelet pools representing 2,188 units of platelets were studied. Platelet pooling was performed under laminar air flow hoods. Triplicate 5 ml samples of each pool were inoculated into tryptic soy broth, brain-heart infusion and thioglycollate and incubated at 37°C for 21 days. During the last half of the study, identical cultures were performed at 25°C as well. Fifty-three of 258 pools were found to contain bacteria as defined by recovery of microorganisms from one or more cultures. Diphtheroids and *S. epidermidis* were the organisms most often recovered, however, other bacteria, including Gram-negative organisms such as *E. cloacae* and *Pseudomonas* sp. were also found. Assuming that only one unit per pool was the source of the bacteria recovered, the calculated incidence of contamination was 1.3, 2.8, 3.4 and 4.9% for units stored 0, 1, 2 and 3 days, respectively.

Culture of 75 bags from 10 different lots of blood packs showed all to be sterile. Supplies and arm preparation materials were also unrelated to the contamination. Although pools, rather than individual untis had been cultured, inadvertent contamination at time of pooling and culture was felt unlikely in view of the correlation between bacterial recovery and storage time. Twenty five of the pools from which bacteria were recovered had been transfused, 13 without room temperature storage. All but five of the remainder contained *S. epidermis* or diphtheroids. The other pools contained *S. aureus, Alcaligenes* sp., *Pseudomonas* sp. [2] and *E. cloacae.* Except for the last (see the second case report) the transfusions were not associated with recognized recipient septicemia. Although quantitative cultures were not performed, the authors speculated that in most instances the number of bacteria present after storage at room temperature was small.

Since inadvertent contamination of platelets could not be totally ruled out when units were pooled in the above study, Buchholz et al. [4] subsequently cultured 3,251 individual fresh units of platelet concentrate using samples obtained from segments after thorough mixing with bag contents. Samples from each unit were cultured on blood agar plates at 37°C and 25°C for 96 hours. Units demonstrating bacterial growth by the time needed for transfusion were excluded from use. Pool cultures were also performed using trypticase soy broth, thioglycollate and brain-heart infusion. In addition, duplicate 0.5 ml samples were incubated on blood agar plates at 25°C and 37°C to quantify the degree of contamination in the pool.

Forty-five of 3,251 (1.4%) individual fresh units of platelet concentrate cultured without pooling were found to contain bacteria. Usually only 1-2 colonies were found, suggesting that the number of bacteria present was small. The 1.4% value compared favorably with a calculated estimate of 1.6% contamination (74 of 4,560 units) based upon earlier culture studies of platelet pools. In pool culture studies bacterial recovery again increased with the time of storage prior to pooling (0.9, 2.1, 2.5 and 4.3%, respectively for pools comprised of units stored 0, 1, 2 and 3 days). Semi-quantitative cultures of pools revealed that in the majority of instances the number of bacteria present per ml of platelet concentrate was low. Of 45 positive pools cultured in this manner, 34 contained fewer than 50 organisms per ml, two contained between 50 and 200/ml and five contained organisms too numerous to count. In four instances, the colony count was not recorded. Thus, in most instances, the number of organisms present was small; this likely accounts for the low rate of recognized clinical septicemia. The authors also presented data which suggested that presumed 'skin plugs' induced by needle coring during phlebotomy may have played a role in entry of bacteria into blood collection systems.

Four additional instances of recipient septicemia took place during or following these studies. In each instance, bacteria were recovered from the patient and the platelet pooling bag. The organisms involved included *Flavobacterium* sp., *Serratia* sp. and *S. epidermis*. Patients who were transfused with the first two organisms eventually recovered. A third patient with acute leukemia and profound granulocytopenia developed a shaking chill, fever to 41°C and severe hypotension after being given platelets stored 24 hours. He developed acute tubular necrosis and died 9 days following the transfusion. The remaining patient displayed nearly identical symptoms, also developed acute tubular necrosis and died 12 days following transfusion.

Mallin et al. [5] cultured 110 units of platelets, 42 prepared under closed system conditions and 68 with deliberate aseptic (open) transfer of platelet-rich plasma to and from a transfer pack prior to cell concentration. Triplicate one ml samples of platelet concentrate were removed from each container at 0, 24, 48 and 72 hours of storage and cultured in thioglycollate, tryptic soy broth and brain-heart infusion. In addition, 1-5 ml aliquots removed from platelet-poor plasma on day 0 were cultured in the same three media. Microorganisms were not recovered from any of the 110 units.

In a large study, Cunningham and Cash [6] cultured one thousand individual units of platelet concentrate following up to 3 day storage at 20°C. Aliquots (1 ml each) were inoculated into cooked meat medium and cultured at 37°C and 20°C for 48 hours. Each was then subcultured on nutrient agar plates maintained anaerobically and aerobically at either 37°C or 20°C (depending upon the original culture temperature) for 48 hours.

Sixty-three of 1000 units (6.3%) were found to contain bacteria. *S. albus (S. epidermidis)* was recovered 52 times, coliforms 6 times, *Cl. welchii* 3 times, and *S. aureus* and *Micrococcus* sp. once each. Plate count studies indicated that in 78% of instances, the number of bacteria present was less than 10/ml, although as many as 585 organisms/ml were recovered from one unit. Culture of 100 units of platelets prepared in platelet packs obtained from a different manufacturer showed a bacterial contamination rate of 6%. In this study, there was no statistically significant correlation between length of storage time prior to culture and percent contamination.

Goddard et al. [7] prepared platelet concentrates with a long length of tubing left attached to the bag to permit respresentative sampling of bag contents without direct entry. After mixing with bag contents, segments (0.6 ml sample size) were obtained from 350 consecutive bags of fresh concentrate and incubated for 18 hours at 4°C, 22°C and 37°C. The contents of each segment were then Gram-stained and cultured overnight at 37°C on blood agar plates. All samples from segments maintained at 4°C and 22°C were sterile. A coagulase negative *Staphylococcus* sp. was recovered from one of the 37°C segments which had been defectively sealed.

Additional studies were performed to qualitatively assess growth of various organisms in platelet concentrate maintained at 4°C, 22°C and 37°C. Small inocula (2-14 organisms) of coagulase-positive and -negative staphylococci, *Ps. pyocyanea, E. coli* and an unidentified spore-forming bacillus were introduced to 2 ml samples of platelet concentrate. After 18 hours of incubation, no growth was seen in any sample maintained at 4°C and heavy growth was seen in all samples maintained at 37°C except those containing the bacillus. In the 22°C group, only *Ps. pyocyanea* showed significant growth by 18 hours. In addition to the above studies, 2,511 segments from fresh units of PC were incubated overnight and Gram-stained. Microorganisms were seen upon microscopic examination in a single instance.

Rhame et al. [8] reported seven cases of *Salmonella cholerae-suis* septicemia that occurred in immunocompromised patients during a 7 month period. One patient died and two had long-term disease recurrences. Epidemiologic data implicated platelet transfusion as the means of bacterial dissemination. The organism was traced to an asymptomatic platelet donor with chronic *Salmonella* osteomyelitis of the tibia. The organism was subsequently isolated from the donor's plasma on three separate occasions. Platelet concentrates had been prepared from platelet-rich plasma maintained at ambient temperature and transfused within 10 hours of collection.

Four hundred units of platelet concentrate were cultured by Wrenn and Speicher [9] following 72-96 hour ambient temperature storage. Triplicate 1 ml samples were injected into 10 ml of thioglycollate broth and incubated at 4°C, 24°C and 37°C, respectively. Four of 1,200 cultures were found to contain bacteria (2 *Corynebacterium* sp. and 2 coagulase-negative staphylococci). In each instance organisms were recovered from only 1 of the 3 triplicate cultures and growth was attributed to accidental contamination during culturing.

Myhre et al. [10] cultured two hundred units of platelet concentrate and reported all to be sterile. Units of concentrate were then deliberately inoculated with variable numbers of *S. epidermidis, S. aureus*, or *Ps. aeruginosa*. Samples were obtained at 0, 4, 12, 24, 30, 38 and 48 hours for culture on blood agar. When fewer than 10^3 *S. epidermidis* or *Ps. aeruginosa* organisms were introduced, no growth of microorganisms was seen. With introduction of 10^4 to 10^6 bacteria, growth was suppressed for 24 hours after which it slowly increased. Progressive growth occurred with inoculation of 10^7 organisms. In contrast, when concentrates were contaminated with *S. aureus*, progressive growth was noted, irrespective of inoculum size.

Studies were also performed to evaluate the role of skin contamination as a mechanism for bacterial entry. After phlebotomy site preparation with green soap, 70% of alcohol and 3% aqueous iodine followed by 70% alcohol, 7 ml of blood was drawn into sterile tubes containing 1 ml of ACD. Approximately 0.5 ml aliquots were dispersed to 16-20 blood agar plates which were incubated at 32°C for 24 hours. Blood obtained from 10 phlebotomies was studied. Bacteria were recovered from all ten and ranged in number from 1 to >200 colonies per 7 ml blood sample.

Kahn and Syring [11] also deliberately inoculated units of whole blood with known numbers of selected bacteria (*E. coli, S. epidermidis, E. cloacae, Ps. aeruginosa*) prior to component preparation. Platelet concentrates were then stored for three days at room temperature or 4°C and samples were removed at 24 hour intervals. During room temperature storage, *E. coli* and *E. cloacae* (initial average numbers of 3 and 11 organisms/ml in Pc, respectively) grew rapidly (>300/ml by 24 hours). *S. epidermidis* grew only slowly during the first 24 hours but then underwent significant proliferation (>300/ml by 48 hours). *Ps. aeruginosa* did not multiply. None of the four organisms increased in numbers during 4°C platelet storage; however, bacteria were *recovered* from all units kept at 4°C.

Blajchman et al. [12] reported three episodes of *Serratia marcescens* sepsis in 1979, one of which resulted in death. A fourth unit of platelet concentrate contaminated with the same organism was detected prior to transfusion. Platelets had been stored at 22°C for up to 72 hours. Sixty units of PC stored up to 72 hours were cultured. One ml samples were divided and cultured on blood agar plates, MacConkey agar and in Robertson's cooked meat medium (48 hours at 35°C). Thirty-two plastic packs (10 ml of thioglycollate/bag) and 550 EDTA vacuum tubes (3 ml blood culture broth/tube) were also cultured. No growth was seen in platelets or blood packs. *Serratia marcescens* was isolated from 14 of 550 vacuum tubes. Simulated blood collection procedures in which EDTA tubes were filled via the phlebotomy needle showed recovery of *Serratia marcescens* in 5 of 6 instances. Contaminated vacuum tubes were felt to be the most likely source of product contamination.

Hogge et al. [13] noted a patient who developed a shaking chill and fever following platelet transfusion which rapidly resolved without therapy. A Gram-positive bacillus was recovered from a culture of the pooled platelets. Culture studies were performed during the course of evaluation of a new polyvinyl chloride 7-day platelet container. One hundred ninety-four units of platelets stored 3 days in standard plastic containers were compared with 195 units collected in 7-day containers. Cultures were performed after units were pooled following 3 or 7 days of storage. Bacteria were recovered from 4 of 39 cultures (3 from 3-day and 1 from 7-day bags). Recovered organisms included *Micrococcus* sp., *Klebsiella pneumonia, Bacillus brevis*, an unidentified Gram-negative rod and a Gram-positive bacillus. Where quantified, the number of organisms recovered was small.

Four cases of transfusion-associated sepsis were reported by Braine et al. [14] in 1986. Platelets, prepared in containers from two different manufactures had been stored at room temperature; at least one unit in each pool had been stored for five or more days. Reactions consisted of chills, fever and hypotension in one patient, chills alone in a second and chills and fever in the remaining two. Three of the four were receiving concurrent antibiotic therapy at the time of the contaminated platelet transfusion. *Staphylococcus epidermidis* was recovered singly in two instances and with *Flavobacterium* sp. in another. The fourth reaction was caused by *Streptococcus viridans*.

Culture studies in platelet concentrates were performed using two examples of *S. epidermidis*, one of *S. aureus* and one of *Corynebacterium* JK group. Each unit was cultured on day zero (immediately after inoculation) and following 7 days of storage at 24°C. Introduction of one *S. epidermidis* organism/unit resulted in a 24-48 hour lag growth phase followed by log-phase growth in three of four units. Inoculation of 7 and 55 organisms resulted in growth in all containers. By 6 days, bags contained from 10^8 to 10^9 organisms per ml. Similar results were seen with *S. aureus* and a second example of *S. epidermidis*. Relatively poor growth was seen in samples inoculated with *Corynebacterium* sp.

Salmonella heidelberg sepsis was reported by Heal et al. [14] following transfusion of 7 units of platelets stored for five days. The organism was recovered from the recipient as well as the platelet container. The transfusion was associated with chills, fever (40.6°C), hives and severe hypotension. Development of shock-induced renal and hepatic failure lead to death six days later. The same organism was recovered from stool culture of one of the platelet donors.

These investigators also studied the rate of bacterial growth in platelet products by directly inoculating 10^1, 10^2, 10^3, 10^4 or 10^5 organisms in the log phase of growth into 50 ml units of platelet concentrate [15]. Cells were maintained at 24°C on a mechanical rotator for 7 days with daily removal of samples for bacterial quantification. When 1000 or more organisms were introduced per unit, 88% (7 of 8) supported bacterial growth. When the inoculum size was 100 organisms or less, 50% of cultures (5 of 10) were sterile by 24 hours and remained so for 7 days. Twenty percent showed logarithmic growth while in the remainder growth was temporarily suppressed for 5-6 days. The authors concluded that bacterial contamination which was not clinically significant following 3 days of storage could become so during 7 days of storage.

Arnow et al. [17] described a transfusion of 12 units of platelet concentrate which resulted in nausea, vomiting, chills, tachypnea and shock. *E. coli* was recovered from the patient as well as a container used for platelet pooling. *E. coli* was also recovered from a unit of red cells corresponding to one of the units of platelet concentrate implicated in the transfusion. The platelets had been stored 3 days at 22°C.

Culture of 500 arbitrarily selected units of concentrate was performed over an 18 month period. One ml aliquots were aspirated aseptically from indiidual units and cultured on sheep blood-Columbia agar plates (36°C for 72 hours). Thirty-five of 500 units (7%) were found to contain bacteria. Nearly all isolates were common skin bacteria (coagulase-negative staphylococci, *Corynebacterium* sp.); however, in two instances *S. aureus* was recovered and in another *Enterobacter aerogenes* was found. All but one of the contaminated units contained fewer than 20 colony-forming units per ml. The remaining unit contained $\cong$1000 viable microorganisms/ml. Bacterial recovery appeared to increase in proportion to the length of time platelets were stored (Table 1).

The authors concluded that the bacterial presence was of relatively little clinical significance due to the fact that

(1) the level of contamination was low; and
(2) most of the organisms were Gram-positive skin flora, bacteria not usually considered pathogenic.

Table 1. Recovery of bacteria from platelet concentrates stored on to five days at 22°C.

Storage time (days)	**No. cultured**	**No. (%) contaminated**
1	33	0 (0)
2	55	3 (5.5)
3	87	5 (6.9)
4	145	11 (7.6)
5	180	15 (8.3)

The above studies suggest that bacteria can be recovered from one to seven percent of platelet units when large scale culture studies are performed. The studies remain controversial in that episodes of clinical sepsis are far less common than would be expected based upon culture data. There may be several reasons for this. In the first place the inoculum size appears to be small in most instances. A likely mechanism for bacterial entry would appear to be the phlebotomy procedure. The care with which the intended site of phlebotomy is cleansed is of obvious importance as is the avoidance of the temptation to repalpate the cleansed area immediately prior to venipuncture. Less well appreciated is the possibility that bacterial resident in sweat and sebaceous gland pores may not come in contact with solutions used to cleanse the skin surface but may in fact be transferred to the blood collection container as the venipuncture is performed. The studies of Buchholz et al. [4] and Myhre et al. [10] suggest that bacteria are present in initial volumes of blood obtained just after venipuncture. The fact that skin organisms such as *S. epidermidis* and diphtheroids were the predominant organisms recovered in a number of studies further suggests this possibility.

Skin bacteria such as *S. epidermidis* are generally not regarded as pathogens although this may not be the case if patients have been severely compromised by the effects of aggressive cancer chemotherapy. Infusion of platelets containing 'nonpathogens' may result only transient chills and fever, often ascribed to platelet or leukocyte alloimmunization of the recipient. Thus, a number of platelet-induced septicemias may not be recognized unless bacterial cultures of recipient and platelet containers are performed. Other organisms, considered pathogenic, may not multiply to numbers sufficient to cause severe problems in the recipient. Proliferation is likely related to the type of organism, the time and temperature of platelet storage and certain donor-specific factors such as opsonins, bacterial species-specific antibodies and residual monocytes/granulocytes which are present in platelet concentrates, residual monocytes may play a significant but unappreciated role in controlling bacterial proliferation during ambient temperature storage. Heal et al. [16] clearly demonstrated 'donor specific' factors in her studies of deliberate inoculation of known numbers of bacteria. When the same strain of organisms was added (≅100/container) to platelets prepared from 10 different donors, in two instances there was immediate logarithmic growth, in three there was a 5-6 day delay in growth and the remainder became sterile by 24 hours. Thus donor to donor differences may play important roles in regulating bacterial proliferation.

In closing, bacterial contamination of platelets does occur and likely occurs at greater frequency than is clinically appreciated. In most instances the initial inoculum size is small, the organisms are 'nonpathogenic' skin bacteria which frequently do not proliferate extensively. The presence of variable numbers of phagocytic cells as well as host-specific opsonins/antibodies further act to prevent or inhibit bacterial multiplication in many instances. That proliferation does occasionally occur suggests that a review of skin-cleansing and phlebotomy procedures should be a regular part of blood bank quality control programmes. In addition, since bacterial proliferation is time dependent, recipient risk can be further reduced by minimizing room temperature and the time of platelet storage prior to transfusion.

References

1. Murphy S, Gardner FH. Platelet preservation: effect of storage temperature on maintenance of platelet viability – deleterious effect of refrigerated storage. N Engl J Med 1969;280:1094-8.
2. Silver H, Sonnenwirth AC, Beisser LD. Bacteriologic study of platelet concentrates prepared and stored without refrigeration. Transfusion 1970;10:315-6.
3. Buchholz DH, Young VM, Friedman NR, Reilly JA, Mardiney MR. Bacterial proliferation in platelet products stored at room temperature. Transfusion-induced enterobacter sepsis. N Engl J Med 1971;285:429-33.
4. Buchholz DH, Young VM, Friedman NR, Reilly JA, Mardiney MR. Detection and quantitation of bacteria in platelet products stored at ambient temperature. Transfusion 1973;13:268-75.
5. Mallin WS, Reuss DT, Brack JW, Roberts SC, Moore GL. Bacteriological study of platelet concentrates stored at 22°C and 4°C. Transfusion 1973;13:439-42.
6. Cunningham M, Cash JD. Bacterial contamination of platelet concentrates stored at 20°C. J Clin Path 1973;26:401-4.
7. Goddard D, Jacobs SI, Manohitharajah. The bacterial screening of platelet concentrates stored at 22°C. Transfusion 1973;13:103-6.
8. Rahme FS, Root RK, MacLowry JD, Dadisman TA, Bennett JV. Salmonella septicemia from platelet transfusions. Study of an outbreak traced to a hematogenous carrier of *Salmonella cholerae-suis*. Ann Intern Med 1973;78:633-41.
9. Wrenn HE, Speicher CE. Platelet concentrates: sterility of 400 single units stored at room temperature. Transfusion 1974;14:171-2.
10. Myhre BA, Walker LJ, White ML. Bacteriocidal properties of platelet concentrates. Transfusion 1974;14:116-23.

11. Kahn RA, Syring RL. The fate of bacteria introduced into whole blood from which platelet concentrates were prepared and stored at 22 or 4°C. Transfusion 1975;15:363-7.
12. Blajchman MA, Thornely JH, Richardson H, Elder D, Spiak C, Racher J. Platelet transfusion-induced *Serratia marcescens* sepsis due to vacuum tube contamination. Transfusion 1979;19:39-44.
13. Hogge DE, Thompson BW, Schiffer CA. Platelet storage for 7 days in second-generation blood bags. Transfusion 1986;26:131-5.
14. Braine HG, Kickler TS, Charache P, et al. Bacterial sepsis secondary to platelet transfusion: an adverse effect of extended storage at room temperature. Transfusion 1986;26:391-3.
15. Heal JM, Forey J, Shadry N. Fatal Salmonella septicemia following platelet transfusion. Transfusion 1984;24(abstract):433.
16. Heal JM, Singal S, Sardisco E, Mayer T. Bacterial proliferation in platelet concentrates. Transfusion 1986;26:388-90.
17. Arnow PM, Weiss LM, Weil D, Rosen NR. *Escherichia coli* sepsis from contaminated platelet transfusion. Arch Intern Med 1986;146:321-4.

PREPARATION OF LEUKOCYTE-POOR BLOOD

B. Brozovic

When transfused, HLA antigens, expressed on granulocytes and lymphocytes, are capable of stimulating the production of HLA alloantibodies in the recipient. These antibodies are responsible for two distinct clinical syndromes: non-hemolytic febrile transfusion reaction (NHFTR), seen in patients receiving multiple blood transfusions, and refractoriness platelet, seen in patients on long-term platelet support.

It has been known that, in those patients in whom antibodies can be detected, NHFTR can be prevented or its severity ameliorated by the transfusion of blood that has been depleted of leukocytes [1-4]. Also, it has been shown that transfusion of leukocyte depleted blood in patients receiving long-term platelet support delays the onset of platelet refractoriness and reduces its overall incidence [5-6]. Therefore, the indications for use of leukocyte depleted blood now include not only prevention of NHFTR but also prevention or immunization to HLA antigens in patients receiving multiple transfusions and in patients on long-term platelet support. Whether other undesirable effects of leukocytes on the recipient, such as immunosuppression in a patient with a malignant disease, can also be prevented by transfusion of leukocyte depleted blood still remains to be elucidated. The aim of this paper is, first, to present an outline of available methods for leukocyte depletion of blood (for details see reviews [7,8]) secondly, to highlight recent developments in this field.

A number of techniques can be used alone or in combination to deplete a unit of blood of leukocytes (and platelets, and sometimes plasma). They are based on one of the following principles.

(i) Separation of red cells and leukocytes by centrifugation. Centrifugation of blood packs and subsequent removal of the buffy coat is technically straightforward. Packs can be centrifuged in an upright position and the plasma and buffy coat expressed manually, or in an inverted position and the red cells removed by draining into a transfer pack. Satisfactory results have been achieved using these techniques (Table 1). Addition of saline to the red cells enables the procedure to be repeated several times, improving leukocyte depletion with the highest reported mean value of 93% [9,10]. Platelet depletion of approximately 90% and a considerable loss of plasma proteins is usual with centrifugation alone or combined with saline washing.

Washing of red cells is carried out much more easily using one of the several commercially available blood cell processors. Results obtained using the system with continuous washing in a bowl and fixed speed centrifugation (Haemonetics Models 15, 102 and 115, and Elutramatic) have been on the

Table 1. Comparison of methods for leukocyte depletion of blood.[1]

Method	Leukocyte depletion[2] (%)	Platelet depletion[2] (%)	Red cell loss[2] (%)	Cost	Comments
Centrifugation and buffy coat removal	65-88	87-90	12-42	Cheap	
Centrifugation and manual washing	up to 93	about 90	20	Cheap	Tedious
Washing with blood cell processor	up to 90	over 90	11-25	Moderately expensive	Red cell loss may reach 40%
Sedimentation of red cells	82-95	over 90	3-9	Cheap	Time-consuming
Freezing and thawing of red cells					
3.8M glycerol	over 98	98	10-22	Expensive	
6.2M and 8.6M glycerol				Moderately expensive	
Filtration					
Imugard IG-500	98	68			Filtration time about 30 minutes
Erypur	98	81	≤10	Moderately expensive	
Cell Select	99	87			
Sepacell R-500	99	83			Filtration time less than 10 min
Microaggregate filter					
Ultipor SQ 40S[3]:					
Alone	15	15	about 5		
Following centrifugation of blood	47	45	about 8		
Following centrifugation and cooling of blood	85		about 8	Cheap	May be labour intensive
Following centrifugation, cooling of blood and exclusion of buffy coat	95		20		

1. Compiled from Hughes and Brozovic [7], Meryman and Hornblower [8] and Polesky et al. [9].
2. Range of mean values reported.
3. Quoted from Mijovic et al. [30] and Parravicini et al. [31].

whole disappointing producing about 60% leukocyte depletion, although they can be improved when blood is centrifuged and buffy coat removed prior to washing [10,11]. The variable speed centrifugation (Dideco Progress 90 Cell Separator) can produce leukocyte depletion greater than 80% [11,12]. Serial centrifugation using the COBE (IBM) 2991 Blood Cell Processor can produce depletion of 90% or better, though red cell losses have varied from 11% to 25% and may be even as high as 40% [10,11,13-15]. The COBE 2991 Blood Cell Processor probably produces the best and the most consistent results and has the added advantage of a fully automated operation. Both manual and machine red cell washing techniques remove more than 90% of platelets and almost all the plasma. In general, centrifugation and saline washing of red cells is inexpensive, while washing with blood cell processors is moderately expensive and can be time-consuming.

(ii) Sedimentation of red cells with high molecular weight polymers such as dextran, gelatin (Plasmagel) and hydroxyethyl starch (HES) have been used to provide better separation between red cells and leukocytes [9,16,17]. Using sedimentation excellent leukocyte and platelet depletion can be achieved (Table 1). Though no special equipment is required the technique can be time-consuming particularly if saline washing is included to remove the sedimenting agent prior to transfusion. In practice, however, this may not be necessary as the incidence of allergic reaction to dextran is exceptionally rare, the rate of accumulation of HES is negligible, and the volume of sedimenting agent administered with blood too small to interfere with coagulation [7].

(iii) Freezing and thawing produces units of red cells almost entirely depleted of leukocytes. The cryopreservative, glycerol, can be used at the concentration of 3.8 M with a rapid rate of freezing of the red cells and storage in liquid nitrogen [18] or at higher concentrations of 6.2 M [19] and 8.6 M [20] with a slow rate of freezing and storage at $-85°C$ in mechanical freezers. With both protocols thawing is rapid and it is followed by extensive washing of red cells with electrolyte solutions in a cell washer. During washing more than 95% of leukocytes (Table 1), and most of the platelets and plasma are removed [9,19,21, Johnson, personal communication]. Red cell losses are usually less than 10%. In contrast to high capital and revenue costs required for freezing and storage of frozen red cells with liquid nitrogen the recently reported method by Valeri et al. [22] for freezing red cells in the primary collection pack employing high glycerol concentration and mechanical freezers is much cheaper and is likely to be widely used. It is of interest that addition of glycerol to the red cells and subsequent washing without freezing is sufficient to remove 98% of both lymphocytes and platelets [23].

(iv) Filtration of blood to achieve leukocyte depletion has been known since 1962 when Greenwalt et al. [24] described the removal of granulocytes from blood passed through the nylon fiber filter. Since then several types of 'specific' leukocyte depleting filters have become commercially available. Nylon fiber filters (Leuko-Pak, Travenol Laboratories) have been superceded by filters made of tightly packed fibres of combed cotton (Imugard IG-500,

Terumo Corporation), cellulose-acetate (Erypur, Organon-Teknika Ltd. and Cellselect, NPBI) or polyester sheets (Sepacell R-500, Asahi Medical Corporation Ltd.). Their mode of action is not quite clear as the fibers retain not only the adhering granulocytes but also non-functional granulocytes, lymphocytes, monocytes and platelets. Cotton wool and cellulose-acetate filters are capable of removing on average 98% of the leukocyte (Table 1) and about 75% of the platelets [25-28]. Red cell losses caused by filtration with 'specific' leukocyte depleting filters are on average 10%. Plasma is not removed unless centrifugation and plasma removal is carried out before and after filtration. Filtration is a simple but moderately expensive procedure, which can be usually completed in less than half an hour. Cellselect and Sepacell are also available as 'in line' filters for bed-side use. Their performance has not been affected by the slow flow of blood (personal observation), and furthermore they can be used for filtering two units of blood.

Recently Wenz et al. [29] have drawn attention to the fact that microaggregate filters, in widespread use for the prevention of pulmonary microemboli due to microaggregates present in stored whole blood, can also deplete blood of leukocytes. Several types of microaggregate filters are commercially available with pore size between 20 and 40 μm, all of which have a similar capacity to reduce leukocyte numbers in stored blood regardless of whether they are of a screen or depth type. The leukocyte depletion achieved with microaggregate filters is on average 40% (Table 1), and can be increased to approximately 55% by centrifugation of blood prior to filtration [29,30]. Depletion of platelets is also about 40%, and red cell losses are negligible. This has been further improved using Ultipor SQ 40S (Pall) filter, firstly, by keeping the units of blood for 3 hours at 4°C following centrifugation, and secondly, by excluding the buffy coat from filtration [31]. These procedures enabled the removal of 93% of the units' leukocytes. In spite of relatively poor leukocyte depletion, Wenz et al. [29] have previously found that filtration of stored blood has caused a 95% reduction in the incidence of febrile reactions among 45 previously sensitized patients. The clinical effectiveness of these filters appears to be due to the fact that the microaggregates removed are largely composed of granulocytes which are the most immunogenic cells involved in the causation of NHFTR.

Combined techniques, for example centrifugation and saline washing prior to filtration of blood or prior to freezing and thawing of red cells, can be used with the aim of increasing the degree of leukocyte depletion. Although the leukocyte depletion is slightly improved by this approach the benefit is outweighed by the greater red cell loss, which can be as high as 40%, the increased complexity of preparation with the possibility of bacterial contamination, and the increased cost.

Although the leukocytes in platelet concentrates are present only in small numbers they may still be capable of immunizing the recipient on long-term platelet support against HLA antigens [32]. Platelet concentrates collected from multiple donors as well as those obtained by a cell separator can be leukocyte depleted by one of the following methods: (i) Platelet concentrates can be pooled in a specially designed transfer pack with a pouch at the bottom, Leukotrap (Cutter Biological), and centrifuged. Leukocytes and

red cells are trapped in the pouch and remain separated from the platelets.
(ii) Platelet concentrates can be filtered using Imugard filter, the procedure which will remove all the leukocytes, at the cost of an average platelet loss of 10% [33].
(iii) Freezing and thawing of platelet concentrates renders them free of leukocytes (Johnson, personal communication). However, the platelet loss, on average 24%, is too high to recommend the procedure for routine use.

In conclusion, the available techniques for leukocyte depletion are capable of removing most of the leukocytes present in the unit of blood. It seems, however, that no procedure can render blood completely non-immunogenic as even transfusions of frozen and thawed red cells have led to the formation of granulocyte and platelet specific antibodies and to HLA antibodies [34].

Acknowledgements

It is a pleasure to acknowledge help and advice received from Miss Jane Johnson and Dr. Valerie Mijovic. It is also a pleasure to thank Mrs Margeret Evans for secretarial help.

References

1. Brittingham TE, Chaplin H. Febrile transfusion reactions caused by sensitivity to donor leukocytes and platelets. JAMA 1957;165:819-25.
2. Payne R. The association of febrile transfusion reactions with leuko-agglutinins. Vox Sang 1957;2:233-41.
3. Perkins HA, Payne R, Ferguson J, Wood M. Nonhemolytic febrile transfusion reactions. Quantitative effects of blood components with emphasis on isoantigenic incompatibility of leukocytes. Vox Sang 1966;11:578-600.
4. Sirchia G, Rebulla P, Mascaretti L, Greppi N, Rivolta S, Parravicini A. The clinical importance of leukocyte depletion in regular erythrocyte transfusions. Vox Sang 1986;51(suppl.):2-8.
5. Eernisse JG, Brand A. Prevention of platelet refractoriness due to HLA antibodies by administration of leukocyte-poor blood components. Exp Hematol 1981;9:77-83.
6. Murphy MF, Metcalfe P, Thomas H, et al. Use of leukocyte-poor blood components and HLA-matched platelet donors to prevent HLA alloimmunisation. Brit J Haemat 1986;62:529-34.
7. Hughes ASB, Brozovic B. Leukocyte depleted blood: an appraisal of available techniques (Annotation). Brit J Haemat 1982;50:381-6.
8. Meryman HT, Hornblower M. The preparation of red cells depleted of leukocytes. Review and evaluation. Transfusion 1986;26:101-6.
9. Polesky JF, McCullough J, Helgeson MA, Nelson C. Evaluation of methods for the preparation of HLA antigen poor blood. Transfusion 1973;13:383-7.
10. Meryman HT, Bross J, Lebovitz R. The preparation of leukocyte-poor red blood cells: a comparative study. Transfusion 1980;20:285-92.
11. Hughes A, Mijovic V, Brozovic B, Davies TD. Leukocyte depleted blood: a comparison of cell washing techniques. Vox Sang 1982;42:145-50.

12. Reverberi R, Fabbri L. A modified procedure for washing liquid stored packed red cells in a continuous flow centrifuge. Riv Emoterapia ed Immunoemat 1979; 26:23.
13. Bryant LR, Holland I, Corkern S. Optimal leukocyte removal from refrigerated blood with the IBM 2991 Blood Cell Processor. Transfusion 1978;18:469-71.
14. Buchholz DH, Charette JR, Bove JR. Preparation of leukocyte-poor red blood cells using the IBM 2991 Blood Cell Processor. Transfusion 1978;18:653-62.
15. O'Connor Wotton MJ. Use and analysis of saline washed red blood cells. Transfusion 1976;16:464-8.
16. Chaplin H, Brittingham TE, Cassell M. Methods for preparation of suspensions of buffy-coat-poor red blood cells for transfusion. Amer J Clin Path 1959;31: 373-83.
17. Dorner I, Moore JA, Collins JA, Sherman LA, Chaplin H. Efficacy of leukocyte-poor red blood cell suspensions prepared by sedimentation in hydroxyethyl starch. Transfusion 1975;15:439-48.
18. Rowe AW, Eyster E, Kellner A. Liquid nitrogen preservation of red blood cells for transfusion: a low glycerol-rapid freeze procedure. Cryobiology 1968;5:119-28.
19. Meryman HT, Hornblower M. A method for freezing and washing red blood cells using a high glycerol concentration. Transfusion 1972;12:145-56.
20. Huggins CE. Frozen blood: principles of practical preservation. Monographs in the Surgical Sciences 1966;3:133-73.
21. Amer KA, Pepper DS, Urbaniak SJ. Lymphocyte, granulocyte and platelet contamination of blood frozen by the low glycerol liquid nitrogen technique. Brit J Haemat 1980;44:253-61.
22. Valeri CR, Valeri DA, Anastasi J, Vecchione JJ, Dennis RC, Emerson CP. Freezing in the primary polyvinylchloride plastic collection bag: a new system for preparing and freezing nonrejuvenated and rejuvenated red blood cells. Transfusion 1981;21:138-49.
23. Kurtz SR, Valeri DA, Melaragno EJ, et al. Leukocyte-poor red blood cells prepared by the addition and removal of glycerol from red blood cell concentrates stored at 4°C. Transfusion 1981;21:435-42.
24. Greenwalt TJ, Gajewski M, McKenna JL. A new method for preparing buffy coat-poor blood. Transfusion 1961;12:23-6.
25. Diepenhorst P, Sprokholt R, Prins HK. Removal of leukocytes from whole blood and erythrocyte suspensions by filtration through cotton wool. Vox Sang 1972; 23:308-20.
26. Kikugawa K, Minoshima K. Filter columns for preparation of leukocyte-poor blood for transfusion. Vox Sang 1978;34:281-90.
27. Sirchia G, Parravicini A, Rebulla P, Fattori L, Milani S. Evaluation of three procedures for the preparation of leukocyte-poor and leukocyte-free red blood cells for transfusion. Vox Sang 1980;38:197-204.
28. Johnson J, Mijovic V, Brozovic B. Evaluation of a new filter for leukocyte depletion of blood. J Clin Path 1983;36:1200-1.
29. Wenz B, Gurtlinger KF, O'Toole AM, Dugan EP. Preparation of granulocyte-poor red blood cells by microaggregate filtration. Vox Sang 1980;39:282-7.
30. Mijovic V, Brozovic B, Hughes ASB, Davies TD. Leukocyte-depleted blood: a comparison of filtration techniques. Transfusion 1983;23:30-2.
31. Parravicini A, Rebulla P, Apuzzo J, Wenz B, Sirchia G. The preparation of leukocyte-poor red cells for transfusion by a simple cost-effective technique. Transfusion 1984;24:508-9.
32. Fisher M, Chapman JR, Ting A, Morris PH. Alloimmunisation to HLA antigens following transfusion with leukocyte-poor and purified platelet suspensions. Vox Sang 1985;49:331-5.

33. Sirchia G, Parravicini A, Rebulla P, Bertolini F, Morelati F, Marconi M. Preparation of leukocyte-free platelets for transfusion by filtration through cotton wool. Vox Sang 1983;44:115-20.
34. Minchinton RM, Waters AH, Baker LRI, Cattell WR. Platelet, granulocyte and HLA antibodies in renal dialysis patients transfused with frozen blood. Brit Med J 1980;281:113-4.

USE OF HEMAPHERESIS-DERIVED HEMOPOIETIC STEM CELLS FOR TRANSPLANTATION IN MALIGNANT LYMPHOHEMOPOIETIC DISORDERS

M. Körbling, W. Hunstein, H. Martin, R. Haas, P. Reichardt

Introduction

The usual source of hemopoietic stem cells for transplantation is the bone marrow. However, evidence in rodents, canines and non-human primates indicates that stem cells with marrow repopulating ability also circulate in the peripheral blood [1-4]. To use the circulating blood as the primary source of stem cells to repopulate an aplastic bone marrow is a concept which reflects the physicological pattern in which fetal hemopoiesis develops. The fetal bone marrow becomes a site of hemopoiesis after pluripotent hemopoietic stem cells immigrate into its stromal matrix via the circulating blood. Thus transfusing blood-derived stem cells in adults may be considered to repeat the prenatal seeding of hemopoiesis into the bone marrow [5,6].

In man the repopulating ability of circulating stem cells is less well established. Goldman et al. [7] were the first who showed that blood-derived hemopoietic stem cells can re-establish hemopoietic function after myeloablative treatment for blast crisis in CML. However, in these patients most stem cells collected and eventually transfused originate from a Ph[1]-positive tumor cell clone. Their repopulating capability does not necessarily mean that 'normal' stem cells act the same way. In 1980 in the Oncology Center of the Johns Hopkins Hospital Baltimore we collected blood stem cells in a transient chemotherapeutically induced Ph[1]-negative phase. The retransfusion of those 'normal' stem cells into the patient after myeloablative treatment resulted in the complete hemopoietic reconstruction without reappearance of the Ph[1]-positive cell clone, but the follow-up was too short to evaluate the reconstitutive potential of the transfused stem cells on a long-term basis [8].

There are other reports on autologous blood stem cell transplantation (ABSCT) in patients with malignant lympho-hemopoietic disorders other than CML or with solid tumors, performed as an alternative approach to bone marrow transplantation [9-22]. These provide clear evidence that hemopoietic engraftment can be achieved with human stem cells collected from the circulating blood rather than from the marrow site. Here we describe the reconstitutive potential of blood derived hemopoietic stem cells in patients with malignant lympho-hemopoietic disorders and we discuss approaches to mobilize stem cells into the peripheral blood in order to optimize the stem cell collection procedure.

Methods

Stem cell harvest

Peripheral blood stem cells were collected by 'stem cell apheresis' using a continuous-flow blood cell separator (Fenwal CS-3000, Fenwal Laboratories, Deerfield, Ill.). The total blood volume processed per run was 10 litres at a flow rate of 50-70 ml per min (Table 1). The interval between stem cell harvests was between one and three days [23]. To optimize the stem cell yield stem cell aphereses were performed in most cases after transient myelosuppression during the subsequent expansion of the circulating blood stem cell pool.

The details of the stem cell apheresis procedure using the Fenwal system are given in Table 2 [24]. This procedure particularly describes the collection of a mononuclear cell product with low RBC contamination.

Table 1. Methodological aspects of stem cell apheresis.

– Donor blood volume processed per run: 10 litres	
– Blood flow rate:	60-70 ml per min
– Centrifuge speed:	1,000-1,600 rpm
– Anticoagulants:	– 5,000 IU heparin (bolus at start of apheresis) – ACD-A continuous infusion (500 ml per run) – 5,000 IU heparin injection into the cell collection bag after completion of apheresis

Table 2. Stem cell apheresis parameters using the Fenwal CS-3000 Blood Cell Separator.

- A 35 Collection Chamber, Granulo-Separation Chamber
- Procedure number 1 (platelets)
- Modification of the basic computer program dependant on the blood flow rate (L-68 is changed to 0750, *not* dependant on the patient's hematocrit)
- The secondary spin procedure to remove the platelets from the collected mononuclear cells is omitted to minimize possible cell loss.

Cryopreservation of apheresis-derived stem cells

The 200 ml cell suspension collected per run was concentrated to 100 ml and mixed with the same volume of Spinner-minimum essential medium (S-MEM) supplemented with 20% dimethyl sulfoxide (DMSO). The final 200 ml cell suspension was distributed into two 100 ml-polyolefine bags (DELMED, Canton, MA) and frozen to −100°C in a computerized freezer (CRYOSON BV-6, Cryoson Deutschland GmbH, Schöllkrippen, West Germany) (Fig. 1). The frozen cells were stored in the liquid phase of nitrogen until use.

Thawing and transplantation of apheresis-derived stem cells

The frozen bags were thawed by immersing them into a 40°C waterbath. The cell suspension was immediately injected into the patient using a central line. Post thaw washing and spinning of cells was avoided to minimize the risk of cell clumping and stem cell loss. The total volume of cell suspension injected into the patient was in the range of 1,500 ml and was given over 2 hours. Forced diuresis was started after infusing 500 ml. The transfusion of remaining free hemoglobin transiently impaired renal function (creatinine was raised to 2.0-2.5 mg/dl for 24-48 hours). In our experience this was without any major risk to the patient, nor caused the infusion of a cooled 6-8°C cell suspension into the right atrium of the heart any cardiac arrhythmia.

Pretransplant conditioning regimens

Regimen 1: Total body irradiation (TBI) using a linear accelerator, superfractionated over four days at 120 rad single dose up to a total of 1320-1440 rad (lungs 900 rad). Three single doses were administered per day at 8 am, noon, and 4 pm. Following irradiation, cyclophosphamide (CY 50 mg/kg) was given on each of four consecutive days (total dose 200 mg/kg; patient 1, 3 and 6).
Regimen 2: TBI, superfractionated over 3 days up to a total of 1200 rad followed by a single dose of melphalan (120 mg/m^2; patient 4).
Regimen 3: CY (1.5 g/m$^2 \times 4$), carmustine (300 mg/m^2) and etoposide (125 mg/m$^2 \times 3$) (CBV regimen [25]; patient 2).
Regimen 4: Mitoxantrone (12 mg/m$^2 \times$ 2d), carmustine (300 mg/m^2), etoposide (125 mg/m$^2 \times$ 3d; patient 5).
Regimen 5: Melphalan 200 mg/m^2 (patient 7).

ABSCT was performed 48 hours after completion of chemotherapy in regimens 1 and 3, and 24 hours thereafter in regimen 2, 4 and 5.

In vitro stem cell assay

To determine the concentration of hemopoietic progenitor cells in each harvested cell suspension and in the peripheral blood before and after ABSCT we used the human multilineage in vitro assay in methylcellulose (CFU-GEMM) previously described by Fauser and Messner [26] and modified according to Ash et al. [27].

Results

Blood stem cell collection

Stem cell yield in 7 patients pretreated and subsequently transplanted with blood stem cells

All patients were treated with various chemotherapeutic regimens before stem cell apheresis was started.

Table 3. Cell yield by leukoapheresis in 7 patients subsequently transplanted with autologous blood stem cells.

	MNCx10^9							CFU-GMx10^3						
Run no.	**pt.1**	**pt.2**	**pt.3**	**pt.4**	**pt.5**	**pt.6**	**pt.7**	**pt.1**	**pt.2**	**pt.3**	**pt.4**	**pt.5**	**pt.6**	**pt.7**
1	6.8	4.2	2.1	2.1	2.1	12.3	2.4	2000	620	130	6	10.5	272	4.8
2	4.5	4.8	1.5	1.6	3.8	4.8	2.7	900	300	62	63	–	114	5.4
3	6.4	4.1	2.4	2.0	2.45	3.0	2.4	N.D.	650	230	108	–	48	36
4	5.0	2.6	1.27	1.7	2.5	5.0	2.1	2600	340	100	10	45	20	17.8
5	15.0	3.9	1.2	3.5	0.75	2.3	2.1	3900	370	91	10	39	34	40
6	7.5	3.1	2.1	2.7	4.5	2.8	3.0	3800	1070	50	10	194	3	45
7	10.0	1.5	4.4	2.0	8.5	5.6	6.2	1900	180	490	32	68	66	37
8		5.6		0.6	4.8	4.9	3.8		530		14	9.6	68	12
9		6.3			6	4.8	2.7		210			6	34	11
10					0.95	5.9	2.9					3.8		37
11					2.5							5		
12					3.7							11		
13					4.3							39		
14					1.1							3		
Total/ kg b.w.	0.77	0.53	0.20	0.65	0.75	0.58	0.5	210	60	16	10	6.7	7.5	4

N.D. = not done

In *patient 1* with NHL, 7 apheresis were performed from 2 to 4 weeks after completion of the second cycle of COMP chemotherapy.

Patient 2 with recurrent Hodgkin's disease was heavily pretreated with irradiation and polychemotherapy (6×COPP, 1×CHOP, 6×ABVD) and received 3 cycles of HOAP-Bleo subsequent to his 3rd relapse. Aphereses were performed in early 4th remission (4 runs 3-4 weeks after the 1st cycle of HOAP-Bleo and 5 runs 2-3 weeks after CY (15 mg/kg×4 days) given 4 weeks after the 3rd cycle of HOAP-Bleo).

Patient 3 with end-stage AML was pretreated with 2×TAD, 2×Amsacrin, 2×Mitoxantrone/VP-16+1×high dose Ara-C. Stem cells were collected by 7 aphereses in early 3rd CR, 3-5 weeks after completion of the last cytotoxic treatment (2nd course of mitoxantrone/VP-16).

Patient 4 with sarcoma (Askin tumor) had 4 VAIA cycles (VCR, Adri, Ifo, Act-D) 8 leukaphereses were performed 4 to 7 weeks after completion of the 4th block of VAIA.

Patient 5 with recurrent Hodgkin's disease was pretreated with irradiation and polychemotherapy (6×COPP and 5×ABVD). A total of 14 aphereses were performed in 3rd remission, 6 runs 2-5 weeks after a course of cyclophosphamide (15 mg/kg×4d) and another 8 runs 4 months later without further intermittent chemotherapy.

Patient 6 with newly diagnosed AML was treated with 2×TAD within 4 weeks. 10 aphereses were performed in early first remission 2-7 weeks after completion of the 2nd TAD cycle.

Patient 7 with rhabdomyosarcoma was pretreated with polychemotherapy (2×VAIA+2×PIAV (Platinex, Ifo, Adri, VCR)). A total of 10 leukaphereses was performed, 6 runs 2-5 weeks after a course of cyclophosphamide (15 mg/kg×4d) and another 4 runs 4 months later without further intermittent chemotherapy.

The number of leukaphereses and the cell yield per run is shown in Table 3 for each of the 7 patients. The highest total stem cell number was reached in patient 1 with 15.1×10^6 CFU-GM, the lowest in patient 4 (a 9 year old boy of 25 kg) with 0.25×10^6 CFU-GM.

Stem cell yield in heavily pretreated patients after cyclophosphamide treatment

In 9 heavily pretreated patients aphereses were performed after a course of cyclophosphamide (CY 15 mg/kg×4 days).

Five of them had end stage Hodgkin's disease and were pretreated at least with C-MOPP and ABVD regimens. One patient with rhabdomyosarcoma received prior polychemotherapy (2×VAIA+2×PIAV). These patients underwent a total of 37 aphereses. The average number harvested per run was 3.1×10^4CFU-GM.

Three patients with non Hodgkin's lymphoma who had been pretreated with standard multiple chemotherapy underwent a total of 16 runs. The average number harvested per run in those patients was 10.4×10^4CFU-GM.

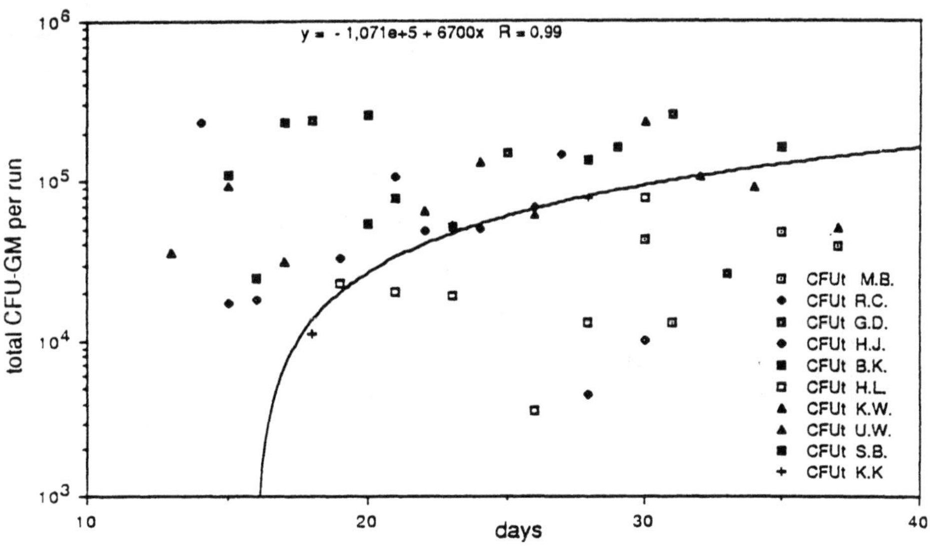

Figure 1. CFU-GM yield per run in heavily pretreated patients after a course of cyclophosphamide (15 mg/kg b.w.×4 days). Abscissa: days after begin of CY-treatment.

In Figure 1 the stem cell yield per run following treatment with cyclophosphamide (CY 15 mg/kg×4 days) is shown. Stem cell apheresis was started 2 to 3 weeks after CY treatment. Usually 6-8 runs were performed over a period of 2-3 weeks. As one can see, in this group of heavily pretreated patients, prior cytotoxic treatment with CY did not result in a subsequent CFU-GM overshooting as seen in early remission patients [28-32]. The most likely explanation is an exhaustion of the mobilizable progenitor cell pool by heavy and prolonged cytotoxic treatment.

Reconstitution of leukocytes and platelets after ABSCT

Blood cell reconstitution after ABSCT occurred very rapidly in patients 1 and 2, and reached 1,000 leukocytes per μl on day 9 (patient 1) and day 10 (patient 2), 500 granulocytes per μl on day 12 on day 10, resp. and 40,000 platelets per μl on day 10 for both (Figs 2,3). Normal blood counts were reached within 2 weeks. Both patients show complete and permanent trilineage engraftment at 21+ (patient 1) and 10+ months (patient 2) post transplantation.

Patient 3 to 7 were transplanted with 0.4-1.6x10^{4}CFU-GM per kg b.w., a stem cell dose believed to be at the lower limit for safe engraftment. Compared to patients 1 and 2 leukocyte and platelet reconstitution was variably delayed. Patient 3 reached 1000 leukocytes and 500 neutrophils on day 14 and 16 after ABSCT, respectively (Figs 3,4). On day 120 his bone marrow is still slightly hypocellular and his WBC is around 1800 with 1000 neutrophils. Patient 4 reached 1000 leukocytes on day 14 and 500 neutrophils on day 14. On day +70 he has 2300 WBC. Patient 3 (day +120) and patient 4 (day +70) did not yet reach 50,000 platelets without platelet support.

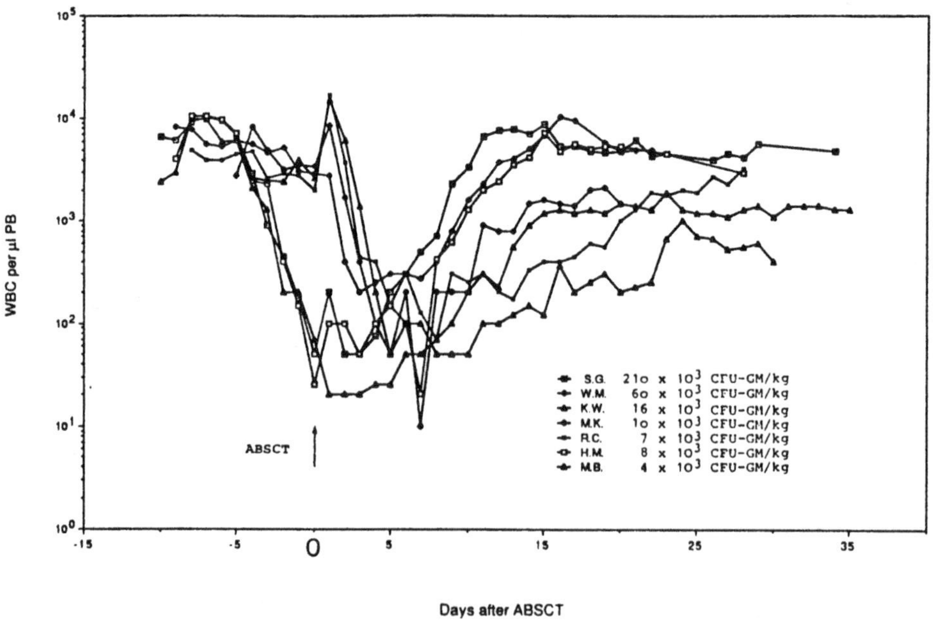

Figure 2. Early reconstitution of WBC after ABSCT.

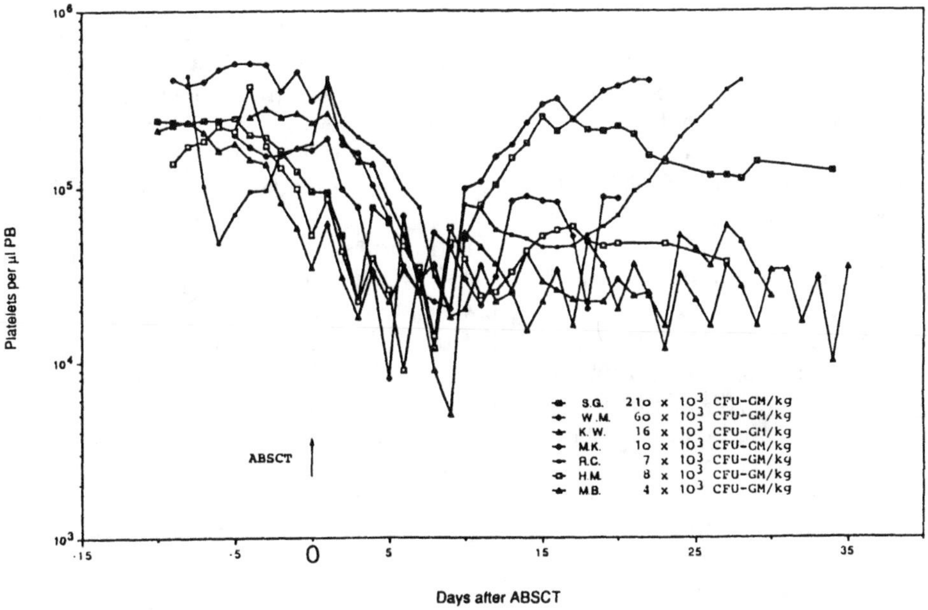

Figure 3. Early reconstitution of platelets after ABSCT.

Patients 5 and 6 reached 1000 leukocytes on day 20 and on day 10, and 50,000 platelets on day 18 and on day 15, respectively. The cell count on day +28 is 3300 and 4600 leukocytes, and 405,000 and 50,000 platelets, respectively. Follow-up is too short to assess long-term engraftment.

Patient 7 has about 600 leukocytes on day +26 and still needs regular platelet support.

Discussion

Successful blood stem cell transplantation to restore hemopoietic function after myeloablative treatment has to fulfill two major requirements: (1) hemopoietic reconstitution (including the lymphopoietic system) must be complete; and (2) the reconstituted hemopoietic function must be permanent.

In our cases transplanted with hemopoietic precursor cells in excess of 2×10^4 CFU-GM per kg b.w. hemopoietic recovery after ABSCT occurred very rapidly and resulted in complete and permanent trilineage reconstitution. Peripheral blood counts reached normal values within less than two weeks. Both patients were in a condition to be discharged from the hospital three weeks post transplantation. Although the total number of CFU-GM transfused per kg b.w. differed by a factor of 3.5, there was no significant difference in the kinetics of cellular reconstitution (Figs 2,3). Follow-up at 21+ and 10+ months after ABSCT shows normal peripheral blood counts and normal bone marrow cellularity in both patients. This demonstrates that blood derived stem cells autotransfused after myeloablative treatment are capable of sustaining long-term hemopoiesis.

In 5 patients transplanted with 0.4×10^4 to 1.6×10^4 CFU-GM per kg b.w. hemopoietic recovery after myeloablative therapy and ABSCT was variably delayed except in patient 6. Patient 3 and 4 stayed thrombocytopenic for 4 and 2 monts after ABSCT and still need platelet support once a week. Both have leukocytes around 1600-2300. Patients 5 and 6, who received only 0.67 and 0.75×10^4 CFU-GM/kg b.w., but high numbers of 7.5 and 5.8×10^8 MNC/kg b.w., had good early reconstitution, despite transfusing such low CFU-GM numbers. Long-term reconstitution remains to be evaluated.

Thus the minimal number of CFU-GM needed for safe engraftment seems to be in the range of 1×10^4 per kg b.w., a stem cell dose which is confirmed by data in the canine blood stem cell transplantation model [31].

As to our knowledge another 25 cases of ABSCT have been reported from 7 other centers [10-21] (Table 4). Patients who survived ABSCT for more than 4 months showed complete hemopoietic engraftment; stable engraftment has also been noted by Reiffers et al. [11], Bel et al. [10], Juttner et al. [16], Castaigne et al. [17,18] and by Tilly et al. [19] with a follow-up of 4+ to 12+ (median 8+) months. The CFU-GM transfused per kg b.w. in those cases ranged from 2.3×10^4 to 230×10^4.

Of particular interest is the rapid hemopoietic reconstitution after ABSCT in patients who received more than 5×10^4 CFU-GM per kg b.w.: 1000 leukocytes, including 500 granulocytes were reached within 2 weeks after ABSCT.

The rapid early rise in peripheral leukocyte counts may be explained by transfusing large numbers of committed progenitor cells which take about 10-14 days to differentiate to mature cells as do CFU-GM in the in vitro assay. Transfusing these committed progenitors which differentiate early and subsequently appear as the first cohort of circulating neutrophils is of clinical importance. It will significantly reduce time of isolation and hospitalization due to treatment induced neutropenia.

Long-term hemopoiesis, however, is re-established by early pluripotent stem cells; they will take longer to eventually give rise to differentiated progeny. Hence the pattern of hemopoietic reconstitution of platelets appears to be composed of successive cohorts of cells which differentiate from various progenitor and stem cells.

Figure 4 illustrates the correlation between numbers of MNC and CFU-GM transfused and early hemopoietic recovery in evaluable patients from Table 4. Early hemopoietic recovery seems to correlate more with the number of MNC transfused ($r=0.65$ for 1000 WBC and $r=0.54$ for 50,000 platelets) than with the number of CFU-GM transfused ($r=0.43$ for 1000 WBC and $r=0.28$ for 50,000 platelets).

Our experience further strongly suggests that the cytotoxic treatment prior to leukaphereses influences both the yield and the repopulating ability of progenitor and stem cells.

Whereas rapid early engraftment appears to be predictable by transfusing sufficient CFU-GM which can be assayed in vitro, the stability of long-term hemopoiesis after ABSCT cannot yet be assessed by in vitro tests but remains dependant on clinical studies.

Table 4. Synopsis of ABSCT reported so far.

Leukocytes/kg CFU-GM/kg Leukocytes 500/ul immunothrombo-

Institution	Diagnosis (status prior to ABSCT)	Pre-transplant regimen	Leukocytes/kg transfused	CFU-GM/kg transfused	Cell concentration after ABSCT: Leukocytes 1.000/μl	PMN 500/μl	Platelets 50.000/μl	Follow-up
Körbling et al. [9] (Heidelberg, West Germany)	Burkitt's lymphoma (CR 1)	CY 200 mg/kg + TBI 13.2 Gy	7.2×10^8	21.0×10^4	d9	d10	d10	alive (22 mo+ in CR 1
	Hodgkin's lymphoma (CR 4)	CY 6.0 g/m² carmustine 300 mg/m² + etopside 600 mg/m²	15.0×10^8	6.0×10^4	d10	d12	d10	alive (11 mo+)
	Hodgkin's lymphoma (CR 3)	mitoxantrone 24 mg/m² carmustine 300 mg/m² etoposide 600 mg/m²	7.5×10^8	0.67×10^4	d20	d22	d18	alive in CR (d +59)
	AML (CR 1)	CY 200 mg/kg TBI 14.4 Gy	5.8×10^8	0.75×10^4	d10	d10	d16	alive in CR (d +51)
	AML (CR 1)	CY 200 mg/kg + TBI 14.4 Gy	12×10^8	12×10^4	d7	d9	d11	alive in CR
	AML (CR 3)	CY 200 mg/kg + TB'i 14.4 Gy	2.0×10^8	1.6×10^4	d14	d16	d120	alive (5 mo+) in CR 3
	Sarcoma (CR 1) (Askins tumor)	TBI 12 Gy melphalan 120 mg/m²	6.5×10^8	1.0×10^4	d14	d14	d70	alive (3 mo+)
	Rhabdomyo-sarcoma (CR 1)	melphalan 200 mg/m²	5×10^8	0.4×10^4	d38	d48	d50	alive (d +50)
Bell et al. [10] (Bournemouth, UK)	cc-NHL (resist.)	melphalan 140 mg/m² + carmustine 600 mg/m² + ara-C 400 mg/m² etoposide 600 mg/m2	5.1×10^8	6.0×10^4	d10	d10	d14	alive (9 mo+)

Table 4. Synopsis of ABSCT reported so far. (Continued)

Institution	Diagnosis (status prior to ABSCT)	Pre-transplant regimen	Leukocytes/kg transfused	CFU-GM/kg transfused	Cell concentration after ABSCT: Leukocytes 1.000/μl	PMN 500/μl	Platelets 50.000/μl	Follow-up
Reiffers et al. [10-13] (Bordeaux, France)	AML (Rel.1)	etoposide 600 mg/m^2 + CY 120 mg/kg + TBI 10 Gy	7.8×10^8	9.5×10^4		d16	d35	death in relapse (7 mo)
	AML (CR 2)	etoposide 600 mg/m^2 + CY 120 mg/kg + TBI 10 Gy	5.6×10^8	30×10^4	d9	d10	d34	alive in CR 2 (12 mo+)
	AML (CR 2)	etoposide 600 mg/m^2 + CY 120 mg/kg + TBI 10 Cy	6.1×10^8	13.7×10^4	d14	d16	immunothrombocytopenia day 11	death due to rel. (3 mo+)
	AML (CR 4)	busulphan 60 mg/kg + melphalan 140 mg/m^2	3×10^8	2.75×10^4	d17	d18	never	early relapse (d45)
	AML (CR 2)	busulphan 60 mg/kg + melphalan 140 mg/m^2	7.6×10^8	12.4×10^4	d12	d14	megakaryocyte engraftment failure	death due to hemorrhage (d69) without leukocytes
	AML (Rel.1)	etoposide 600 mg/m2 + CY 120 mg/kg + TBI 10 Gy	10×10^8	49.7×10^4	d8	d9	d11	alive in CR (4 mo+)
	AML (Rel.1)	busulphan 60 mg/kg + CY 200 mg/kg	4×10^8	5.3×10^4	d10	d15	d14	alive in CR (3 mo+) 55.000 platelets
Juttner et al. [14-16] (Adelaide, Australia)	AML (Rel.1)	melphalan 200 mg/m^2	1.3×10^8	29.0×10^4	d14	d14	TETE	death in relapse (ca. +2 mo)
	AML (Rel.1)	CY 120 mg/kg + TBI 12 Gy	3.0×10^8	23.0×10^4	d16	d16	d16	death in relapse (d111)
	AML (Rel.1?) relapse?	CY 120 mg/kg + TBI 12 Gy	2.3×10^8	24.0×10^4	'early trilineage engraftment'			
	AML (Rel.1)	CY 120 mg/kg + TBI 12 Gy	2.8×10^8	230×10^4		d10	d11	alive (7 mo+)

Table 4. Synopsis of ABSCT reported so far. (Continued)

Institution	Diagnosis (status prior to ABSCT)	Pre-transplant regimen	Leukocytes/kg transfused	CFU-GM/kg transfused	Cell concentration after ABSCT: Leukocytes 1.000/μl	PMN 500/μl	Platelets 50.000/μl	Follow-up
Castainge et al. [17,18] (Paris, France)	AML (CR 1)	CY 100 mg/kg + TBI 10 Gy	1.9×10^8	2.3×10^4	d16		d75	alive (8 mo+)
	AML (CR 1)	CY 100 mg/kg TBI 10 Gy			ABSCT engraftment failure			dead after subsequent allogeneic BMT
	ALL (Ph 1)(CR 1)	CY 100 mg/kg TBI 10 GY				d21	d19	relapse d 60 death
	ALL (Ph 1)(CR 1)	CY 100 mg/kg TBI 10 Gy				d30	d19	alive d 30+
	T-ALL (CR 1)	CY 100 mg/kg TBI 10 Gy				d36	d120	alive in CR with VOD d +120
	ALL (CR 3)	CY 100 mg/kg TBI 10 Gy				d25	d42	relapse d50 death
Tilly et al. [19] (Rouen, France)	ALL (CR 1)	CY 120 mg/kg TBI 10 Gy		77×10^4		d11	d16	alive in CR (6 mo+)
	AML (CR 2)	CY 120 mg/kg TBI 10 Gy		36×10^4		d12	d50	alive in CR (4 mo+)
Kessinger et al. [20] (Omaha, Nebraska, USA)	breast cancer (metastatic)	cis-platinum 125 mg/m² + CY 120 mg/kg + TBI 11 Gy	8.4×10^8	10.0×10^4	d10		TETE	death due to hepatic failure (d12)
	breast cancer (metastatic)	cit-platinum 125 mg/m² + CY 120 mg/kg + TBI 11 Gy	6.3×10^8	6.62×10^4		d16	immunothrombocytopenia 41,000 day 43	death due to pneumonia (d104)
Stiff et al. [21] (Springfield, Illinois USA	small cell lung cancer ($\times \pm$SD of 3 patients)	BCNU 900 mg/m² CY 4 g/m² etoposide 500 mg/m² cis-platin 100 mg/m²	$3.8 \pm 2.0 \times 10^8$	$11.9 \pm 9.9 \times 10^4$	d14	d14	d269 d129 d48	

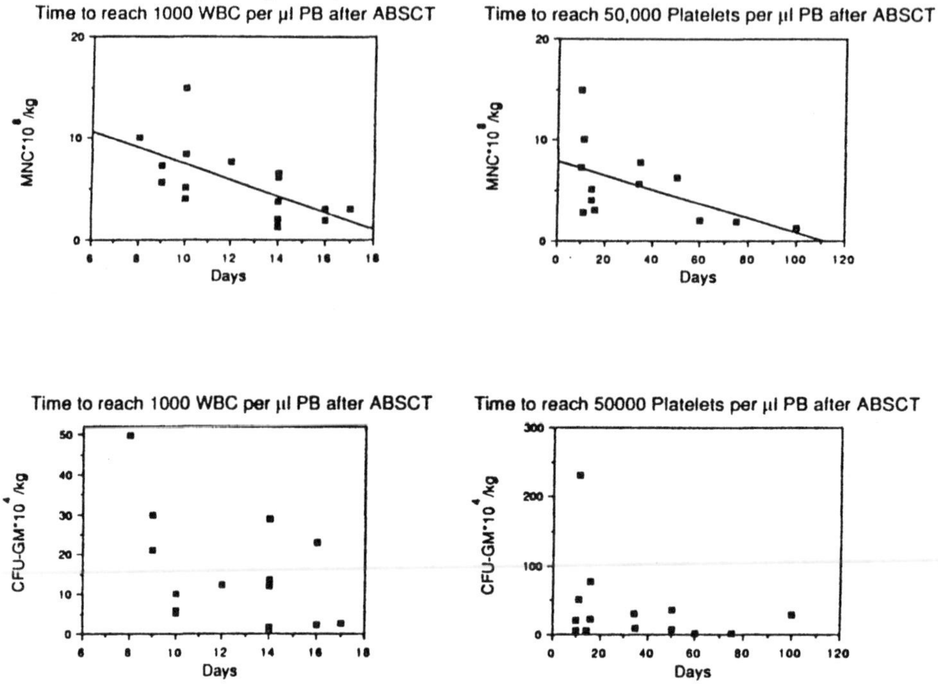

Figure 4. Correlation between cell number transfused and hemopoietic recovery after ABSCT.

Table 5. Platelet recovery after ABSCT (data from 32 patients shown in Table 4).

Recovery		No of patients
– Very rapid	(50,000 plts within 16 days)	9
– Slow	(50,000 plts within 34-50 days)	5
– Delayed (CFU-GM transfused $<2.5\text{x}10^4$/kg		6
– Delayed without explanation (all 3 patients in one center [20])		3
– Immunothrombocytopenia		2
– Megakaryocytic engraftment failure		1
– Early relapse		1
– TETE due to early death/data not available		3

In contrast to consistent early leukocyte reconstitution platelet recovery after ABSCT varied (see Table 5). In our patients 1, 2 and 5 platelet recovery was very rapid. They reached 50,000 platelets within 2 weeks after ABSCT. Nine of the patients reported so far showed such rapid platelet recovery. Delayed platelet recovery for various reasons which are detailed in Table 6 was seen in our patients 3, 6 and 7 and was reported by Reiffers et al. [10-13], Castaigne et al. [17,18], Kessinger et al. [20] and Stiff et al. [21]. Patients who were transplanted with less than 2.5x10^4 CFU-GM/kg b.w. except our patients 6 consistently had delayed platelet recovery. Two cases of immunothrombocytopenia and one case of megakaryocytic engraftment failure were also reported.

Five of the patients receiving ABSCT in AML [10-16] who were transplanted in overt relapse eventually died in subsequent relapse. In three of his four patients Juttner et al. [14-16] reported a consistent rapid early, but later incomplete engraftment despite transfusing 23-29x10^4 CFU-GM per kg b.w. collected in the very early first remission phase of AML [29]. Late incomplete engraftment seen in 3 of the patients may be due to underlying leukemia. Alternatively the pattern of engraftment may be explained by the transfusion of abundant numbers of committed but insufficient numbers of pluripotent stem cells. It must be re-emphasized, however, that stable long-term engraftment was achieved in all patients, who survived ABSCT disease free for more than 4 months.

It is well known that circulating progenitor cells in man are increased during recovery from myelosuppressive chemotherapy [28]. Large numbers of CFU-GM circulate also in very early remission after induction therapy for AML [29-32]. The CFU-GM compartment in these patients is preferentially expanded 10-25 fold, but CFU-GEMM are increased only about 3 fold [15,31]. In all centers performing ABSCT for leukemia or lymphoma [9-19] hemopoietic progenitor and stem cells were collected during the recovery phase after various chemotherapy regimens.

Mobilization of progenitor cells, however, appears to depend very much on the patients' pretreatment. In our series of heavily pretreated patients with lymphoma we could not observe an expansion of the circulating progenitor cell pool after a course of cyclophosphamide (15 mg/kg per b.w. $\times$ 4 days), a finding not previously reported in man. Heavy and prolonged cytotoxic treatment seems to exhaust the mobilizable progenitor cell pool. This is in agreement with canine data [33-37]. Consequently circulating progenitors should be collected as early as possible after diagnosis or achieving first complete remission, respectively.

Besides cytotoxic treatment with subsequent expansion of the peripheral blood stem cell pool a number of other approaches to increase the peripheral blood stem cell concentration have been reported (see Table 6).

Table 6. Factors that increase the number of circulating stem cells.

- Endotoxin
- Pyran copolymer and related agents
- Low molecular weight dextran-sulphate

- Exercise, ACTH, prednisone, hydrocortison
- Stem cell overshooting after transient chemotherapy-induced myelosuppression
- Recombinant human GM-CSF (?)

Table 7. Indications for autologous blood stem cell transplantation.

Supportive approach
- Augmenting the reconstitutive potency of quantitatively inadequate autologous marrow collections

Therapeutic approach
- Acute leukemia in CR
- Non Hodgkin's lymphoma
- Resistant multiple myeloma (?)

Prophylactic approach
- In persons who are at risk for severe radiation exposure
- In persons with genetic predisposition for malignant lymphohemopoietic disorders

The administration of endotoxin [38,39], pyran copolymer [40] and related agents or low molecular weight dextran sulphate has been studied in animal models. These compounds have not yet been approved for clinical use. Results not yet conclusive or reproducible have been published using corticosteroids or activators of endogenous steroid production to mobilize peripheral stem cells [43-45].

Transplantation of circulating stem cells may have advantages over the use of marrow derived stem cells, such as:

(1) In patients at risk for general anesthesia, continuous-flow apheresis offers an alternative and safe way for stem cell harvest.
(2) Blood stem cell harvest, processing, and freezing is simple and can basically be done in blood banks, like the handling of any other blood component. Besides collecting stem cells from patients already affected by malignant disease blood stem cells may be harvested as a prophylactic approach from normal individuals known to be at risk for acquiring malignant lymphohemopoietic disorders such as twins, or persons at risk of severe radiation exposure.
(3) Stem cell harvest is feasible in case of damage to the marrow collection site by previous radiotherapy or tumor involvement.
(4) hemopoietic reconstitution after myeloablative treatment and ABSCT seems to be more rapid for the WBC line, and therefore the aplasia-related risks in the early post transplantation period are lowered, provided sufficient numbers of stem cells are transplanted.
(5) The ratio between normal hemopoietic stem cells and clonogenic tumor cells in the peripheral blood of patients with malignant lymphohemopoietic disorders in remission may be in favor of the former, a hypothesis yet to be proven.

ABSCT after myeloablative chemo/radiotherapy promises an alternative approach to autologous bone marrow transplantation which provides additional safety because of low aplasia-related risks. The possible long-term benefit to those patients, however, has to be proven in further clinical trials.

Table 8. Conclusions.

– Apheresis-derived hemopoietic stem cells are able to reconstitute hemopoiesis *completely* and *permanently.*
– Hemopoietic reconstitution after ABSCT occurs rapidly provided sufficient numbers of stem cells are transfused (more than 1-2x10^4 per kg b.w.)
– The efficiency of hemopoietic stem cell collection depends on the patient's cytotoxic pretreatment
– New and more effective approaches for mobilizing hemopoietic stem cells into the peripheral blood are needed resp. under investigation

Acknowledgement

The excellent technical assistance of Mrs Monika Baumann and Mrs Eva Holdermann is fully acknowledged.

References

1. Goodman JW, Hodgson GS. Evidence for stem cells in peripheral blood of mice. Blood 1962;19:702-14.
2. Cavins JA, Scheer SC, Thomas ED, Feerebee JW. The recovery of lethally irradiated dogs given infusions of autologous leukocytes preserved at −80°C. Blood 1964;23:38-43.
3. Fliedner TM, Calvo W, Körbling M, Nothdurft W, Pflieger H, Ross W. Collection, storage and transfusion of blood stem cells for the treatment of hemopoietic failure. Blood Cells 1979;5:313-28.
4. Storb R, Graham RC, Epstein RB, Sale GE, Thomas ED. Demonstration of hemopoietic stem cells in the peripheral blood of baboons by cross circulation. Blood 1977;50:537-42.
5. Keleman E, Calvo W, Fliedner TM. Atlas of human hemopoietic development. Heidelberg/New York: Springer Verlag 1978.
6. Fliedner TM, Calvo W. Hematopoietic stem-cell seeding of a cellular matrix: a principle of initiation and regneration of hematopoiesis. In: Differentation of normal and neoplastic hematopoietic cells. Cold Spring Harbor Laboratory 1978:757-73.
7. Goldman JM, Catovsky D, Goolden AWG, Johnson SA. Galton DAG: Buffy coat autografts for patients with chronic granulocytic leukemia in transformation. Blut 1981;42:149-55.
8. Körbling M, Burke P, Braine H, Elfenbein G, Santos BW, Kaizer H. Successful engraftment of blood derived normal hemopoietic stem cells in chronic myelogenous leukemia. Exp Hematol 1981;9:684-90.
9. Körbling M, Dörken B, Ho AD, Pezzutto A, Hunstein W, Fliedner TM. Autologous transplantation of blood-derived hemopoietic stem cells after myeloablative therapy in a patient with Burkitts lymphoma. Blood 1986;67:529-32.
10. Bell AJ, Figes A, Oscier DG, Hamblin TJ. Peripheral blood stem cell autografting. Lancet 1986;i:1027(letter).
11. Reiffers J, Broustet A, David B, et al. Successful autologous transplantation with peripheral blood hemopoietic cells in a patient with acute leukemia. Exp Hematol 1986;14:312-5.

12. Reiffers J, Marit G, Bernard P, et al. Autologous transplantation with circulating stem cells in patients with acute non-lymphoblastic leukemia. Book of Abstracts, XXI Congress ISH. Sydney 1986:371.
13. Reiffers J. Personal communication 1986.
14. Juttner CA, To LB, Haylock DN, Branford A, Kimber RJ. Circulating autologous stem cells collected in very early remission from acute non-lymphoblastic leukemia produce prompt but incomplete haemapoietic reconstitution after high dose melphalan or supralethal chemoradiotherapy. Brit J Heamatol 1985;61: 739-45.
15. Juttner CA, To LB, Dyson P, Haylock DN, Branford A, Kimber RJ. The peripheral blood CFU-mix: CFU-GM ratio during very early remission from acute non-lymphoblastic leukemia. Brit J Haematol 1986;62:598-9.
16. Juttner CA, To LB, Haylock DN, Branford A, Dyson P, Kimber RJ. Hemopoietic reconstitution using circulating autologous stem cells collected in very early remission from acute non-lymphoblastic anemia. Exp Hematol 1986; 14(abstract):465.
17. Castaigne S, Calvo F, Douay L, et al. Successful haemopoietic reconstitution using autologous peripheral blood mononucleated cells in a patient with acute promyelocytic leukemia. Brit J Haematol 1986;63:209-11.
18. Castaigne S, Tilly H, Leverger G, et al. Autologous blood derived hemopoietic stem cell (BHSC) transplantation in acute leukemia. Abstract, 28th Annual Meeting of the American Society of Hematology 1986.
19. Tilly H, Bastit D, Lucet JC, Esperou H, Monconduit M, Piguet H. Haematopoietic reconstitution after autologous peripheral blood stem cell transplantation in acute leukemia. Lancet 1986;ii:154-5(letter).
20. Kessinger A, Armitage JO, Landmark JD, Weisenburger DD. Reconstitution of human hemopoietic function with autologous cryopreserved circulating stem cells. Exp Hematol 1986;14:192-6.
21. Stiff PJ, Koester AR, Lanzotti VJ. Autologous transplantation using peripheral blood stem cells. Exp Hematol 1986;14(abstract):465.
22. To LB, Dyson PG, Juttner CA. Cell dose effect in circulating stem-cell autografting. Lancet 1986;ii:404-5(letter).
23. Körbling M, Fliedner TM, Pflieger H. Collection of large quantities of granulocyte-macrophage progenitor cells (CFU-c) in man by means of continuous flow leukapheresis. Scand J Haematol 1980;24:22-8.
24. Fenwal CS3000 blood cell separator LAK cell procedure book. Fenwal Laboratories, Deerfield, Illinois, USA 60015.
25. Jagannath S, Dicke KA, Armitage JO, et al. High-dose cyclophosphamide, carmustine, and etoposide and autologous bone marrow transplantation for relapsed Hodgkin's disease. Ann Int Medicine 1986;104:163-8.
26. Fauser AA, Messner HA. Identification of megakaryocytes, macrophages, and eosinophils in colonies of human bone marrow containing neutrophilic granulocytes and erythroblasts. Blood 1979;53:1023-7.
27. Ash RC, Detrick RA, Zanjani ED. Studies of human pluripotential hemopoietic stem cells (CFU-GEMM) in vitro. Blood 1981;58:309-16.
28. Richman CM, Weiner RS, Yankee RA. Increase in circulating stem cells following chemotherapy in man. Blood 1976;47:1031-9.
29. To LB, Haylock DN, Kimber RJ, Juttner CA. High levels of circulating haemopoietic progenitor cells in very early remission from acute non-lymphoblastic leukemia and their collection and cryopreservation. Brit J Haematol 1984;58: 399-410.

30. Bernard PH, Reiffers J, Vezon G, et al. Collection of circulating haemopoietic cells after chemotherapy in acute non-lymphocytic leukemia. Brit J Haematol 1985;61:577-94.
31. Geissler K, Hinterberger W, Lechner K. Increased ratio of granulocyte/macrophage progenitor cells (CFU-GM) to multilineage progenitor cells (CFU-mix) in the peripheral blood from patients with acute non-lymphoblastic leukemia in early remission. Brit J Haematol 1986;62:596-7.
32. Tilly H, Vannier JP, Bastit D, Monconduit M, Pugiet H. Daily evaluation of circulating granulocyte-monocyte progenitors during bone marrow recovery from induction therapy in acute leukemia. Leuk Res 1986;10:353-6.
33. Nothdurft W, Fliedner TM, Calvo, et al. CFU-c populations in blood and bone marrow of dogs after lethal irradiation and allogeneic transfusion with cryopreserved blood mononuclear cells. Scand J Haematol 1978;21:115-30.
34. Haen M, Grilly G, Nothdurft W, Fliedner TM. Studies on the repopulating ability of blood stem cells of dogs given a single dose of cyclophosphamide. Exp Hematol 1980;8(suppl.7; abstract):26.
35. Haen M, Grilli G, Fliedner TM. Characterization of blood and bone marrow derived CFU-c after a single high dose of cyclophosphamide. Blut 1982; 45(abstract):213.
36. Raghavachar A, Prümmer O, Fliedner TM. The effect of cyclophosphamide treatment in canine long-term survivors after autologous bone marrow transplantation. Exp Hematol 1984;12(abstract):439.
37. Raghavachar A, Prümmer O, Fliedner TM, Steinbach KH. Progenitor cell (CFU-c) reconstitution after autologous stem cell transfusion in lethally irradiated dogs: decreased CFU-c populations in blood and bone marrow correlate with the fraction mobilizable by dextran sulphate. Exp Hematol 1983;11:996-1004.
38. Vos O, Buurman WA, Ploemacher RE. Mobilization of hemopoietic stem cells (CFU) into the peripheral blood of the mouse; effects of endotoxic and other compounds. Cell and Tissue Kinetics 1972;5:467-79.
39. Cline MJ, Golde DW. Mobilization of hemopoietic stem cells (CFU-C) into the peripheral blood of man by endotoxin. Exp Hematol 1977;5:186-90.
40. Zander AR, Templeton J, Gray KN, Spitzer G, Verma DS, Dicke KA. Mobilization of canine hemopoietic stem cells by pyran copolymer (NSC 46015). Biomedicine and Pharmacotherapy 1984;38:107-10.
41. Ross WM, Calvo S, Fliedner TM, Körbling M, Nothdurft W. Hemopoietic blood stem cell mobilization by dextrane sulphate. Exp Hematol 1977;5:13-6.
42. Ross WM, Körbling M, Nothdurft W, Fliedner TM. The role of dextrane sulphate in increasing the CFU-c concentration in dog blood. Proc Soc Exp Biol Med 1978;157:301-5.
43. Morra L, Ponassi A, Parodi GB, Caristo G, Bruzzi P, Sacchetti C. Mobilization of colony-forming cells (CFU-c) into the peripheral blood of man by hydrocortisone. Biomedicine 1981;35:87-90.
44. Lasky LC, Ascensao J, McCullough J, Zanjani ED. Steroid modulation of naturally occurring diurnal variation in circulating pluripotential haematopoietic cells (CFU-GEMM). Brit J Haematol 1983;55:615-22.
45. Barrett AJ, Longhurst P, Sneath P, Watson JG. Mobilization of CFU-C by exercise and ACTH induced stress in man. Exp Hematol 1978;6:590-4.

PURGING OF BONE MARROW

M.K. Brenner, J-P. Grob, H.G. Prentice

Bone marrow transplantation (BMT) is an effective adjunct in the treatment of a number of malignant and non-malignant hematological conditions [1]. Bone marrow (BM) may be obtained from a gentically matched donor (allogeneic BMT) or – for the treatment of malignant disease – from the patient himself (autologous BMT), and is used to rescue the patient from the intensive treatment given for the underlying disease. The major disadvantage of allografting is that donor T-lymphocytes may cause graft-versus-host disease (GvHD) in the recipient; conversely the major problem associated with autologous BMT is that marrow may be contaminated with malignant cells contributing to relapse. Thus in both types of BMT, success may be compromized by the presence of unwanted cells in the graft and BM purging is the name given to the process of their removal.

Table 1. Methods of BM purging.

Principle	**Method**
I Physical	Density gradients, elutriation
II Pharmacological	*In vitro chemotherapy:*
	Cyclophosphamide derivates
	4-HC
	Asta Z-7557
	Deoxycoformycin
	Etoposide (VP-16)
	Merocyanin
III Immunological	*Target removal:*
	Magnetic microspheres + magnetic fields
	Target killing:
	Complement mediated
	Toxin mediated

Three approaches to BM purging have been adopted (Table 1), biophysical, pharmacological and immunological:

(1) Biophysical purging is based on differences in cell density and/or size between malignant cells (or mature T-cells) and hemopoietic progenitors, which thereby permit separation on density gradients. These techniques are cumbersome and are not now widely used [2,3].

(2) Pharmacological purging has been used mainly in autografting and is based on the possibility of a difference in sensitivity to chemotherapeutic agents between leukemic cells or mature T-cells and hemopoietic progenitors [reviewed in 4]. Two cyclophosphamide derivates, 4-hydroperoxycyclophosphamide (4-HC) and INN mafosfamide (Asta Z-7557), currently dominate this area [5,6], but other agents such as the podophylotoxins [7] and deoxycoformycin [8] have also been used, as well as photoreactive intercalating dyes including merocyanin [9]. However, the human pluripotent stem cell has not yet been identified, and there is no proof that it is any more resistant than the leukemic clonogenic cell to these agents.

A few centers have adopted a pharmacological approach to T-cell depletion of allografts: incubation with high doses of steroids [10] or deoxycoformycin plus deoxyadenosine [11] may provide effective depletion.

(3) Immunological purging exploits the selective targeting of specific antigeneic structures present on either leukemic cells or mature T-cells which are absent from hemopoietic progenitors [reviewed in 12]. This technique usually employs monoclonal antibodies directed against surface antigens. The bound Ab is then used either to remove these cells physically or to lyse them. Physical removal of T-cells or residual malignant cells has been achieved by coupling the antibodies to magnetic microspheres which are separated with the target cells in magnetic fields [13]. Target-cell killing is usually achieved either with human or rabbit complement mediated lysis (C'-mediated cytotoxicity) [14]. Alternatively the McAb may be coupled to a toxin (toxin-mediated cytotoxicity) [15], most frequently ricin. Ricin is derived from castor beans and is composed of 2 chains. The A chain causes cell death once it has entered the cell by inactivating elongation factor 1 and thereby blocking protein synthesis at the polysome level, while the B chain binds to galactose-containing glycoproteins present on the surface of all human cells and orientates the A chain so that penetration into the cell is facilitated [16]. The antibodies selected may be coupled either to the A chain alone, utilizing ammonium chloride during incubation to increase cytotoxicity [17], or to an intact ricin molecule providing that the binding of the B chain to non-relevant cells is avoided by adding lactose to the system [15] or by modifying the B chain itself.

Table 2 gives a list of antigens which have been or could be used as targets for immunologic purging.

Table 2. Target antigens for BM purging with McAb.*

	Antigen	MW	CD number
I. T-cell depletion			
a. T-associated	T_1-like	(p 67)	(CD5)
	T_2-like	(p 41)	(CD7)
	T_3-like	(p 19-29)	(CD3)
	T_8-like	(p 32)	(CD8)
	T_{11}-like	(p 50)	(CD2)
	T_{12}-like	(p 100)	(CD6)
b. T and B + monocyte associated	Campath-1-like	(p 44)	–
II. ABMT			
T-cell disorders	T_1-like	(p 67)	(CD5)
	T_2-like	(p 41)	(CD7)
	T_{11}-like	(p 50)	(CD2)
B-cell disorders	$Y_{29/55}$	(p unknown)	–
	B_1-like	(p 35)	(CD20)
	B_4-like	(p 87)	(CD19)
Common ALL	cALLA	(p 100)	(CD10)
	BA_1-like	(p 30)	(CD24)
	BA_2-like	(p 24)	(CD9)
	B_4-like	(p 87)	(CD19)

* Reviewed in [12].

Clinical applications of BM purging

Allogeneic BMT

Experiments in a number of animal species in the late 60's and early 70's [18-20] showed clearly that graft-versus-host disease (GvHD) after allogeneic BMT could be totally abolished by removing mature T-cells from the donor graft, a procedure which did not significantly affect marrow engraftment. Although in man some successes were subsequently reported by removing unwanted T-lymphocytes with polyclonal rabbit antisera [21] or cell elutriation [3], it was not until the introduction of monoclonal antibodies to clinical medicine that T-cell depletion could be undertaken with sufficient ease, reliability and reproducibility for the procedure to enter into general use. Most published series of T-cell depleted BMT report the use of monoclonal antibody mediated lysis of T-cells with either mouse anti-human T-cell monoclonal antibodies and rabbit complement [22] or Campath-1, a rat pan-lymphocyte IgM antibody which fixes human complement [23]. More recently reports have been published describing the use of toxin conjugated antibodies [24] or antibody coupled magnetic beads [25]. Improvements in elutriation technology have also led to a renewed interest in this physical approach to T-cell removal [3]. Whatever technique of T-cell removal is used there is now no doubt that the procedure effectively abolishes significant

GvHD. In previous series between 25 and 50% of patients develop grade II or greater GvHD and about half of those so affected, subsequently perished [26,27]. In addition the acute form of GvHD progressed to chronic GvHD in at least half of the survivors to produce fibrosis of skin, liver and bowel, profound immunodeficiency and consequent mortality from opportunistic infections [28]. In contrast in our own series of 70 patients transplanted using T-cell depletion or sole method of GvHD prophylaxis, 51 developed no GvHD at all, 13 developed grade I GvHD and only 4 patients developed grade II or grade III GvHD. The incidence of chronic GvHD was less dramatically reduced but occurred in only 19% of patients surviving. These excellent results have been matched by other groups [29,30].

Problems of T-cell depletion

While there is now no doubt that T-cell depletion is the most effective way of preventing GvHD new problems have evolved in its wake.

1. Graft rejection (GvHD)

Recipients of bone marrow grafts are conditioned with cytotoxic agents with or without total body irradiation (TBI) before transplantation. For all recipients this has the purpose of eliminating residual marrow and host immunity, allowing the allografted marrow to 'take'. Where the recipient suffers from leukemia, conditioning has the additional purpose of eliminating residual leukemic cells and it is therefore correspondingly more intense than that undertaken for non-malignant disease. The different intensity of conditioning was reflected in the different rates of GvHD in the two groups of recipients. HvG was rare when BMT was undertaken for leukemia but occurred in about 25% or more of patients transplanted for aplastic anemia or thalassemia [31]: not only do such patients receive less intensive conditioning, but the multiple transfusions they require serve to immunize them against a wide range of alloantigens, some of which may well be present on donor marrow progenitor cells. When T-depletion was introduced as GvHD prophylaxis, however, many centers were surprised by a relatively high incidence of rejection even after transplantation for leukemia [32]. It seems likely that under normal circumstances infused donor T-lymphocytes interact with the recipient immune system to block graft resistance/rejection. The implication of this is that if the donor marrow is T-depleted then the recipient must receive more intensive or more immunosuppressive conditioning [33]. Fortunately it appears that relatively minor changes in the conditioning protocol are sufficient to permit engraftment of T-cell depleted marrow [29,32,34]. Thus, of patients transplanted in a collaborative study using the Royal Free Hospital McAb treated marrow, 9 of 13 (69%) rejected bone marrow if total body irradiation was given in fractions to a total dose between 1000 and 1200 Gy, but only 1.5% rejected when radiation was given as a single prescribed fraction of 750 Gy at a dose rate of 26 Gy/min in air (15-18 Gy/min mid-plane received dose rate), a regimen which in animal models is more potently immunosuppressive than fractionated TBI [33]. Similar, graft rejection by the recipients of Campath-treated marrow can be prevented by using total lymphoid irradiation [29]: this modification to conditioning is effective in allowing engraftment even in thalassemic and aplastic anemia recipients.

Clearly, increasing or modifying radiotherapy is not ideal for patients transplanted for non-malignant conditions and in such individuals we have found that increased pretransplant cytotoxic conditioning in combination with anti-lymphocyte globulin (ALG) reduces the rate of rejection. Nonetheless it remains unsatisfactory that all the methods so far adopted to augment recipient immunosuppression before T-depleted BMT have utilized more rigorous conditioning schedules with TBI or cytotoxic agents. These modified regimens increase the morbidity and mortality due to the conditioning protocol, thus partially offsetting some of the benefits of a low rate of GvHD. A more elegant approach to the abolition of HvG disease would be destroy or disable specifically the components of the recipient immune system responsible for rejecting the donor marrow by in vitro treatment of the recipient with McAb. One such monoclonal antibody that appears to have the appropriate characteristics is anti-lymphocyte function associated antigen 1 (LFA-1) [35]. This antigen is a two-chain structure on the surface of lymphocytes and neutrophils and is responsible for ensuring tight apposition of cells in the immune system. Blockade of this molecule using anti-LFA-1 prevents the binding of cytotoxic effector cells to their target and has been used successfully in rodents and in man to reduce the risk of marrow rejection [36]. As yet it has been applied only to HLA-mismatched transplants in whom the problem of rejection is correspondingly more severe, but there is little doubt that this or related antibodies will prove equally effective at preventing rejection in HLA-matched transplants without the need for more intensive and therefore more toxic conditioning.

2. Prolonged immunodeficiency

Even after conventional BMT, immune infection is poor for 6-18 months [37,38]. T-cells play a central role in all immune functions, so that one potential problem associated with T-cell depletion for GvHD prevention is that the recipient – deprived of his own T-cells by conditioning (see 1 above) and lacking donor T-cells in the transplanted marrow – might remain immunoincompetent for even longer. Paradoxically T-depletion actually seems to enhance the speed at which immune function is restored in the recipient, so that CD4 (helper) to CD8 (suppressor) ratio is less deranged than that seen with conventional BMT and the usual CD8 'overshoot' is prevented [39], immunoglobulin levels do not fall from pretransplant levels [40], antibody responses can be made in the immunized transplant recipient [41] and natural killer function rapidly reappears [42]. This improved immune function may, in part, be a consequence of the reduction in the incidence and severity of GvHD so that patients do not regularly require immunosuppressive drugs after BMT. Reconstitution of NK and T-cell function following Campath-1 treatment follows a similar pattern [43].

3. Leukemic relapse

GvHD occurs when donor alloreactive T-cells recognize alloantigens on recipient cells. Residual leukemic blasts are obviously also of recipient origin and it is possible that GvHD would therefore also have a graft-versus-leukemia effect. If this were so then one would predict that patients with acute or chronic GvHD would have a lower incidence of leukemic recurrence than patients who did not suffer this complication. Early studies investigating the probability of disease-free survival after BMT tended to confirm the presence of graft-versus-leukemia effect: patients with acute chronic GvHD had a lower recurrence rate than those who did not [44]. Subsequent studies have not confirmed these data for all types of leukemia [45,46], and only in children transplanted for acute lymphoblastic leukemia in second or later remission is a statistically significant evidence of graft-versus-leukemia effect convincingly demonstrated [47]. The possibility, however, remains an important one; if T-cells are implicated in the prevention of leukemic recurrence, then patients receiving purged marrow for the treatment of leukemia would be expected to have a high relapse rate. At the moment the position is unclear. Two groups carrying out bone marrow transplants for chronic granulocytic leukemia claim a higher incidence of recurrence after using marrow depleted of T-cells or treated with Campath-1 [48,49]. Other groups including our own have not found any increased incidence of relapse and, indeed, in our own series of 36 patients transplanted in first remission there has been only one possible leukemic recurrence (focal brain lesion of undetermined origin) over a 40 month period. The incidence of leukemic relapse in second or subsequent remission transplants is high regardless of whether the marrow is first T-cell depleted and, at the moment, it is not possible to say whether there is any overall increase in risk in the recipients of purged marrow. It seems likely that this issue will be hotly disputed for some time to come. Nonetheless, it is also clear that the ultimate aim of transplantation for leukemia is to avoid relapse altogether and we believe that T-cell depletion, which will allow us to safely explore the use of biological response modifiers, offers the best hope of achieving this end (see below).

Overall value of T-cell depletion and future prospects

At the moment Kaplin Meyer plots show a 73% probability of disease-free survival to 3½ years for patients receiving T-cell depleted BMT for acute leukemia in first remission. Other centers using T-cell depletion have reported even better results [29]. Because of the wide confidence limits associated with Kaplin Meyer plots of data from relatively small numbers of patients, it is not yet possible to say that T-cell depletion BMT offers a long term survival advantage over transplantation with unmanipulated marrow. But even if it were ultimately shown that T-cell depletion only reduced acute and chronic GvHD without influencing overall survival, it would still represent a major advance: many of the patients who survive conventional transplants have chronic GvHD and this produces poor quality of life, while death from severe acute GvHD is an horrific experience for patients, relatives and staff. However, T-cell depletion offers enormous potential for improving marrow grafting. The most obvious benefit is that transplants between MHC-mismatched donor and recipient become feasible since T-cell purging prevents significant GvHD even where donor and recipient are haploidentical or of treating marrow recipients with immuno-enhancing agents such as Interleukin 2 in an attempt to overcome the profound immunodeficiency that follows transplantation. Studies in animals have shown that Il-2 accelerates and potentiates GvHD when given to the recipients of convential allografts. In contrast, when animals are given T-cell depleted marrow grafts, GvHD does not occur even in the presence of high doses of IL-2, while there is increased recovery of cell mediated immune responses [50]. It is more difficult to assess the place of T-cell depleted transplantation for the treatment of non-malignant disease like aplastic anemia and thalassemia, since fewer centers have experience with these conditions and the risk of rejection is thought to be greater. But here too, with appropriate conditioning, it seems likely that high survival figures can be obtained which should be further improved as methods of immunological conditioning are explored.

Problems and outcome of autologous BMT

White T-cell depletion may present us with new problems to solve, at least it offers one benefit – the abolition of significant GvHD. Claims for the benefits of purging in autologous transplantation, however, are obstructed by two problems. First the effectiveness of purging on the patient marrow cannot readily be determined and, second, trials directly comparing the outcome of purged vs. unpurged BMT have not been undertaken.

1. Does purging remove residual blasts?

Whatever method of purging is used, alone or in combination, in preclinical models removal of 3-6 logs of malignant cells mixed with normal BM may be achieved without significant damage to BM progenitors [51]. These models are, however, somewhat artificial, as they use leukemic cell lines of known sensitivity to the purging method tested, and they might not therefore apply to clinical situations. In fact there is already evidence to support the contrary view: (1) leukemic blasts from patients with AML are no more sensitive to cyclophosphamide derivatives than normal BM progenitors and (2) immunologic methods using monoclonal antibodies and rabbit complement for lysing blasts from patients with ALL induces significant lysis (>2 logs) in only 75% of cases expressing the relevant antigen [53]. Effective lysis seems to be dependent on the density of the target antigen on the blasts and can be predicted by previous estimations of this parameter [54]. Unfortunately assessment of the efficiency of any form of BM purging at the time of transplant is not possible as recognizable blasts in BM harvested during remission are usually absent and up to now there has been no reliable cloning system for most leukemias/lymphomas.

2. Does purging increase patient survival?

The clinical value of any form of purging is similarly difficult to assess in the absence of any reported results from trials comparing purged to nonpurged autologous BMT. In addition the question of whether relapse after BMT is due to infused malignant cells or to resistant disease in the patient is always difficult to answer. Present experience in autologous BMT for lymphomas has emphasized the importance of residual disease [55], and this problem, of course, minimizes the possible impact of purging.

3. Outcome of purged BMT

Biophysical purging using discontinuous density gradients has been tried by a group in Houston in patients in relapse and was found not to be superior to unpurged BM [56,57]. At this stage of the disease the probability of resistant disease in the patient is, however, high and no patient remained disease-free.

Pharmacological purging is being used in many ongoing studies and has already produced some interesting results. The Johns Hopkins' group have used 4-hydroxyperoxy-cyclophosphamide to purge marrows from 25 patients with AML in second or third CR [58]. Four patients died early after BMT and another died later while persistently aplastic. Nine patients relapsed less than one year after BMT but eleven remained disease-free at 230 to 1650 days posttransplant. A group from Paris used another cyclophosphamide derivative, INN Mafosfamide, to purge the BM of 24 patients with ALL or AML at various stages of their disease [59]. Of 13 patients transplanted in first CR, 2 relapsed at 6 and 15 months, 2 died from transplant related complications and 9 remained disease-free at 8 to 26 months after BMT. In contrast 6 of 11 patients transplanted with more advanced diseases relapsed less than 5 months after BMT and only 2 remained disease-free, at 9 to 10 months.

Immunologic purging is presently restricted to eliminating malignant cells expressing surface antigens thought to be absent from the hemopoietic stem cells, and so it is used mainly for ALL and lymphoma BMT, although marrow from patients with non-hematologic tumors such as neuroblastoma may also be treated [60]. Most centers use cell killing techniques (predominantly complement-mediated cytolysis), but removal using immunomagnetic procedures is also under investigation, mainly in neuroblastoma. The two largest studies have used monoclonal antibodies and rabbit complement for the BM purging of children with common-ALL in second or subsequent CR. The Boston group used 2 antibodies J5+/−J2 in 34 patients [61]. Twelve patients died during the prolonged aplasia, 10 patients relapsed within 8 months and 12 remained disease-free at 4-50 months (median 22 months). The Minneapolis group used 3 antibodies BA1+BA2+BA3 and 1 or 2 incubations in 23 patients [62]. Only one patient died of infection, 15 relapsed and 7 remained disease-free 6-32 months after transplant (median 21 months).

4. Future prospects

These studies, as well as many smaller ones not reported here, support the view that BM purging is feasible in autologous BMT. Improvements in techniques to detect minimal residual disease will become available. These will permit more accurate assessment of the efficiency of BM purging and so reduce the risk of reinfusing a contaminated marrow. Nonetheless, the relapse rate after autologous BMT may remain higher than that observed after allogeneic BMT, perhaps due to the absence of a graft-versus-leukemia effect: improvements in pretransplant therapeutic regimens may therefore be needed in addition. Finally the problem of delayed engraftment will need to be overcome, as this leads to an unacceptably high incidence of infection related morbidity and mortality. Delay in engraftment could be due simply to previous patient chemotherapy but it may also be exacerbated by ex vivo BM purging. One potential means of accelerating engraftment will be to use recombinant GM-CSF in vivo, assuming that responsive precursors are present, and this agent may also prove of benefit to recipients of T-cell depleted allografts.

Conclusions

There is no doubt that marrow purging for both auto- and allogeneic transplantation offers major advantages in the treatment of hematological disease. The next 5 years should establish much more clearly (i) how the choice should be made between autograft and allografting, (ii) what procedure of purging should be adopted and (iii) how purging can be integrated with administration of recombinant cytokines such as Interleukin-2 and CSF to obtain optimum results.

References

1 Good RA, Kapoor N, Reisner Y. Bone marrow transplantation – an expanding approach to the treatment of many diseases. Cell Immunol 1983;82:36-54.
2. Hagenbeek A, Martens ACM. Cell separation studies in autologous bone marrow transplantation for acute leukemia. In: Gale RP (ed). Recent advances in bone marrow transplantation. New York: Alan R Liss Inc 1983:717-25.
3. De Witte T, Hoogenhout J, de Pauw B, et al. Depletion of donor lymphocytes by counterflow centrifugation successfully prevents acute graft-versus-host disease in matched allogeneic marrow transplantation. Blood 1986;67:1302-8.
4. Santos GW, Colvin OM. Pharmacological purging of bone marrow with reference to autografting. Clin Haematol 1986;15:67-84.
5. Douay L, Gorin NC, Lopez M, et al. Study of ASTA Z7557 on human hemopoietic stem cells: Application to autologous bone marrow transplantation. Exp Heamtol 1984;12:135-42.
6. Kaizer H, Stuart RK, Brookmeyer R, et al. Autologous bone marrow transplantation (BMT) in acute leukemia: a phase I study of in vitro treatment of marrow with 4-hydroperoxycyclophosphamide (4HC) to purge tumor cells. Blood 1985; 65:1504-10.
7. Stiff PJ, Wustrow T, DeRisi M, et al. An in vivo murine model of bone marrow (BM) purification of tumor by VP-16-213. Blood 1982;60(abstract):17a.
8. Prentice HG, Ganeshaguru K, Bradstock KF, et al. Remission induction with adenosine-deaminase inhibitor 2'-deoxycoformycin in Thy-lymphoblastic leukemia. Lancet 1980;i:170-3.
9. Sieber F, Spivak JL, Sutcliffe AM. Selective killing of leukemic cells by merocyanine 540-mediated photosensitization. Proc Natl Acad Sci USA 1984;81:7584-91.
10. Zander AR, Chow H, Yau J, et al. Pharmacological treatment of bone marrow grafts. In: Dicke KA, Spitzer G, Zander AR (eds). Autologous bone marrow transplantation – Proceedings of the First International Symposium. Houston: University of Texas, M.D. Anderson Hospital and Tumor Institute 1985:467-70.

11 Russell NH, Carron J, Hoffbrand AV, Bellingham AJ. The relative sensitivity of peripheral blood T-lymphocyte colony forming cells and bone marrow CFU-GM to deoxyadenosine and 2'-deoxycoformycin. Leuk Res 1985;9:315-22.

12. Jansen J, Falkenburg JHF, Stepan DE, Le Bien TW. Removal of neoplastic cells from autologous bone marrow grafts with monoclonal antibodies. Seminars in Haematol 1984;21:164-81.

13. Dicke KA, Poynton CH, Reading CL. Elimination of leukemic cells from remission marrow suspensions by an immunomagnetic procedure. In: Löwenberg B, Hagenbeeck J (eds). Minimal residual disease in acute leukemia. The Hague: Martinus Nijhoff Publ 1984:209-15.

14. Ritz J. Use of monoclonal antibodies in autologous and allogeneic bone marrow transplantation. Clin Haematol 1983;12:813-4.

15. Thorpe PE, Ross WCJ. The preparation and cytotoxic properties of antibody-toxin conjugates. Immunol Rev 1982;62:119-45.

16. Neville DM Jr, Chang TM. Receptor-mediated protein transport into cells. Entry mechanisms for toxins, hormones, antibodies, viruses, lysosomal hydrolases, asialoglycoproteins and carrier proteins. Cur Topics in Membranes and Transport 1978;10:65-84.

17. Casellas P, Canat X, Fauser AA, et al. Optimal elimination of leukemic T-cells from human bone marrow with T 101-Ricin A-chain immunotoxin. Blood 1985; 65:284-97.

18. Dicke KA, van Bekkum DW. Avoidance of acute secondary disease by purification of hemopoietic stem cells with density gradient centrifugation. Exp Hematol 1978;20:126-35.

19. Dicke KA, van Hooft J, van Bekkum DW. The selective elimination of immunologically competent cells from bone marrow and lymphatic cell mixtures. Transplantation 1968;6:562-70.

20. Rodt HV, Thierfelder S, Eulitz M. Anti-lymphocytic antibodies and marrow transplantation. III. Effect of heterologous anti-brain antibodies on acute secondary disease in mice. Eur J Immunol 1974;4:25-9.

21. Rodt H, Kolb HB, Netzel B, et al. Effect of anti-T-cell globulin on GvHD in leukemic patients treated with BMT. Transplantation Proc 1981;13:257-61.

22. Prentice HG, Blacklock HA, Janossy G, et al. Depletion of T-lymphocytes in donor marrow prevents significant graft-versus-host disease in matched allogeneic leukemic marrow transplant recipients. Lancet 1984;i:472-6.

23. Waldmann H, Hale G, Cividalli G, et al. Elimination of graft-versus-host disease by in vitro depletion of alloreactive lymphocytes with a monoclonal rat anti-human lymphocyte antibody (Campath-1). Lancet 1984;ii:483-7.

24. Filipovich AH, Vallera D, Youle RJ, et al. Ex-vivo treatment of donor bone marrow with anti-T-cell immunotoxins for prevention of graft-versus-host disease. Lancet 1984;i:469-72.

25. Albrechtsen D, Gauderbach G, Kvalheim G, et al. Depletion of T-cells from human bone marrow using antibody-coated magnetic polystyrene microspheres. Bone Marrow Transplantation 1986;1(suppl.1):108(Abstract).

26. Powles RL, Clink HM, Spence D, et al. Cyclosporin A to prevent graft-versus-host disease in man after allogeneic bone marrow transplantation. Lancet 1980;i: 327-31.

27. Ringden O, Lindholm A, Lönnqvist B, et al. Preliminary report of a randomized trial comparing cyclosporin and methotrexate for graft-versus-host disease prophylaxis in patients with hematologic malignancies. Exp Hematol 1987 (in press).

28. Glucksberg H, Storb R, Fefer A, et al. Clinical manifestation of graft-versus-host disease in human recipients of marrow from HLA-matched sibling donors. Transplantation 1974;18:295-304.
29. Slavin S, Or R, Weshler Z, et al. The use of total lymphoid irradiation for abrogation of host resistance to T-cell depleted marrow allografts. Bone Marrow Transplantation 1986;1(suppl.1):98(Abstract).
30. Kernan NA, Collins NH, Juliano L, et al. The number of residual T-lymphocytes measured by a limiting dilution assay correlates with the development of GvHD in 32 T-cell depleted bone marrow transplant recipients. J Cell Biochem 1986;(suppl.D):245(Abstract).
31. Storb R, Prentice RL, Thomas ED. Marrow transplantation for treatment of aplastic anemia. An analysis of factors associated with graft rejection. N Engl J Med 1977;296:61-5.
32. Patterson J, Prentice HG, Brenner MK, et al. Analysis of rejection after T-cell depleted allogeneic bone marrow transplantation. Brit J Haematol 1986;63:221-7.
33. Soderling CCB, Song CW, Vallera DA. A correlation between conditioning and engraftment in recipients of MHC-mismatched T-cell depleted murine bone transplants. J Immunol 1985;135:941-6.
34. Burnett AK, Robertson AG, Hann IM, et al. In vitro T-depletion of allogeneic bone marrow: prevention of rejection in HLA-matched transplants by increased TBI. Bone Marrow Transplantation 1986;(suppl.1):121(Abstract).
35. Dongworth DW, McMichael AJ. Inhibition of human T-lymphocyte function. Brit Med Bull 1984;40:154-60.
36. Fisher A, le Deist F, Blanche S, et al. HLA-mismatched bone marrow transplantation: in vivo use of an anti-LFA-1 monoclonal antibody for the prevention of graft failure, preliminary results. Bone Marrow Tranplantation 1986;(suppl.1):167(Abstract).
37. Witherspoon RP, Matthews D, Storb R, et al. Recovery of in vivo cellular immunity after human marrow grafting. Influence of time postgrafting and acute graft-versus-host disease. Transplantation 1984;37:145-50.
38. Crawford DH, Mulholland N, Iliescu V, Powles R. EB virus infection and immunity in bone marrow transplantation patients. Exp Hematol 1985;13(suppl.17):71(Abstract).
39. Janossy G, Prentice HG, Grob JPh, et al. T-cell recovery after T-depleted allogeneic bone marrow transplantation. Clin Exp Immunol 1986;63:577-86.
40. Brenner MK, Wimperis JZ, Reittie JE, et al. Recovery of immunoglobulin isotypes following T-cell allogeneic bone marrow transplantation. Brit J Haematol 1986;64:125-32.
41. Wimperis JZ, Brenner MK, Reittie JE, et al. Transfer of a functional B-cell immune system in T-cell depleted allogeneic bone marrow transplantation. Lancet 1986;i:339-43.
42. Rooney CM, Wimperis JZ, Brenner MK, et al. Natural killer cell activity following T-cell depleted allogeneic bone marrow transplantation. Brit J Haematol 1986;62:413-9.
43. Irle C, Chapuis B, Marini P, Jeannet M. Recovery of T-cells and LAK-cells after transplantation with Campath-1 + complement treated HLA-identical bone marrow. Bone Marrow Transplantation 1986;1(suppl.1):138(Abstract).
44. Weiden kPL, Flournoy N, Thomas ED, et al. Antileukemic effect of graft-versus-host disease in human recipients of allogeneic-marrow grafts. N Engl J Med 1979;300:1068-73.

45. Fefer A, Clift RA, Thomas ED. Allogeneic marrow transplantation for chronic granulocytic leukemia. JNCI 1986;76:1295-9.
46. Sullivan KM, Buckner CD, Weiden P, et al. Antileukemic effect of high-dose fractionated total body irradiation (TBI) and manipulation of graft-versus-host disease (GvHD) immunosuppression following bone marrow transplantation (BMT), Blood 1984;64(suppl.1;abstract 796):221a.
47. Sanders JE, Flournoy N, Thomas ED, et al. Marrow transplant experience in children with acute lymphoblastic leukemia: an analysis of factors associated with survival, relapse, and graft-versus-host disease. Med Ped Oncol 1985;13: 165-72.
48. Goldman JM, Apperley JF, Jones J, et al. Bone marrow transplantation for patients with chronic myeloid leukemia. N Engl J Med 1986;23:202-7.
49. Gale RP. Clinical trials of T-lymphocyte depletion in man. J Cell Biochem 1986; 103:10,210.
50. Malkovsky M, Brenner MK, Hunt R, et al. T-cell depletion prevents potentiation of graft-versus-host disease by IL-2. Cell Immunol 1986;103:476-80.
51. Treleaven JC, Kemshead JT. Removal of tumor cells from bone marrow: an evaluation of the available techniques. Hematol & Oncol 1985;3:65-75.
52. Singer CRJ. Evaluation of cyclophosphamide derivatives as purging agents in autologous bone marrow transplantation for AML. Bone Marrow Transplantation 1986;1(suppl.1):275(Abstract).
53. Campana D, Grob J-P, Coustan-Smith E, Janossy G. Efficacy of purging with monoclonal antibodies and complement in autologous bone marrow transplantation. Brit J Haematol. (In press).
54. Grob J-P, Campany D, Tims A, et al. Purging in autologous BMT: relevance of target antigen density on blasts to the efficiency of complement-mediated lysis. Bone Marrow Transplantation 1986;1(suppl.1);280(Abstract).
55. Anderson KC, Takvorian T, Ritz J, Nadler L. Monoclonal antibody (MA) purged autologous bone marrow transplantation (ABMT) for relapsed non-Hodgkin's lymphoma (NHL). Int J Cell Cloning 1985;3:220-8.
56. Zander AR, Vellekoop L, Spitzer G, et al. Combination of high dose cyclophosphamide, BCNU and VP-16 followed by autologous marrow rescue in the treatment of relapsed leukemia. Cancer Treat Rep 1981;65:366-81.
57. Dicke KA, Spitzer G, Peters L, et al. Autologous bone marrow transplantation in relapsed adult acute leukemia. Lancet 1978;i:514-7.
58. Yeager AM, Kaizer H, Santos CW, et al. Autologous bone marrow transplantation in patients with acute nonlymphocytic leukemia, using ex vivo marrow treatment with 4-hydroperoxycyclophosphamide. N Engl J Med 1986;315:141-5.
59. Gorin NC, Douay L, Laporte JP, et al. Autologous bone marrow transplantation using marrow incubated with ASTA Z7557 in adult acute leukemia. Blood 1986; 67:1367-76.
60. Pinkerton R, Philip T, Bouffet E, et al. Autologous bone marrow transplantation in pediatric solid tumors. Clin Haematol 1986;15:187-211.
61. Takvorian T, Sallan S, Ritza J. Monoclonal antibody purged autologous bone marrow transplantation for relapsed non T-cell acute lymphoblastic leukemia. In: Löwenberg B, Hazenbeek H (eds). Minimal residual disease in acute leukemia. Dordrecht: Martinus Nijhoff Publ 1986:266-74
62. Kersey J, LeBien T, Ballera D, et al. Allogeneic and autologous bone marrow transplantation: ex vivo purging with monoclonal antibody or immunotoxins to remove leukemic cells or to prevent graft-versus-host disease. In: Löwenberg B, Hazenbeek H (eds). Minimal residual disease in acute leukemia. Dordrecht: Martinus Nijhoff 1986:275-81

DISCUSSION

P.C. Das and S. Murphy

P. Rebulla (Milan): Dr. Slichter, how do you standardize the amount of plasma which is left on the platelet concentrate, I mean in routine. Can you comment on the practical aspects of separating platelet concentrates from the buffy coat.

S.J. Slichter (Seattle): The amount of plasma transferred is standardized by putting a wedge in each corner of a plasma expressor. The thickness of the wedge has been determined to leave the desired residual plasma volume on the platelet concentrate. However, to prevent plasma siphoning once the expressor plate has met the wedges, the plasma bag must be placed above the level of the platelet concentrate bag.

P. Rebulla: Well, if I understood properly in The Netherlands there are several centers where the platelet concentrates are separated from buffy coats. I think they make buffy coats and then they make centrifugations in order to sediment red cells and white cells. Do you have any experience?

S.J. Slichter: I have no experience with these procedures.

J.C. Bakker (Amsterdam): Dr. Slichter, you mentioned five methods by which we could measure platelet function or predict platelet function in vivo. You did not comment which method is your method of choice. A lot of investigators in the field of platelet preservation, prefer morphology as seen under the microscope, but it is not an objective method. Which would be your method of choice?

S.J. Slichter: I am one of those who have predominantly relied on in vivo measurements. I think all of us would love to have a standardized way that we could all agree on to do in vitro measurements. Sofar the one we do agree on is pH extremes. There is no good evidence from studies like dr. Murphy has done, that some of the lesions (either morphological changes, aggregation changes, hypotonic shock response, or whatever in vitro parameter you have been evaluating and have found to be abnormal), may well reverse either simply after taking off the plasma, in which the platelets have been stored adding fresh plasma in vitro and then showing that the abnormal parameter improves or in addition by simply putting the platelet in vivo into the patient's plasma. There is increasing evidence, however, that when the disc-sphere transformation measured by whatever technique is irreversible, there is a non-vital cell.

One of the major problems is that we cannot be exactly sure without in vivo transfusion experiments. So, I really believe that the in vitro measurements help us to exclude, but cannot necessarily help us to include platelets in terms of changes and storage to ensure we are delivering a quality product to the patient.

J.C. Bakker: Does dr. Murphy have any further comments?

S. Murphy (Philadelphia): Well, to summarize the situation we have a variety of measurements, which I think often correlate with each other. I think the safest and best thing to do in developmental work is to do a panel of in vitro studies. As a generalization cells that have good maintenance of morphology and therefore good maintenance of results in the more objective reflections in morphology, invariably do well when labelled with chromium. The problem is that some of the changes are more or less slowly reversible. One may have preparations after storage which will do well in vivo, but will not have done so well in the in vitro tests. So I think that as long as the in vitro tests are giving good results, you can feel relatively confident that the in vivo results will be good. But some poor results may still be compatible with good in vivo viability. I fundamentally agree with dr. Slichter that any method in storage has to be confirmed in vivo.

J.C. Bakker: Dr. Arnaud, the propylene glycol as a cryoprotectant seems promising as far as toxicity is concerned. In the beginning of your paper you mentioned a toxicity of dimethyl sulphoxide and glycerol. It would have been nice if you could compare the toxicity of glycerol and dimethyl sulphoxide to propylene glycol.

F.G. Arnaud (Cambridge): I did not do the experiments that way. If you look at the results quoted in the literature they are very difficult to compare because no one uses the same technique of preparation and assay of the cells. It is very difficult to correlate all the results. So, what we can say is just that propylene glycol seems much less toxic than DMSO, as 2.5 PG is tolerated by platelets. The advantage of propylene glycol is that, compared to glycerol for instance, it has to be incubated with platelets for a shorter time. One just has to incubate propylene glycol and platelets for 40 or 50 seconds and the propylene glycol will penetrate the cells. So it is much less toxic in the sense that the period of contact is reduced.

J.C. Bakker: Does DMSO penetrate the cell more slowly?

F.G. Arnaud: No, faster. Propylene glycol penetrates faster than glycerol. Propylene glycol permeation is somewhere in between glycerol and DMSO.

J.C. Bakker: Propylene glycol is not a normal compound of the body, so you would expect to have to remove it to zero levels. Is that possible?

F.G. Arnaud: Well yes, I have checked this by measuring the osmolarity of the final solution, when the cells are resuspended in stored plasma and I have obtained the same osmolarity as platelets suspended in fresh plasma. So, there might be still some propylene glycol, but this is not significant.

G.B. Humphrey (Groningen): Is there an arcadian rythm to circulating peripheral blood stem cells under normal circumstances or during the period of chemotherapy induced overshoot. Are there times when harvesting would be more ideal as a function of the time of the day?

M. Körbling (Heidelberg): Yes there is, but what we do is using this induction chemotherapy treatment just to mobilize the stem cells, that means we can reconstitute hemopoiesis. I think the problem is the pretreatment of the patient himself. If the patient is heavily pretreated we can not mobilize the stem cells at all, for example in the end-stage Hodgkin patients. If the treatment is less it is very well possible to mobilize the stem cells.

C.Th. Smit Sibinga (Groningen): Dr. Brozovic came at the end of his presentation with the bedside practice of leukocyte removal. We now know how crucial it is to have good control of the optimal depletion of white cells from, specifically, red cell concentrates, which are the major transfusion commodity, as well as from platelet concentrates. How do you implement quality control of the bedside practice?

B. Brozovic (London): In experimental trials one can take samples at various points of the giving set. We have done that at the bedside and found that blood which comes through the filter is almost leukocyte free. However, you can simulate this exercise in the laboratory. If you adjust the flow of the blood through the filter to 30 drops per minute, collect samples continuously, and count the white cells, you will find that filters perform well. So it seems that the efficiency of the filter to remove white cells is not dependant on the flow of blood through the filter.

C.Th. Smit Sibinga: I see your point. However, we are now shifting major responsibility from the experts in the field of tissue preservation to the bedside practitioner. Not that I do not have confidence in my clinical colleagues and the nursing staff, but we should realize that there is a danger in shifting this responsibility from the Blood Bank laboratory to the bedside.

B. Brozovic: You are quite right. There are two aspects of this problem. One is the responsibility for the quality of the product and the criteria used for it. The other perhaps more important question is who pays for the filter. Once the filters are used at the bedside, the financing or purchasing of the filters will fall entirely on the hospital.

C.Th. Smit Sibinga: That immediately brings you to the next danger in this practice, because now we rely on the policy of a hospital for buying whatever there is on the market. There are major experiences that not always the hospital buys the best and the most efficient material for optimal clinical use, because of economical impact.

B. Brozovic: You are quite right on that. My personal view is that filtration techniques ought to remain in Blood Transfusion Centers. There is no reason why that cannot be done and it is really just convenience to place them at the bedside.

M.K. Elias (Groningen): Dr. Brozovic, I have a comment on the efficiency of the filter to retain the leukocytes, especially the specific filters. Although called selective for leukocytes they also retain red cells and platelets, but this is not valid for all the products. If I take for example the Imugard filter, the recovery of platelets is 60 or 70% when filtering a unit of whole blood, while the recovery is 90%, when filtering leukocyte-poor blood. We have done a comparative study in Groningen using different leukocyte contamination gradients to determine the capacity of the filter to retain the leukocytes. So we have used the leukocyte-poor platelet concentrates and a pool of standard platelet concentates and a pool of buffy coats. We found that the more the product is contaminated with white and red cells, the less is the recovery of platelets.

B. Brozovic: Well, this is certainly a vary interesting study. We do not know exactly the mechanism of retention of leukocytes and platelets on the filters. There must be a good explanation for your observations, but I can not say.

P. Rebulla: I would like to make a comment on the bedside filtration point. The best quality control of this procedure could be monitoring the febrile transfusion reaction rate in a reactive patient population. We have been quite happy during the last year transferring the whole filtration procedure to the wards with two different filters: the Pall and the Sepacell. The overall reaction rate remained unchanged in thalassemia patients, when it was compared with units filtered in the Blood Bank. So, we are quite happy with the bedside procedure and no problems were seen.

S. Murphy: Dr. Körbling, about the collection of stem cells from the peripheral blood, do you need to do CFU-C and CFU-GM measurements to know whether you have an adequate dose or could you not just count the number of cells which look like lymphocytes to know whether you have had an adequate collection. As I understand it, there is no known necessary correlation between the colony forming cells and the cells that rescue the patient.

M. Körbling: You are totally right. The CFU-C or CFU-GM assay is the best indicator, but what we have learned especially from purging is that the relationship shifts completely. If we do a pharmocological purging, we transplant marrow grafts for example without any evidence for CFU-GM and the patient reconstitutes very well.

C.Th. Smit Sibinga: Dr. Körbling, you see for the future an indication in peripheral stem cell collection for those who are at risk for continuous exposure to irradiation. We see now what comes of Tsernobyl and all know that these disasters might occur anywhere in the world. Do you see this indication limited to only workers in nuclear plants or do you see this broader. How about the mobility of people and how do you see then bone marrow following them around the world.

M. Körbling: We made such a proposal to the German government. First of all the procedure is very expensive, per person about 10,000 DM. Now, that is not the real problem. The real problem is a political one. Nobody would like to admit, especially in Germany, that nuclear power plants are not 100% safe. That is the reason that we cannot proceed with that approach. Even the workers in the plant would not admit that their plant is not 100% safe. The people we would like to apherese and collect stem cells from, are mainly people who have to do with repairment. That is the most risky thing to do in atomic power plants. The government of Baden Würtenberg West Germany, has some 200 names on a list. That means a realistic number of 200 people from whom blood stem cells are to be collected and preserved as a preventive measure.

IV. LABORATORY ASPECTS

HLA-MATCHING AND CROSSMATCHING IN PLATELET TRANSFUSION

J.M. Beelen

Introduction

Repeated platelet transfusion often induces alloimmunization to HLA-antigens resulting in a state of refractoriness of the thrombocytopenic patient. Such patients can be successfully treated with platelet concentrates from an HLA compatible sibling donor [1]. Also matched platelets from unrelated donors can survive normally in the highly sensitized patient [2-4]. The HLA-antigens are coded by a very polymorphic genetic system. Therefore even in a large pool of blood bank donors chances of finding a perfectly matched donor are low. However in the alloimmunized thrombocytopenic recipient the effectiveness of transfusion of platelets from donors selectively mismatched for crossreactive antigens does not differ from the cell increment obtained with HLA fully matched platelets [5,6]. A positive crossmatch as a result of circulating antibodies against donor incompatibilities is associated with a poor transfusion response. HLA-antibody screening enables us to determine which donor HLA-incompatibilities will not lead to a positive crossmatch and therefore can be considered as acceptable mismatches. The aim of this paper is to summarize the methods which are currently used in routine HLA-typing and antibody screening.

HLA-typing techniques

In this review, Moore already discussed the genetics and structure of the HLA molecules [7]. The HLA-ABC (class I) antigens are expressed on all nucleated cells and also on platelets whereas of the periferal blood cells only B-lymphocytes, monocytes and macrophages do express HLA-DR (class II) antigens. The incidence of alloimmunization is principally defined by the degree of class II incompatibility expressed by the contaminating white blood cells in the platelet concentrate [8-10]. Until now, HLA-DR matching has not been applied in platelet transfusion therapy. By the use of leukocyte-poor platelet suspensions the incidence of sensitization is successfully reduced [11-14]. If as a result of alloimmunization antibodies are formed, those responsible for a poor platelet survival are directed against class I antigens and also against platelet specific antigens [15]. However, because the incidence of antibody formation against platelet specific antigens is low, selection of platelet donors for the sensitized patients is primarily based on HLA-ABC compatibility.

HLA-ABC typing

HLA-ABC typing is done by a microlymphocytotoxicity assay. Mononuclear cells are isolated from heparinized or defibrinated blood by Ficoll Isopaque density gradient centrifugation. In 60 wells microtiter plates 1 μl of cell suspension with a concentration of $2 x 10^6$ cells per ml is added to each well containing 1 μl of a specific antiserum. After 30 minutes incubation time 5 μl rabbit complement is added. Cytotoxicity is visualized by eosine or trypan blue dye exclusion. Automatic reading of the trays has become possible by using propidium iodide (red fluorescence) to visualize cell lysis [16]. The most reliable results are obtained when in a double staining technique carboxyfluorescein diacetate (green fluorescence) is used as a viability label simultaneously [17].

HLA-DR typing

In the mononuclear cell fraction isolated by Ficoll Isopaque gradient centrifugation only B-lymphocytes and monocytes/macrophages do express HLA-DR antigens. By the use of an enriched B-lymphocyte suspension, e.g. obtained with a rosetting technique, the standard microlymphocytotoxicity assay can be applied for HLA-DR typing. However, the two-color fluorescence technique, originally described by Van Rood and his coworkers, circumvents the time and cell consuming enrichment procedures [18]. In this technique B-cells and monocytes are specifically labeled by fluorescein (FITC) conjugated anti-human immunoglobulin. Cell lysis is now visualized with ethidium-bromide. In the two-color fluorescence method not only cytotoxicity is measured but this test also shows whether the cell lysis is restricted to the class II positive cells, indicating that the positive reaction is the result of binding of an anti-DR serum.

Typing sera

Numerous typing sera are needed to characterize all of the antigens encoded by the different loci of the highly polymorphic HLA system. Sera of multiparous women, successively alloimmunized by pregnancy against paternal incompatibilities of the foetus, are still the most important source of typing reagents. Since alloimmunization only occurs against a limited number of antigens, the induced antibody is frequently directed against a single antigenic specificity or against a crossreactive group of antigens to which one of the paternal incompatibilities belongs. This is in clear contrast with the antibodies detected in sera of patients alloimmunized by multiple transfusions, which are largely multispecific.

Because of the differences in expression of class I and class II antigens a positive reaction due to HLA-ABC antibodies will overrule cytotoxicity induced by anti-DR sera. By platelet absorption the HLA-ABC antibodies can be selectively eliminated leaving the HLA-DR antibodies in the serum. The introduction of the hybridoma technique by Köhler and Milstein has enabled the production of monoclonal antibodies against HLA-antigens.

Until now, only a limited number of specificities can be defined by monoclonal reagents. A striking feature of some of the monoclonal antibodies is that they may detect antigenic determinants that have not been picked up by alloantisera. For example, antigenic variants of HLA-A2, a specificity by well defined alloantisera, have now been characterized by monoclonal antibodies.

A highly conscientious analysis of the reaction patterns of the alloantisera shows that antibodies against these antigenic splits are only rarely formed. Antigenic determinants shared by the different antigenic splits, detected by antibodies with a broad specificity, seem to be more immunogenic. Therefore these subtypes, although very important from the immunogenetist' point of view, may be of minor relevance in clinical HLA-matching.

Antibody screening

Sensitization to HLA-antigens as the cause of refractoriness of a patient transfused with platelets from a random donor can be confirmed by antibody screening. In the microlymphocytotoxicity assay the patient serum is tested against a panel of lymphocytes. By selecting a panel representing the HLA-specificities in a balanced make up, it is possible to characterize the antibody specificity. In sera of thrombocytopenic patients alloimmunized by multiple cell concentrate transfusions, HLA-antibodies are detected which are frequently multispecific. By testing the patient serum with lymphocytes of panel donors selectively mistmatched for one single HLA-antigen one can determine which HLA-incompatibilities can be considered as acceptable. By this procedure of intelligent mismatching, the number of compatible donors eligible for the strongly alloimmunized patient can be greatly extended.

Crossmatching

Crossmatching is the ultimate test to confirm compatibility between the sensitized patient and the selected platelet donor. An optimal donor selection is achieved with a combination of lymphocytotoxic and platelet specific crossmatching [19,20]. The standard lymphocytotoxicity assay is used for the lymphocytotoxic crossmatch. The platelet crossmatch techniques will be discussed by Von dem Borne [21]. If crossmatching is performed by the microlymphocytotoxicity test only cytotoxic HLA-antibodies will be detected. A positive platelet crossmatch with a corresponding negative lymphocytotoxicity can be caused by non-cytotoxic HLA-antibodies and antibodies directed against crossmatch-specific alloantigens. A chloroquine modification of the platelet crossmatch enables to distinguish between HLA- and platelet-specific antibodies. Chloroquine treated platelets no longer react with HLA-antibodies whereas reactions with platelet-specific antibodies are unchanged or even enhanced [22,23]. A positive platelet crossmatch is always accompanied by a low platelet increment indicating that cytotoxic and non-cytotoxic HLA-antibodies as well as platelet specific antibodies may be responsible for a poor platelet transfusion response [14].

The presence of platelet-specific antibodies will make selection for platelet donors compatible for platelet-specific antigens obligatory.

Concluding remarks

The number of compatible donors available to the alloimmunized patient can be increased significantly by the use of platelets from donors selectively mismatched for HLA-antigens crossreactive with antigens of the patient.

For the highly immunized patient the number of compatible donors can be greatly extended by defining the acceptable mismatches in an antibody screening with lymphocytes of selected panel donors each of which is incompatible for a single antigenic specificity.

Crossmatching is the ultimate test to confirm platelet donor compatibility. A lymphocytotoxic crossmatch in combination with a platelet crossmatch will detect the antibodies responsible for a poor platelet survial in an optimal way.

References

1. Yankee RA, Grunet FC, Rogentine GN. Platelet transfusion therapy, the selection of compatible platelet donors for refractory patients by lymphocyte HLA typing. N Engl J Med 1969;281:1208-12.
2. Thorsby E, Helegesen A, Gjemdal T. Repeated platelet transfusion from HLA compatible unrelated and sibling donors. Tissue Antigens 1972;2:397-404.
3. Yankee RA, Graff KS, Dowling R, Dowling R, Henderson ES. Selection of unrelated compatible platelet donors by lymphocyte HLA-matching. N Engl J Med 1973;15:760-4.
4. Lohrmann HP, Bull MI, Decter JA, Yankee RA, Graw RR Jr. Platelet transfusion from HLA compatible donors to alloimmunized patients. Ann Intern Med 1974;80:9-14.
5. Duquesnoy RJ, Filip DJ, Rodey GE, Rimm AA, Aster RH. Successful transfusion of platelets 'mismatched' for HLA-antigens to alloimmunized thrombocytopenic patients. Am J Hematol 1977;2:19-26.
6. Dahlke MB, Weiss KL. Platelet transfusion from donors mismatched for crossreactive HLA-antigens. Transfusion 1984;24:299-302.
7. Moore SB. The human MHC and its relevance to transfusion practice. In: Smit Sibinga CTh, Das PC, Engelfriet CP (eds). White cells and platelets in blood transfusion. Boston, Dordrecht, Lancaster: Martinus Nijhoff 1987:1-12.
8. Welsh KI, Burgos H, Batchelor JR. The immune response to allogeneic rat platelets: Ag-B antigens in matrix for lacking Ia. Eur J Immunol 1977;7:267-72.
9. Batchelor JR, Welsh KI, Burgos H. Transplantation antigens per se are poor immunogens within a species. Nature 1978;273:54-6.
10. Claas FH, Smeenk RJT, Schmidt R, van Steenbrugge GJ, Eernisse JG. Alloimmunization against the MHC antigens after platelet transfusion is due to contaminating leukocytes in the platelet suspension. Exp Hematol 1981;9:84-9.
11. Eernisse JG, Brand A. Prevention of platelet refractoriness due to HLA-antibodies by the administration of leukocyte-poor blood components. Exp Hematol 1981;9:77-83.

12. Schiffer CA, Dutcher JP, Aisner J, Hogge D, Wiernik PH, Rully JP. A randomized trial of leukocyte-depleted platelet transfusion to modify alloimmunization in patients with leukemia. Blood 1983;52:815-20.
13. Fischer M, Chapman JR, Ting A, Morris PJ. Alloimmunization to HLA-antigens following transfusion with leukocyte-poor and purified platelet suspensions. Vox Sang 1985;49:331-5.
14. Murphy MF, Metcalfe P, Thomas H, et al. Use of leukocyte-poor blood components and HLA-matched-platelet donors to prevent HLA alloimmunization. Brit J Haematol 1986;62:529-34.
15. Pegels JG, Bruynes EC, Engelfriet CP, von dem Borne AEG Kr. Serological studies in patients on platelet and granulocyte-substitution therapy. Brit J Haematol 1982;52:59-68.
16. Bruning JW. Automatic reading of HLA-ABC typing and screening, the propidium iodide (PI) method. Hum Immunol 1982;5:225-31.
17. Bruning JW, Kardol MJ, Arentzen R. Carboxyfluorescein fluorochromasia assays. I. Non-radioactively labeled cell mediated lympholysis. J Immunol Methods 1980;33:33-44.
18. Van Rood JJ, van Leeuwen A. Simultaneous detection of two cell populations by two-color fluorescence and application to the recognition of B-cell determinants. Nature 1976;262:795-7.
19. Brand A, van Leeuwen A, Eernisse JG, van Rood JJ. Platelet transfusion therapy. Optimal donor selection with a combination of lymphocytotoxicity and platelet fluorescence test. Blood 1978;51:781-8.
20. Waters AH, Minchinton RH, Bell R, Foros JM, Lister TA. A crossmatching procedure for the selection of platelet donors for alloimmunized patients. Brit J Haematol 1981;48:59-68.
21. Von dem Borne AEG Kr. Platelet antibody detection. In: Smit Sibinga CTh, Das PC, Engelfriet CP (eds). White cells and platelets in blood transfusion. Boston, Dordrecht, Lancaster: Martinus Nijhoff 1987:261-7.
22. Nordhagen R, Flaatzen ST. Chloroquine removal of HLA-antigens from platelets for the platelet immunofluorescence test. Vox Sang 1985;48:156-9.
23. Metcalfe P, Minchinton RM, Murphy MF, Waters AH. Use of chloroquine-treated granulocytes and platelets in the diagnosis of immune cytopenias. Vox Sang 1985;49:340-5.

CELL CULTURE AND IMMUNE FUNCTION TESTS

J.W. Smit, J.T.M. de Wolf, M.T. Esselink, M.J.A. van Luyn, N.R. Blom, T. Cazemier, H.E. Modderman, W. Huiges, M.R. Halie

Introduction

Concerning the role of white blood cells in blood transfusions different aspects have to be considered:

1. Antibody formation against HLA and cell specific antigens by the patients immune system.
2. The influence of transfusion on the composition of different white blood cell populations in the patient. Several studies have demonstrated that supportive hemotherapy may influence the immune system: improvement of graft rejection in renal transplantation [1]; alterations in lymphocyte subpopulations in hemophilia patients [2].
3. The properties and the function of the white blood cells of the donor, which have been collected for transfusion. For instance granulocytes used in transfusion for granulocytopenic patients. But most important are here perhaps the bone marrow grafts now that bone marrow transplantation has become an established procedure in the treatment of hematological disorders.

Cell separation techniques (density gradient centrifugation, counter flow centrifugation) and monoclonal antibodies make it possible to distinguish and to isolate functionally different cell populations. Functions of granulocytes, monocytes and of lymphocyte subpopulations can be tested separately in the laboratory.

Clonogenic colony assays with their specific growth factors have been developed to demonstrate the presence or absence of progenitor cells of the different hemopoietic cell lineages.

These different techniques can also be applied in the above mentioned aspects of blood transfusion and white blood cells.

Lymphocytes

In the fine-tuned network of interacting cells in the immune system two major functionally different lymphocyte populations can be distinguished: B- and T-cells. These two types of lymphocytes are derived from or processed by two different primary lymphoid organs, the adult bone marrow and the thymus respectively, and can be identified by characteristic membrane surface markers.

B-lymphocyte bear surface membrane-bound immunoglobulins, acting as specific antigen receptors. The surface immunoglobulins are detected by staining a lymphocyte suspension (isolated by density gradient centrifugation) with fluorescein labeled specific antibodies to the appropriate immunoglobulin on the membrane. Since immunoglobulins can also be bound to Fc-receptors for immunoglobulins, also present on other than B-cells, care should be taken in counting the number of B-cells, because the fluorescein labeled anti-immunoglobulin conjugate will also stain these Fc-receptor bound immunoglobulins. Though B-lymphocytes are classically defined by membrane-bound surface immunoglobulins, there are now B-cell specific monoclonal antibodies available, suitable for use in the immunofluorescence technique.

T-lymphocytes were originally identified by the cell marker which binds to sheep erythrocytes. At present these lymphocytes are detected using monoclonal antibodies in the immunofluorescence technique. Hybridoma technology has resulted in the production of many monoclonal antibodies which have been valuable in defining different lineage stages in the maturation of the T-cell in the thymus and in defining different functional T-cell subsets.

Using flow cytometry techniques which allow the simultaneous detection of more than one fluorescent label, it is possible to define the two major T-cell subpopulations, i.e. T-helper and T-suppressor lymphocytes. This is illustrated in Figure 1.

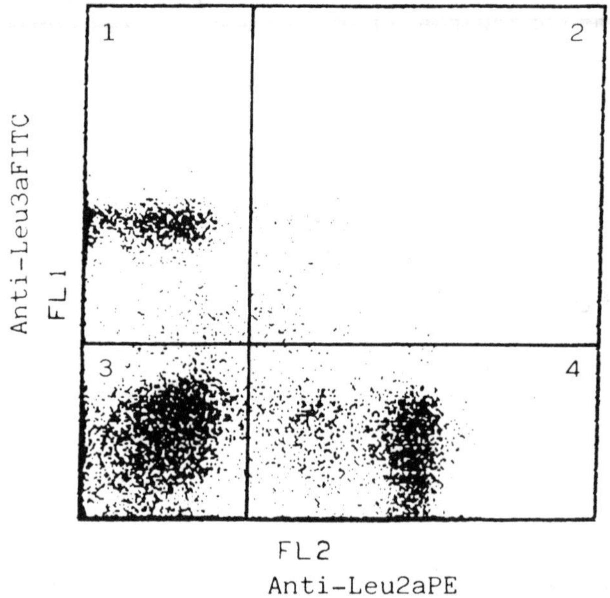

Figure 1. Simultaneous enumeration of T-helper (anti-Leu-3aFITC) and T-suppressor (anti-Leu-2aPE) cells in peripheral blood.
Quadrant 1: T-helper cells; Quadrant 2: Double labeled cells (rare in normal blood); Quadrant 3: Unstained cells; Quadrant 4: T-suppressor cells.

Other techniques to detect cell populations by surface markers are the immunoenzyme techniques, i.e. the immunoperoxidase and the alkaline phosphatase-anti-alkaline phosphatase (APAAP) methods. Especially the latter technique, introduced by the group of Mason [3] in Oxford and combining phenotyping and morphology has been propagated as extremely sensitive. However, in our hands only a selective number of monoclonal antibodies is reacting after the appropriate fixation. For instance the helper/inducer T-cell subset could be detected with the anti-Leu-3a monoclonal antibody but not with the OKT4 monoclonal antibody while until now B-cell specific monoclonal antibodies gave hardly any positive results. Similar findings were reported by Lowenthal et al. [4].

Besides the B- and T-lymphocytes there is in the peripheral blood a population of lymphocytes which do not have markers corresponding to B- or T-lymphocytes. This population is called the Null cell population. The majority of this lymphocyte population is characterized by Fc-receptors and by the monoclonal antibody anti-Leu-11. Morphologically these cells are defined as the large granular lymphocytes (LGL) due to the azurophilic granules in the cytoplasm. At the ultrastructural level part of these granules are characteristic parallel tubular structures (Fig. 2) [5]. It has been suggested that these structures play a role in the function of these cells as effector cells in the natural killer (NK) and antibody dependent cellular cytotoxicity or killer (K) processes [6].

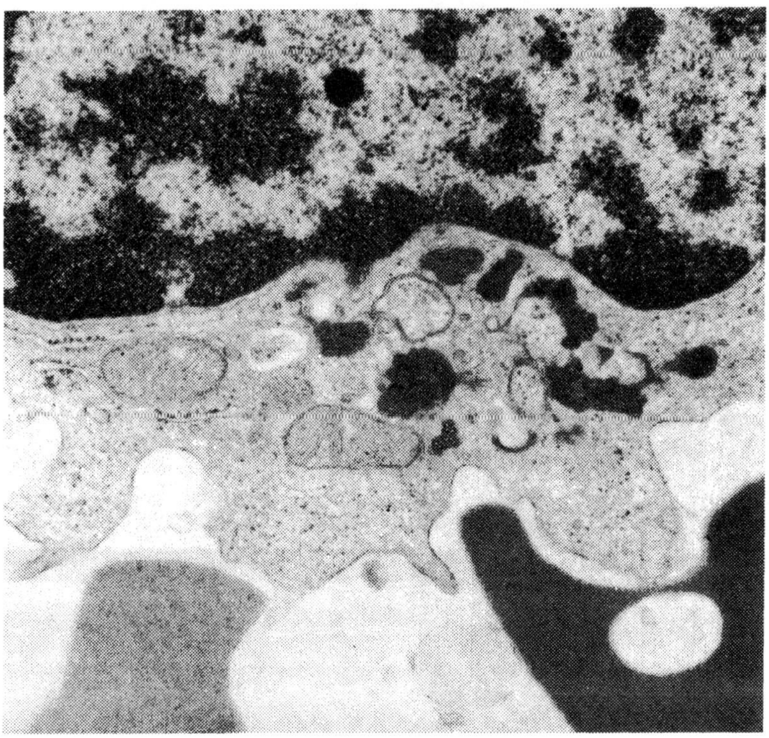

Figure 2. Part of a large granular lymphocyte showing parallel tubular structures.

Immune function tests

The demonstration of the presence of lymphocyte subsets is not always a condition for functional activity. This is illustrated in Table 1, which summarizes the phenotype and functional activity of the peripheral blood lymphocytes in a group of patients with Tγ lymphocytosis. In these patients an expanded population of Tγ lymphocytes has been found. Though these cells are T8 positive they do not possess the suppressor cell activity of normal T8 positive lymphocytes. Therefore it is often necessary to study functional activity in vitro.

Following stimulation by their specific antigen the cells of the B-lineage can proliferate and differentiate into antibody secreting plasmacells, thus mediating humoral immunity. In vitro this process can be mimiced by stimulating lymphocytes with mitogenic lectins, derived from plants or bacteria. Thus the functional activity of human B-lymphocytes has been studied in a pokeweed mitogen (PWM) driven immunoglobulin (Ig) production system. The results can be assessed by means of determining the number of Ig synthesizing cells (by an immunofluorescence technique) or by measuring the Ig levels in the culture supernatant as described by Rümke et al. [7]. The in vivo formation of antibodies against specific antigens can be tested by using patients serum in an in vitro assay, e.g. the detection of antibodies directed against HLA, granulocytes or thrombocytes.

Table 1. Phenotype and functional properties of Tγ cells in most patients with Tγ lymphocytosis.

E_{SRBC}	Fγ	T3	T4	T8	T11	Help	Suppr.	K	NK
+	+	+	−	+	+	−	−	+	−

Because the B-cell stimulation system requires the presence of other cell types, i.e. monocytes and T-lymphocytes, the in vitro regulating activity of the latter cell type and its subsets has also been studied by means of the PWM-driven polyclonal IgM synthesis system. Aspecific T-cell function may be studied by stimulation with the mitogens phytohemagglutin (PHA) and concanavalin A (Con A) using a ^{3}H-thymidin incorporation technique. The same ^{3}H-thymidin uptake is used to evaluate T-cell function in a mixed lymphocyte culture (MLC). In this sytem T-cells are stimulated by contact with allogeneic lymphocytes, resulting in transformation.

NK- and K-cell activities attributed to the normal Leu-11 positive LGL, are measured in an in vitro assay using ^{51}Cr labeled target cells from cultured cell lines. The antibody dependent cellular cytotoxicity (K-cell activity) is often measured with P-815 mouse mastocytoma cells, sensitized with rabbit IgG antibodies [8], the NK-cell activity with the myeloid/erythroblastoid K-562 cell line [9]. However, other target cells are also possible.

Hemopoietic cell culture methods

In the normal peripheral blood several cell types can be demonstrated: erythrocytes, (neutrophilic, eosinophilic and basophilic) granulocytes, monocytes, lymphocytes and thrombocytes. All these cell lines originate – directly or indirectly – from the bone marrow, where in the normal adult human hemopoiesis takes place.

By morphological examination of the bone marrow it is possible to recognize, in addition, most of the immature precursors of these cell lines, however, only of the last five or six cell divisions. More immature precursors, the multipotential stem cells and the committed progenitor cells are too few to be recognized microscopically.

For this purpose in vitro clonal assay systems have been developed, at first in the mouse. Later these systems were modified for growth of human hemopoietic cell lines. Reviews on hemopoietic cell cultures are found in references 10-12. In Figure 3 a schematic representation of the multipotential stem cell and the related precursor cells in each lineage is presented. Clonal assays for different progenitor cells are available, not only for the myeloid and erythroid cells but also for the lymphoid cells.

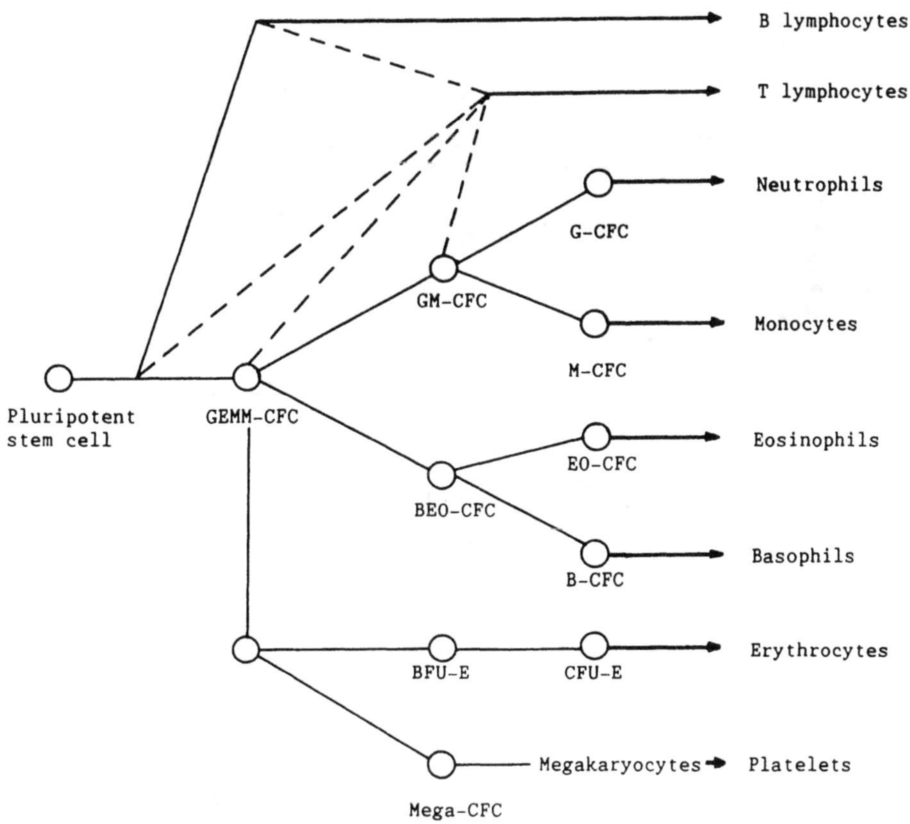

Figure 3. Schematic representation of the hematopoiesis. Some lines are hypothetical.

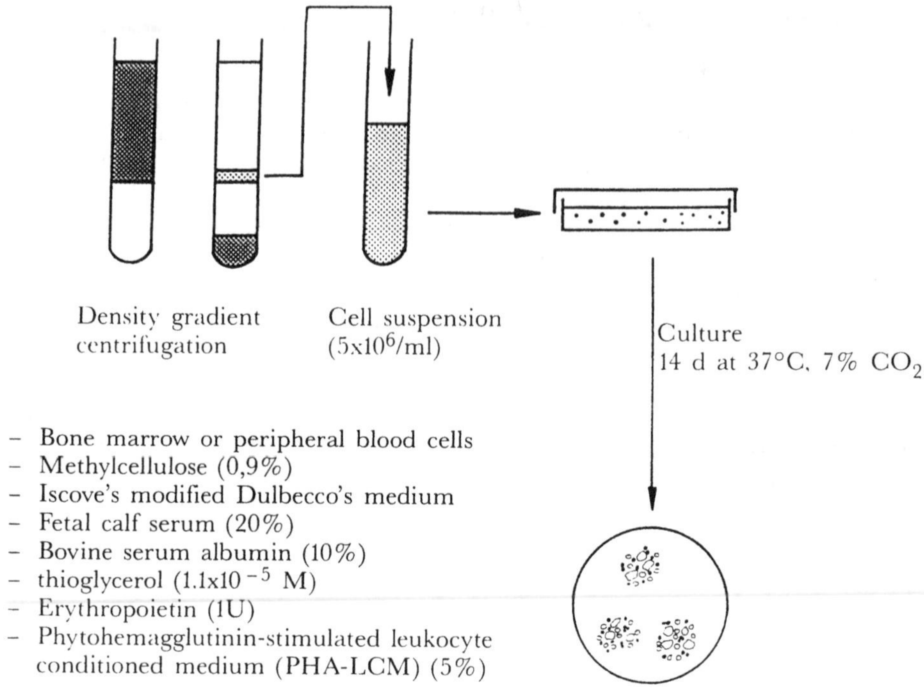

Figure 4. Culture conditions for CFU-GEMM.

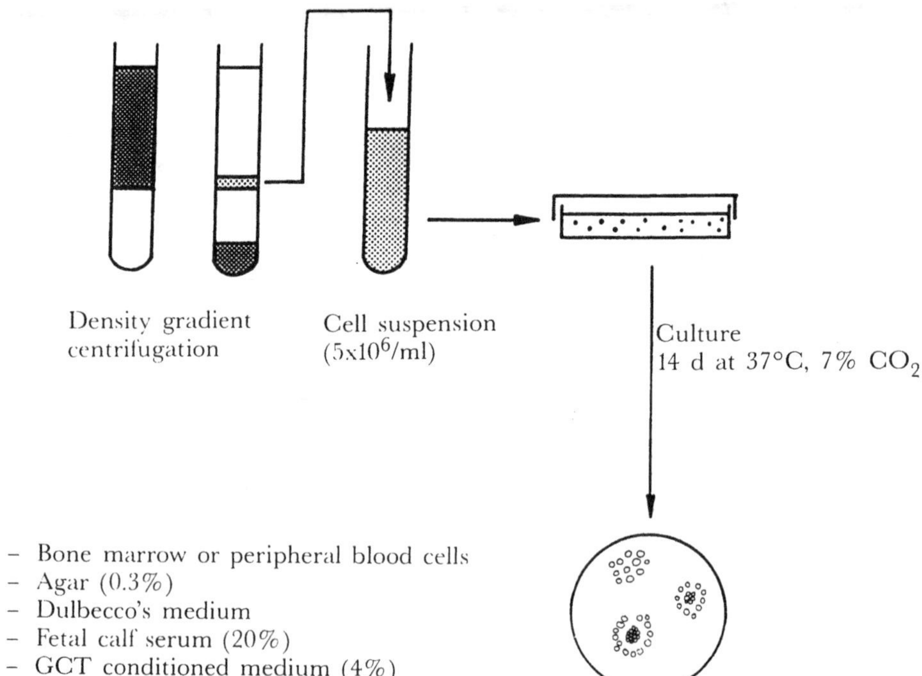

Figure 5. Culture conditions for CFU-C.

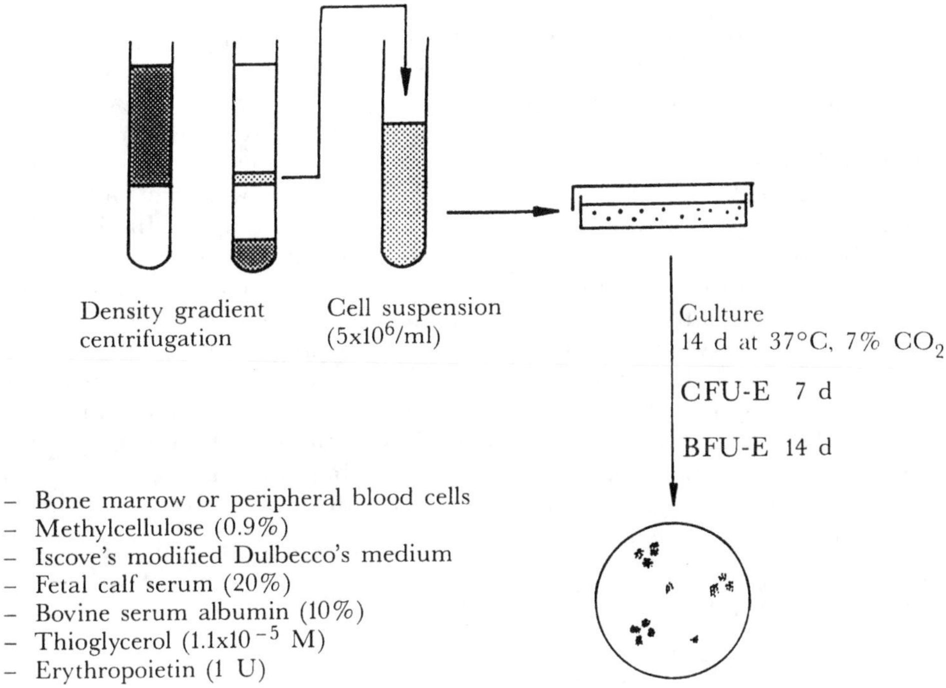

Figure 6. Culture conditions for red cell procursors.

In Figures 4, 5 and 6 the culture conditions are outlined for CFU-GEMM, CFU-C (CFU-GM) and CFU-E and BFU-E respectively. These clonal assays are most often used in clinical situations. The frequency distribution of these various colony types of nine healthy volunteers show a considerable variation as demonstrated in Figure 7.

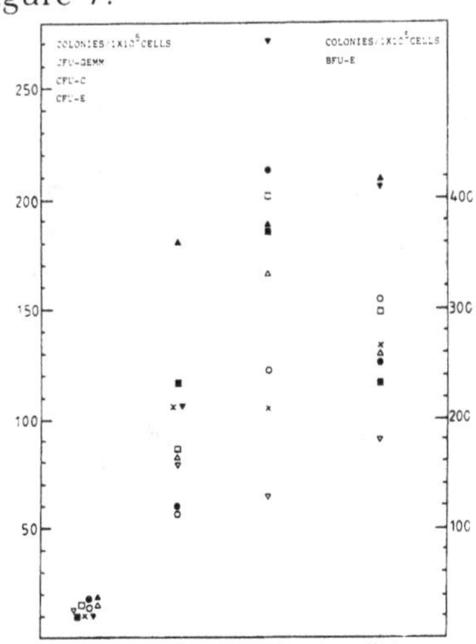

Figure 7. Frequency distribution of CFU-GEMM, CFU-C, CFU-E and BFU-E in the bone marrow of nine healthy volunteers.

Essential in these cultures is the presence of hemopoietic growth factors or colony stimulating activity (CSA). In the originally developed culture system of Pike and Robinson [13] a double agar layer was used. The underlay contained blood leukocytes (feeder cell layer) which produce the CSA, while in the overlay the cells to be cultured were present. CSA is also produced by other cell types, which has led to the commercial production of growth factor containing media, e.g. medium conditioned by the histiocytic cell GCT (giant cell tumor). This medium is used in our CFU-GM assay. In the CFU-GEMM and the CFU-E assays a leukocyte conditioned medium is used, after the leukocyte suspension ahs been stimulated with phytohemagglutin (PHA). Because the use of these CSA containing conditioned media is far from standardized it is very important that considerable progress has been made in identifying and characterizing the different colony stimulating factors (CSF's), glycoproteins in the 20,000-70,000 molecular weight range and active at very low concentrations. Recently several CSF's have been purified and cDNA's have been cloned (Table 2). This may lead to mass-production of recombinant hemopoietic growth factors with possible clinical use in the future [14].

Table 2. Cloned human hemopoietic growth factors.

	Responding cells
GM-CSF	Granulocytes, macrophages, eosinophils
G-CSF	Granulocytes
M-CSF	Macrophages
IL-3	Multilineage
Erythropoietin	Erythroid cells
EPA	Early erythroid cells
IL-2	T-lymphocytes

Another system controlling the hemopoiesis is achieved by the stromal cells in the bone marrow, forming the hemopoietic microenvironment [15]. Though the investigations concerning the role of the microenvironment on the blood cell formation are preliminary, both cell-cell contact and local short range humoral factors are suggested to be of influence. Long-term bone marrow cultures or Dexter cultures [16] are an approach to study both the function of the microenvironmental cells and growth factors necessary for blood cell formation from stem and progenitor cells. These cultures are also propagated by Zanjani et al. [17] to provide a system capable of producing progenitor cells and mature granulocytes, opening the way for clinical use of these cell cultures. Other accessory cells in the bone marrow, i.e. T-lymphocytes and monocytes-macrophages have also been found to influence hemopoiesis. Both cell types are able to produce colony stimulating activity, thus promoting growth of hemopoietic progenitors. However, activated T-lymphocytes and monocytes can also exert an inhibitory effect on blood cell formation, originally demonstrated in diseased states, later on also found in experiments concerning normal hemopoiesis. Therefore these accessory cells with dual function may have important regulating activities on the hemopoietic process. The effect of these cells probably depends on local short range influences, i.e. the presence of activators, differentiation state of the precursor cell and the level of γ-interferon [18-20]. In vitro examination of the mechanisms by which these accessory cells affect blood cell formation in health and disease requires therefore standardized procedures. Variations in experimental conditions may change the interpretation of the results. Such an example is demonstrated in Table 3, where different monocyte fractions exerted different effects on BFU-E in peripheral blood.

Table 3. Effect of different monocyte fractions on BFU-E.

Cell populations	
	– Density gradient centrifugation of peripheral blood cells: lymphocytes + monocytes – Elutriation: – lymphocyte/monocyte fraction = intermediate fraction (I) – monocyte fraction: MON_{EL} – Depletion of monocytes from the intermediate fraction by adherence: $MON_{ADH/I}$ and $lymphocyte_I$ – Separation of T- and non-T-cells from $lymphocytes_I$ (E_{SRBC} rosetting/density gradient centrifugation): T_I and non-T_I-cells

Cell cultures	**BFU-E colonies**
$0.5x10^5$ NON-T_I	108
$0.5x10^5$ NON-T_I + 0.25 $MON_{ADH/I}$	132
$0.5x10^5$ NON-T_I + 0.25 MON_{EL}	210
$0.5x10^5$ NON-T_I + $4.0x10^5$ T_I	126
$0.5x10^5$ NON-T_I + $4.0x10^5$ T_I + $0.25x10^5$ $MON_{ADH/I}$	164
$0.5x10^5$ NON-T_I + $4.0x10^5$ T_I + $0.25x10^5$ MON_{EL}	202

Immune function tests and cell cultures in blood transfusion

In particular situations it could be possible to test immunological disturbances in relation to blood transfusions. For the detection of antibodies against HLA, granulocytes and thrombocytes following transfusion of blood or blood products several serological techniques are available: immunofluorescence, complement-dependent cytotoxicity, cell mediated cytotoxicity.

Table 4. Enrichment of progenitor cells by elutriation of peripheral blood mononuclear cells.

Elutriation fractions	CFU-C	BFU-E
	colonies	
Lymphocyte fraction 10x10^5 cells	3	6
Lymphocyte/monocyte fraction 1x10^5 cells	>200	>200
Monocyte fraction 1x10^5 cells	43	29

Table 5. Elutriation of bone marrow cells: isolation of stem cell fractions depleted of T-lymphocytes.

	Before elutriation	Fraction 1	Fraction 2	Fraction 3
Experiment 1				
% T3	24	40	30	1
% T11	32	50	34	2
CFU-C	150	0	40	200
CFU-GEMM	10	0	6	15
Experiment 2				
% T11	N.D.	70	30	3
CFU-C	160	10	183	296
BFU-E	374	31	594	940
CFU-E	196	0	14	572
Experiment 3				
% T11	13	41	22	1
CFU-C	35	0	3	141
BFU-E	11	1	27	98

As has recently been demonstrated in relation to AIDS, hemotherapy may cause alterations in lymphocyte subpopulations [2]. To measure lymphocyte subpopulations flow cytometry methods have been introduced which enable us collecting reliable results very easily. Cell separation methods using monoclonal antibodies – probably in combination with cell sorting – may be suitable to isolate lymphocyte subsets for immunotherapy. In these situations it may be necessary to apply in vitro lymphocyte function tests, e.g. a NK function test.

Since blood transfusion and bone marrow transplantation are very close to each other it is not surprising that blood banks are involved in bone marrow transplantation programmes. To participate in these transplantation programmes new separation methods have to be present for collecting stem cell enriched fractions together with methods to deplete T-lymphocytes for allogeneic bone marrow transplantation and to remove malignant cells with monoclonal antibodies + complement or immunotoxins as is needed in autologous bone marrow transplantation. In this kind of programmes it is necessary to have access to facilities performing hemopoietic cell cultures. In Table 4 enrichment of progenitor cells from peripheral blood by elutriation (counter flow centrifugation) is demonstrated. The progenitor cells are found in a fraction of lymphoid cells and monocytes with a relatively high percentage of blasts and blast-like cells.

In Table 5 some results of bone marrow elutriation are shown. in these experiments immunophenotyping and cell culture techniques are combined to evaluate T-cell depletion and committed stem cell enrichment. These examples may illustrate that methods measuring immunological imbalances and cell culture techniques may have a place in modern blood banking even if the proposal of Zanjani et al. [17] to produce hemopoietic cells in culture for clinical use is not yet reality.

References

1. Singal DP. Annotation. Blood transfusion and renal transplantation. Br J Haematol 1985;61:595-602.
2. Gjerset GF, Martin BJ, Counts RB, Fast LD, Hansen JA. Immunological status of hemophilia patients treated with cryoprecipitate or lyophilized concentrate. Blood 1984;64:715-20.
3. Erber WN, Mijnheer LC, Mason DY. APAAP labeling of blood and bone marrow samples for phenotyping leukemia. Lancet 1986;i:761-5.
4. Lowenthal RM, Pralle H, Matter HP. A sensitive method for immunophenotyping stored leukemia and lymphoma cells with preservation of morphological detail. Pathology 1985;17:481-7.
5. Smit JW, Blom NR, van Luyn MJA, Halie MR. Lymphocytes with parallel tubular structures: morphologically a distinctive subpopulation. Blut 1983;46:311-20.
6. Henkart MP, Henkart PA. Lymphocyte mediated cytolysis as a secretory phenomenon. In: Clark WR, Goldstein P (eds). Mechanisms of cell mediated cytotoxicity. New York, London: Plenum Press 1982:227-41.
7. Rümke HC, Terpstra FG, Out TA, Vossen JM, Zeijlemaker WP. Immunoglobulin production by human lymphocytes in a microculture system: culture conditions and cellular interactions. Clin Immunol Immunopath 1981;19:338-50.
8. Van Oers MHJ, Zeijlemaker WP, Schellekens PThA. Separation and properties of EA-rosette-forming lymphocytes in humans. Eur J Immunol 1977;7:143-50.
9. Ortaldo JR, Oldman RK, Cannon GC, Herberman RB. Specificity of natural cytotoxic activity of normal human lymphocytes against a myeloid leukemia cell line. J Natl Cancer Inst 1977;59:77-82.
10. McCullock EA. Clinics in hematology. Cell culture techniques. London, Philadelphia, Toronto: WB Saunders 1984;vol.13,nr.2.
11. Metcalf D. The hemopoietic colony stimulating factors. Amsterdam: Elsevier Publ. 1984.
12. Linch D. Role of cell culture in the management of hematological diseases. In: Das PC, Smit Sibinga CTh, Halie MR (eds). Supportive therapy in hematology. Dordrecht: Martinus Nijhoff Publ. 1985:3-22.
13. Pike Bl, Robinson WA. Human bone marrow colony growth in agar gel. J Cell Physiol 1970;76:77-84.

14. Metcalf D. Annotation. Hemopoietic growth factors now cloned. Br J Haematol 1986;62:409-12.
15. Singer JW, Keating A, Wight TN. The human haematopoietic microenvironment. In: Hoffbrand AV (ed). Recent advances in haematology. Edingburgh: Churchill Livingstone 1984;4:1-24.
16. Dexter TM, Allen TD, Lajtha LG. Conditions controlling the proliferation of haematopoietic stem cells in vitro. J Cell Physiol 1977;91:335-44.
17. Zanjani ED, Schulman JC, Lasky LC. Production of hematopoietic cells in culture. In: Smit Sibinga CTh, Das PC, Greenwalt TJ (eds). Future developments in blood banking. Boston, Dordrecht, Lancaster: Martinus Nijhoff Publ. 1985: 131-45.
18. Harada M, Nakao S, Kondo K, et al. Effect of activated lymphocytes on the regulation of hematopoiesis: enhancement of in vitro BFU-E growth by T-cells stimulated by autologous non-T-cells. Blood 1986;67:1143-7.
19. Chicappa G, Phillips PG. Regulation of granulopoiesis by T-cells and T-cell subsets. In: Bond VP, Chandra P, Rai KR (eds). Hematopoietic cellular proliferation. Ann NY Acad Sciences. New York 1985;459:26-39.
20. Zoumbos NC, Djeu JY, Young NS. Interferon is the suppressor of hematopoiesis generated by stimulated lymphocytes in vitro. J Immunol 1984;133:769-74.

PLATELET ANTIBODY DETECTION

A.E.G. Kr. von dem Borne, W.H. Ouwehand, C.M. van Dalen

Introduction

In the past 40 years a plethora of publications has appeared in the literature, which describe methods to detect platelet antibodies in sera or bound to cells of patients in various clinical conditions. These methods can be broadly subdivided by the principle on which they are based into methods that measure:

a. The functional effect that antibodies may have on platelets, such as the induction of aggregation and release or just the opposite, i.e. the inhibition of these processes.
b. The immunologic effect that antibodies may have on platelets such as agglutination, complement fixation, complement dependent cytotoxicity or ^{51}Cr-release, cell mediated cytotoxicity and immunophagocytosis.
c. The binding of immunoglobulins and/or complement to platelets, either directly or indirectly.

In general, tests of the last category have proved to be the most reliable and senstive ones for antibodies of all immunoglobulin classes or subclasses, either complement fixing or non complement fixing.

In 1980 the Expert Panel on Serology of the International Society of Blood Transfusion (ISBT) and the International Committee for the Standardization in Hematology of the International Society of Hematology (ISH) decided to set up a Working Party on Platelet Serology. The aim of this working party was to compare platelet antibody tests in laboratories all over the world and exchange test sera, in order to improve the state of the art.

Till now three workshops have taken place, the last in 1986, leading to a meeting of members of the working party in Sydney, during the International Congress of the ISBT and the ISH May 1986. Also National Workshops have been organized in two countries (Canada and England) by the local Societies for Blood Transfusion.

The conclusions of all these workshops are that the platelet immunofluorescence test (PIFT) [1] is the best test at present available and therefore should be used as a standard method. With this test alloantibodies in sera can be correctly detected, with sufficient sensitivity. Moreover with platelets from typed donors the antigenic specificity of the antibodies can be determined and with properly selected antisera platelet antigen typing can be performed, i.e. for the well defined platelet antigens Zw^a and Zw^b of the $Zw(P1^A)$-system and Bak^a of the Bak-system. The method can be applied on a micro-scale, but is somewhat time consuming (about 2½ hours). Tests for alloantibodies should always be done together with a lymphocytotoxicity test and/or a lymphocyte immunofluorescence test, for the correct interpretation of the results (HLA- and/or platelet specific antibodies). For large scale evaluation of patient's sera and for crossmatching with platelets of large series of donors, the platelet-enzyme-linked-immunosorbent-assay (platelet-ELISA), performed as solid phase assay [2,3] has found to be a reasonable alternative, provided that the test is correctly performed and carefully selected peroxidase-labeled antiglobulin sera are used. For further studies into the nature of platelet reactive antibodies the immunoblot or Western blot has been found to be an interesting additional method [4].

These tests will be discussed in detail. A few laboratories also have had reasonable results with tests such as the ^{125}I-antiglobulin or ^{125}I-Staphylococcus protein A test, but these tests will not be discussed at length.

We also use the platelet agglutinin test [5], but mainly for antigen typing of platelets with agglutinating sera such as anti-Zw^b, anti-Ko^a and anti-Ko^b. The reason for this is that still no suitable sera are available for typing of these antigens in the PIF. The test will be briefly described.

Platelet immunofluorescence test

This method has already been described in 1960 by Silber et al., but was not generally introduced because of lack of specificity. We found that this problem could be largely solved by the use of Na_2EDTA as anticoagulant and platelet anti-aggregant and by fixation of the platelets with a 1% w/v paraformaldehyde solution (PFA) [1]. The role of platelet fixation is not yet entirely clear, but among others it prevents the aggregation of platelets during the test and induces platelet swelling and reduction of the amount of non-immunologically bound immunoglobulins [6]. The test is performed on platelets, isolated by differential centrifugation from Na_2EDTA anticoagulated donor blood, washed (3 times) in phosphate buffered saline (PBS) to which Na_2EDTA (9 mM) has been added. The platelets are fixed for 5 min in 1% w/v PFA (obtained by dilution of a suitably prepared and stored 4% w/v stock solution in PBS), washed and suspended in EDTA-PBS (150-300x10^6/ml platelets). 100 μl of the serum under investigation (neat or in dilutions), is incubated with 100 μl of the platelet suspension, for 30 min at 37°C. The platelets are than washed again (3 times) and incubated with a properly selected and diluted FITC-labeled antiglobulin serum for 30 min at room temperature in the dark. After 2 more washes they are than suspended in glycerol-PBS (3 part of glycerol, 1 part of PBS) and examined under a fluorescence microscope. It is also possible to measure the fluorescence strength in a laser flow cytometer.

As antiglobulin serum FITC-labeled-anti-human-total-Ig may be used. But also anti-IgG, anti-IgM, anti-IgA, anti-IgG-subclass and anti-light chain sera can be applied. The latter sera give the possibility to study the Ig-class and light chain type of the antibodies.

Also anti-complement sera (anti-C4, anti-C3) may be used to study complement fixation by platelet antibodies. But than the platelets should be washed and suspended in PBS without EDTA (which is anticomplementary), or even in Ca^{++} and Mg^{++} containing Veronal buffered saline. Moreover after incubation with the serum, the sensitized platelets should be incubated with normal AB serum (as a complement source) for 30 min at 37°C.

Platelet-enzyme-linked-immunosorbent-assay (Platelet-ELISA)

Many reports have been published on modifications of the standard ELISA to detect platelet antibodies. Untill recently we have used this method in our laboratory only incidently, because we were not able to obtain satisfactory results (in terms of sensitivity and specificity). This was also the general experience during the various international workshops.

However Sintnicolaas et al. [3] have modified the method of Horai et al. [2] in such a way that comparable results are obtained as in the PIFT.

This ELISA method is now applied in our laboratory on a routine scale. The initial steps of platelet preparation and fixation are the same as in the PIFT. However, nonfixed platelets can be applied as well. For the ELISA 50 μl of a freshly prepared platelet suspension ($100 x 10^6$/ml) is pipetted into the well of a microtiter plate, which is than centrifuged for 5 min (300 **g**). The platelet pellet is washed in PBS containing Tween (0.05% v/v) after which 50 μl of serum is added. After incubation for 30 min at 37°C, the platelets are again washed and than incubated with a suitably selected and diluted horse radish peroxidase labeled antiglobulin reagent ($F(ab^1)_2$ fragments of goat-antihuman IgG, Cappel, Cooper Biomedical). After incubation for 30 min at 37°C, the platelets are again washed, 100 μl of fresly prepared solution of substrate (ortho-phenylenediamine/H_2O_2) is added and after 10 min incubation at room temperature in the dark, the reaction is stopped with 4M H_2SO_4. The optical density is read in an automated micro-ELISA reader at 492 nm.

The selection of a peroxidase-labeled reagent of acceptable quality is of crucial importance. We compared reagents from eight different companies, and found only the Cappel conjugate to be satisfactory (in terms of sensitivity and specificity). Untill now we have not found any anti-Ig-, anti-IgM- or anti-IgA conjugate that gave satisfactory results. This is a limitation of the ELISA, because only IgG- and not IgM-platelet antibodies are detected. IgM platelet antibodies may cause platelet destruction as well.

Possibly an interesting new development in this respect is that monoclonal antibody conjugates can be constructed, directed against all possible Ig-classes, subclasses and light chain types, for use in the ELISA.

Lansdorp et al. [7] in our laboratory produced monoclonal rat anti-mouse IgGl antibodies, which could form stable tetrameric complexes with mouse IgGl monoclonal antibodies (Mab's). When added to a mixture of two different IgGl Mab's, stable tetramers containing only one as well as both mouse antibodies were formed, i.e. mono- and bispecific tetramers. In this way, for instance with mouse monoclonal IgGl anti-horseradish peroxidase and mouse IgGl anti-human IgG or IgM, stable bispecific tetramers are obtained, which upon addition of horseradish peroxidase can be used for

ELISA tests. In our hands these tetrametric constructions appeared to be superior anti-IgG and anti-IgM reagents in the platelet-ELISA.

Platelet agglutination test [5]

Platelets are prepared from EDTA anticoagulated blood by differential centrifugation, washed with EDTA-PBS three times and suspended in EDTA-PBS (concentration 500x10^6/ml). To the serum under investigation extra EDTA is added (1 volume of 55 mM Na_2EDTA to 9 volumes of serum). 100 μl of the serum, and 50 μl of the platelet suspension are mixed in the well of a Kline plate, which is covered and rotated on a shaker for 30 min at 4°C. The reaction is read microscopically. A microtiter modification of this method can also be used.

Immunoblot (Wester blot) [4]

This interesting, but complicated method is not useful for large scale routine investigations. However, it may play an important role in the unravelling of the specificity of platelet reactive antibodies and the analysis of the antigens involved in platelet antibody-reactions. Washed platelets are dissolved in a lysis buffer (containing tris, EDTA, the detergent Nonidet-P40 (NP40) and some enzyme inhibitors). The lysate, containing the platelet proteins, is cleared by centrifugation and boiled in a tris-glycerol-sodium dodecylsulphate (SDS) solution. The SDS-polyacrylamide gel-electrophoresis is carried out. Subsequently the platelet proteins, separated by electrophoresis, are electrophoretically transferred to nitrocellulose. After treatment of the nitrocellulose with a NP40 and gelatin containing solution, it is incubated with antiserum, diluted in PBS containing gelatin and Tween. After incubation, the nitrocellulose is washed with this solution and incubated with ^{125}I-labeled anti-human IgG or IgM, diluted in the same solution. After washing and blotting with filter paper, autoradiography (film and intensifying screen) takes place to visualize binding of the antibodies to one or more of the platelet proteins.

Antigen specificity of platelet antibodies

The above described methods not only can be used to detect platelet reactive antibodies, but also to determine their specificity. Platelets carry two types of antigens. These are the antigens of the HLA-ABC system, which they share with all nucleated cells, and antigens which are specific for platelets. Platelet-specific antigens belong to four different antigen systems: Zw, Yuc(Pen), Bak and Ko. The antigens of the HLA-ABC system are antigenic determinants of membrane glycoproteins with a molecular weight of 44 kDa, bound to the 12 kDa glycoprotein β_2-microglobulin. The two known Zw antigens, Zw^a and Zw^b are allelic antigens of the platelet membrane glycoprotein IIIa, with a molecular weight of 95 kDa. The only known Bak antigen, Bak^a, is an antigen of platelet glycoprotein IIb, with a molecular weight of 135 kDa. Preliminary findings indicate that the two Yuc-antigens (Yuc^b and Yuc^a) are also on glycoprotein IIIa. The localization of the Ko-antigens, Ko^a and Ko^b, is not yet known.

To show that platelet antibodies are directed against HLA-ABC antigens, two approaches are generally used. The first is to show that the antibodies react not only with the platelets, but also with the lymphocytes of an individual. This is done by lymphocytotoxicity and lymphocyte immunofluorescence tests.

The second is to show that the antibodies do not react anymore with platelets that have been incubated at 37°C with a chloroquine solution ('stripping'). By this treatment HLA-ABC glycoproteins, but not other glycoproteins, are eluted from the platelet membrane [8].

To further determine the specificity of the HLA-antibodies, studies with panels of lymphocytes and platelets from HLA-typed donors are necessary. The specificity of antibodies against platelet specific antigens is determined with a panel of platelets from donors, typed for these antigens. When these antibodies are present in the sera together with HLA-antibodies, chloroquine stripping is again of great help. Platelet specific antigens are not eluted by chloroquine.

Also of help is immunoblotting, in which reactivity of antibodies with HLA- or platelet specific glycoproteins can be easily differentiated.

Antibodies against platelet cryptantigens

A special problem in platelet serology is the occurrence in sera of antibodies against hidden or cryptic antigens present on the protein complex, formed by glycoprotein IIb and IIIa [9,10]. Such antibodies have been found in the serum of many patients, and sometimes also of normal donors. Why such antibodies are present in the blood is not clear, but they could be directed against antigens expressed during activation of platelets or during platelet aging.

The antibodies cause false positive direct and indirect platelet antibody tests, because they react with platelets in the presence of EDTA and/or after paraformaldehyde fixation. They also may cause agglutination of platelets in EDTA anticoagulated blood, which leads to false low platelet counts or pseudothrombocytopenia.

Antibodies against platelet cryptantigens are probably not affecting platelet survival of the patient's own platelets nor of transfused donor-platelets.

Postive reactions due to this type of antibodies can be excluded by using platelets isolated from citrate anticoagulated blood, which are not fixed with PFA and are washed with and suspended in PBS without EDTA. This is not routinely done because platelets, isolated from citrate anticoagulated blood, are much less stable and are difficult to handle and to store. Aggregation and activation may occur, with as a result loss of platelets and aspecific positive test results.

Applications of platelet serology

At present platelet serology is used nearly as widely as red cell serology. It is applied in the blood transfusion field, to study the causes of transfusion reactions (such as fever and posttransfusion purpura) and of refractoriness to platelet transfusions. It is also used to diagnose diseases such as alloimmune thrombocytopenia of the newborn, autoimmune thrombocytopenia and drug induced immune thrombocytopenia. The possibility to detect alloimmunization as a cause of refractoriness to platelet transfusions has attracted much interest in the last few years. This because it is possible to select platelets from donors which are compatible and when transfused give suitable platelet increments and good platelet survival.

When alloimmunization occurs in patients on platelet transfusion therapy, this is often due to HLA-immunization, although also antibodies against platelet specific antigens may be produced [11,12]. Thus an approach to select compatible platelet-donors is by HLA-typing.

The lymphocytes of the patient are typed for the antigens of the HLA-ABC system, HLA-typed donors which match with the patient's HLA-typing are traced via a computer file and their platelets tested in a crossmatch with serum of the patient. Platelets from compatible donors are than obtained by thrombocytapheresis. However, this is an expensive approach, which is only possible in specialized centers, with sufficient facilities for HLA-typing. It is more simple and less expensive to select compatible platelets by a crossmatch procedure directly. This can be done in every blood bank with sufficient amounts of platelet concentrates in stock.

Summary

Nowadays platelet serology is sufficiently advanced to be applied on a routine scale in blood bank laboratories. Platelet immunofluorescence appears to be the standard method, but for screening the solid-phase-platelet ELISA is a suitable alternative.

Platelet agglutination and immunoblotting are tests for special investigations.

Alloimmunization against platelet antigens is an important cause of refractoriness for platelet transfusions. The antigens involved are often of the HLA-ABC system, but may be also platelet specific. Selection on HLA-matching is used to find compatible donors in case of refractoriness, but selection by a direct platelet crossmatch is an interesting and less expensive alternative.

References

1. Von dem Borne AEG Kr, Verheugt FWA, Oosterhof F, von Riesz E, Brutel de la Rivière A, Engelfriet CP. A simple immunofluorescence test for the detection of platelet antibodies. Br J Haematol 1978;39:195-207.

2. Horai S, Claas FJ, van Rood JJ. Detection of platelet antibodies by enzyme-linked immunosorbent assay (ELISA) on artificial monolayers of platelets. Immunology Letters 1981;3:67-72.
3. Sintnicolaas K, van der Steuyt KJB, van Putten WLJ, Bolhuis RLH. A microplate ELISA for the detection of platelet alloantibodies; comparison with a platelet immunofluorescence test. Br J Haemat 1987.
4. Huisman JJ. Immunoblotting: an emerging technique in immunohematology. Vox Sang 1986;50:129-36.
5. Van der Weerdt ChM, Veenhoven-von Riesz E, Nijenhuis LE, van Loghem JJ. The Zw blood group system in platelets. Vox Sang 1963;8:513-30.
6. Vos JJE, Huisman JG, Winkel IN, Risseeuw-Bogaart NG, Engelfriet CP, von dem Borne AEG Kr. Quantification of platelet-bound alloantibodies by radioimmunoassay. A study on some variables. Vox Sang 1987 (in press).
7. Lansdorp PM, Aalberse RC, Bos R, Schutter WG, van Bruggen EFJ. Cyclic tetramolecular complexes of monoclonal antibodies: a new type of cross-linking reagent. Eur J Immunol 1986;16:672-83.
8. Nordhagen R, Flaathen ST. Chloroquine removal of HLA-antigens from platelets for the platelet immunofluorescence test. Vox Sang 1985;48:156-9.
9. Pegers JG, Bruynes ECE, Engelfriet CP, von dem Borne AEG Kr. Pseudothrombocytopenia: an immunologic study on platelet antibodies dependent on ethylene diamine tetra-acetate. Blood 1982;59:157-61.
10. Von dem Borne AEG Kr, van der Lelie J, Vos JJE, et al. Antibodies against cryptantigens of platelets. Characterization and significance for the serologist. Karger, Basel: Curr Stud Hematol Blood Transf. Platelet Serology, research progress and clinical implications 1986;52:33-46.
11. Brand A, van Leeuwen A, Eernisse JG, van Rood JJ. Platelet transfusion therapy. Optimal donor selection with a combination of lymphocytotoxicity and platelet fluorescence test. Blood 1978;51:781-8.
12. Pegels JG, Bruynes ECG, Engelfriet CP, von dem Borne AEG Kr. Serological studies in patients on platelet- and granulocyte-substitution therapy. Br J Haematol 1982;52:59-68.

DECREASED FLUIDITY OF HUMAN PLATELET MEMBRANES AFTER INTERACTION WITH AN ANTI PL^{A1} ANTIBODY

P. Champeix, C. Kaplan, M. Roche, C. Motta

Introduction

Neonatal alloimmune thrombocytopenia (NAITP) is primarily due to a foeto-maternal incompatibility of a specific platelet alloantigen. When the PL^{A1} antigen [1] is involved, its incidence has been recently evaluated to 1/3000 births [2]. The PL^{A1} antigen has been located on the platelet membrane glycoprotein IIIa [3]. This glycoprotein is mainly involved in the platelet aggregation system. The Glanzmann thrombasthenia is due to a lack of this protein [4] and in this disease patients can have severe hemorrhages. In vitro it was shown that the platelets were unable to adhere after activation [5]. Von dem Borne et al. [6] have shown that the antibody anti-PL^{A1} interacts in the normal platelet aggregation process. So it was of interest to study the effect of the interaction of such an antibody on the membrane platelet fluidity and order. For this purpose fluorescence polarization was used. The method allows a submacroscopic level of investigation in membrane fluidity studies which is directly correlated with physicological events [7].

Material and methods

The serum containing the anti-PL^{A1} antibody was from a PL^{A1}-negative mother, who gave birth to a neonatal alloimmunized thrombocytopenic child. HLA antibodies or irregular blood cell agglutinins were not detectable and the antibody was IgG in nature. The serum was tested at different dilutions (from 1/2 to up to 1/128) against normal blood platelets from healthy volunteers. (All were without any treatment for at least two weeks). The incubation was at room temperature for 30 min without agitation. The classical aggregation tests with ADP, collagen and ristocetin sulfate were performed at 37°C on an aggregometer according to Born [8]. Part of the platelets (after the serum incubation) were treated in PBS containing the fluorescence probes 1,6-diphenyl-1,3,5-hexatriene (DPH) and trimethylammonium-DPH (TMA-DPH) [9]. The DPH was deeply hidden in the platelet membranes, while the TMA-DPH, because of its surface location [10] reported surface events. Fluorescence polarization was used to monitor the fluidity of the membrane, by studying the probe movements [8].

The fluorescence anisotropy r was calculated [8] and the degree of order estimated from these measurements [11]. The fluorescence anisotropy was directly related to the fluidity of the membrane in the neighbourhood of the probe. As r increased, the fluidity decreased and reversely [8]. The S parameter describes the molecular order (as S increased toward 1, the molecular order increased and reversely).

Results and discussion

The binding of the anti-PL^{A1} antibody to the membrane receptors was followed by an increase of both r and S. Figure 1 shows the significant increase of r and S from the original platelets for a 1/2 dilution and below. As shown, this increase was reported both for DPH and TMA-DPH. For dilution factors from 2 to 64, a plateau was reached and then followed at 128 by a net decrease. These results suggest a rapid rigidification of the membrane upon the binding of the antibody. For more important dilution factors the phenomenon disappears and the values obtained were similar to the original ones.

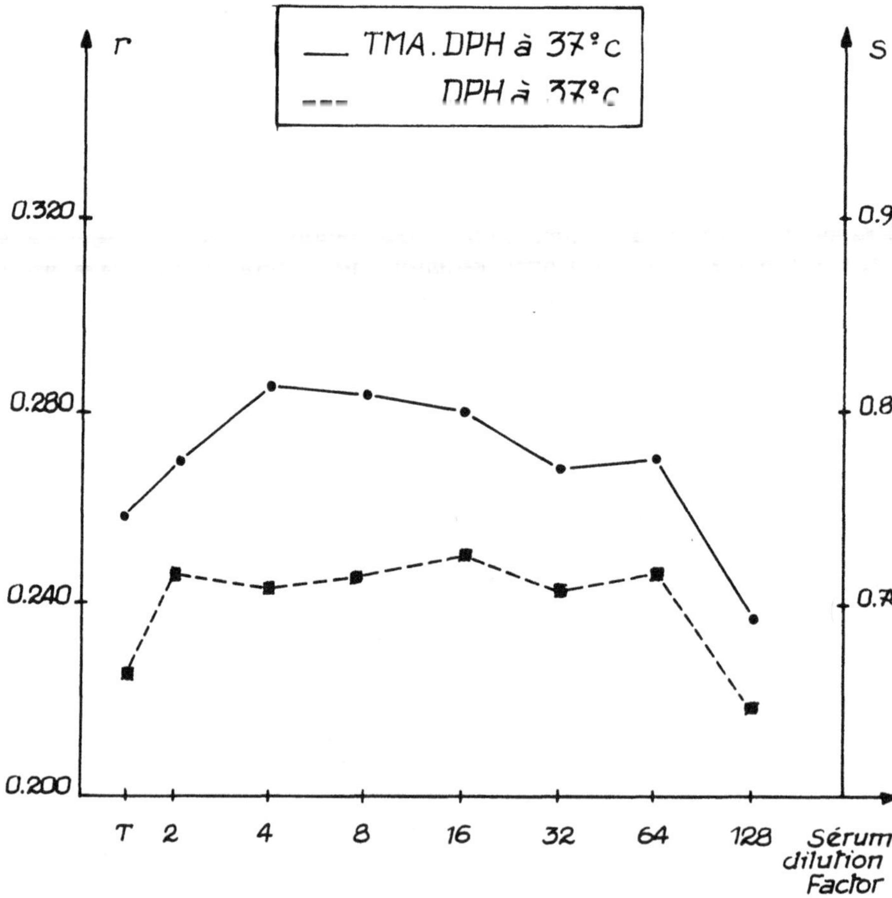

Figure 1. PL^{A1} membrane lipid fluidity after interaction with an anti-PL^{A1} antibody fluorescence anisotropy (r) and degree order (S) using two fluorescent probes DPH and TMA-DPH.

As sensed by the two probes (with different membrane locations) the rigidification phenomenon observed affects the whole membrane bilayer and not only the outer hemileaflet. This could be due to a membrane receptor conformation change, resulting in increased phospholipid-protein interaction forces. This has been already observed for other antibodies binding on membrane platelets [12].

All these changes could result in modifications in the lateral and transverse diffusion of proteins and lead to modified aggregation properties of platelets. This preliminary work is under current development with other serum samples containing anti-PL^{A1} antibodies in order to confirm these findings.

Associated to membrane studies by fluorescence polarization with different fluorescence probes, glycoprotein interactions with the bilayer have to be studied in order to understand the phenomenon observed.

The method used offers a good sensitivity and could be proposed as a convenient means to detect anti-PL^{A1} antibodies in the maternal serum which are commonly undetected by conventional techniques.

Acknowledgement

We thank miss Gatignol Raymonde for her help in the preparation of the manuscript.

References

1. Shulman NR, Marder VJ, Hiller MC, Collier EM. Platelet and leukocyte isoantigens and their antibodies: serologic, physiologic and clinical studies. In: Progress in Hematology. New York: Grune and Stratton 1964:222.
2. Blanchette V, Hogan V, McMurray S. Canadian Pediatric Society, Annual Meeting, Quebec City. 1983 (abstract).
3. Kunicki TJ, Aster RH. Isolation and immunologic characterization of the human platelet alloantigen PL^{A1}. Mol Immunol 1979;16:353-60.
4. Nurden AT, Caen JP. An abnormal platelet glycoprotein pattern in three cases of Glanzmann's thrombasthenia. Br J Haemat 1974;28:253-60.
5. Caen JP, Castaldi PA, Leclerc JC, et al. Congenital bleeding disorders with long bleeding time and normal platelet count. Glanzmann's thrombasthenia (report of fifteen patients). Am J Med 1966;41:4-26.
6. Van Leeuwen EF, Leeksma OC, van Mourik JA, Engelfriet CO, von dem Borne AEG Kr. Effect of the binding of anti-Zw^{a} antibodies on platelet function. Vox Sang 1984;47:280-9.
7. Schinitzky M, Yuli I. Lipid fluidity at the submacroscopic level: determination by fluorescence polarization. Chem Phys Lipids 1982;30:261-75.
8. Born GVR, Cross MJ. The aggregation of blood platelets. J Physiol 1963;168: 178-95.
9. Shinitzky M, Inbar M. Microviscosity parameters and protein mobility in biological membranes. Biochim Biophys Acta 1976;433:133-49.
10. Prendergast FG, Haugland RP, Callaman PJ. 1[4-(Trimethylamino-phenyl)]-6-phenylhexa-1,3,5-triene: synthesis fluorescence properties, and use as a fluorescence probe of lipid bilayers. J Biol Chem 1980;255:7333-8.

11. Van Blitterswisk WJ, van Hoeven RP, van der Meer BW. Lipid structural order parameters (reciprocal of fluidity) in biomembranes derived from steady-state fluorescence polarization measurements. Biochim Biophys Acta 1981;644:323-32.
12. Kowalska MA, Cierniewsky CS. Microenvironment changes of human blood platelet membranes associated with fibrinogen binding. J Membr Biol 1983;75: 57-64.

ROLE OF WHITE CELLS IN REAGENTS FOR AIDS

F. Rey, F. Barre-Sinoussi, J.C. Chermann

It is now known that HIV-I is the agent of AIDS (Fig. 1)

Particularly conditions for the culture in vitro of T-lymphocytes were at the origin of the isolation of LAV-I, from peripheral blood lymphocytes of a patient with a persistent lymphadenopathy. The T4-lymphotropism and the cytopathic effect of this retrovirus on the susceptible cells were rapidly observed in vitro and were related to the immune deficiency which characterizes patients with AIDS.

For virus production, premature T-cell lines like H9 or CEM were infected successfully. Despite the apparent T4 lymphotropism of HIV-I and the role played by this molecule on the binding of the virus on the target cells, it has been possible to infect other white cells like B-lymphocytes, macrophages and bone marrow cells. HTLV-I-infected cells are also permissive to HIV-I. The effect of superinfection depends on the cell-strain. The radically cytopathic effects observed on MT4 leads to a rapid test for titration of neutralizing antibodies which will be useful on the way to the vaccine.

Infection of peripheral blood lymphocytes

Long-term growth of T-lymphocytes in vitro

The white cells are classically separated from the other blood cells by centrifugation on a Ficoll Hypaque density gradient. Since the discovery and the purification of TCGF (T-cell growth factor) in 1976 [1] it is now possible to grow T-lymphocytes in vitro for 4 to 6 weeks. The white cells are usually cultured in RPMI 1640 containing 10% of foetal calf serum, at a concentration of 10^6 cells/ml. The T-cells have to be stimulated by PHA (phytohemagglutinin) to be able to use TCGF and grow. After a decrease in the total number of cells, on day 3, which corresponds to the selection of T-lymphocytes between all the white cells, a good cellular division can be observed up to day 20 (Fig. 2). Then, the cells grow more slowly and stop growing on day 30. They are then resistent to a PHA stimulation.

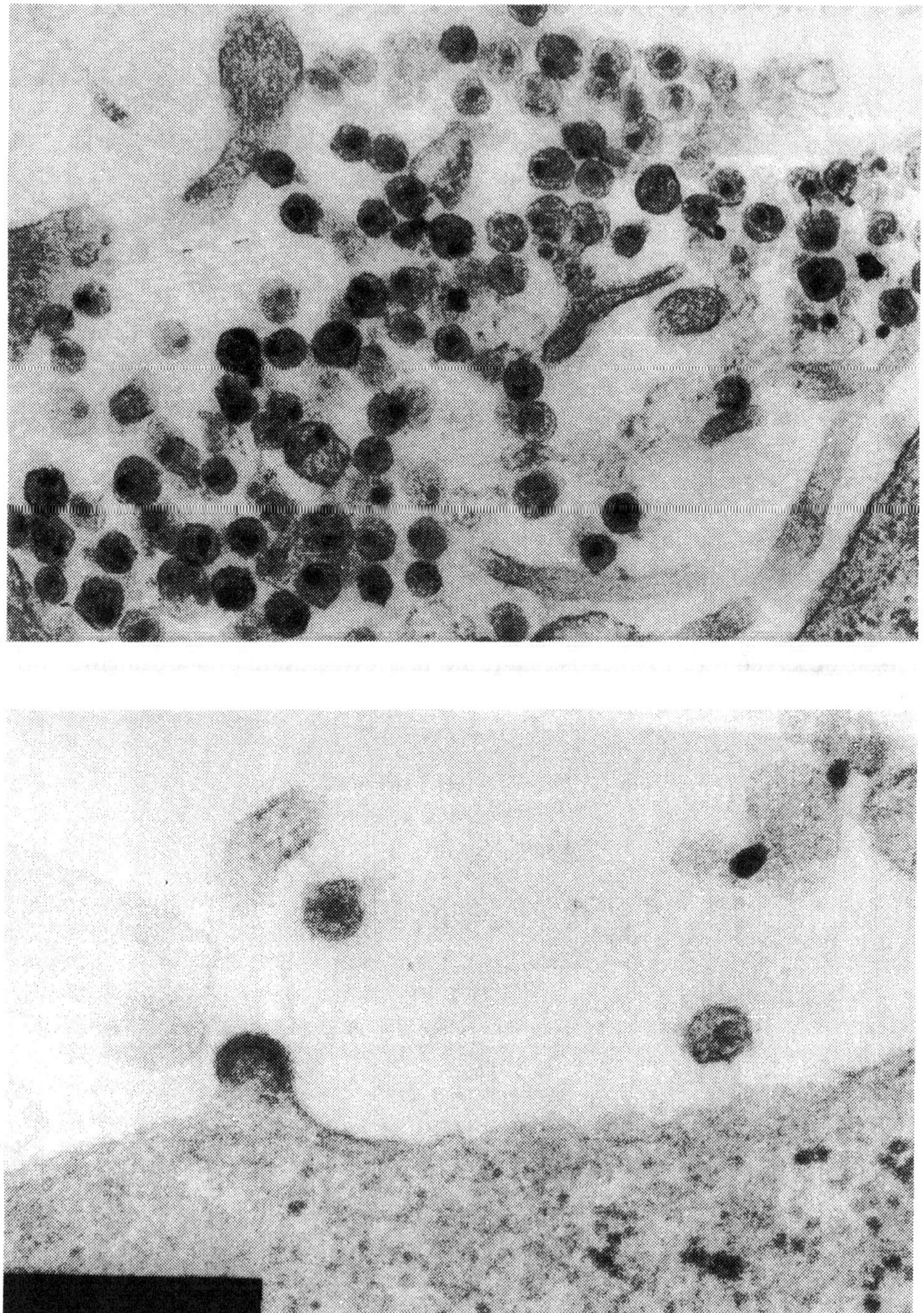

Figure 1. Morphology of the virus: electron microscopy.

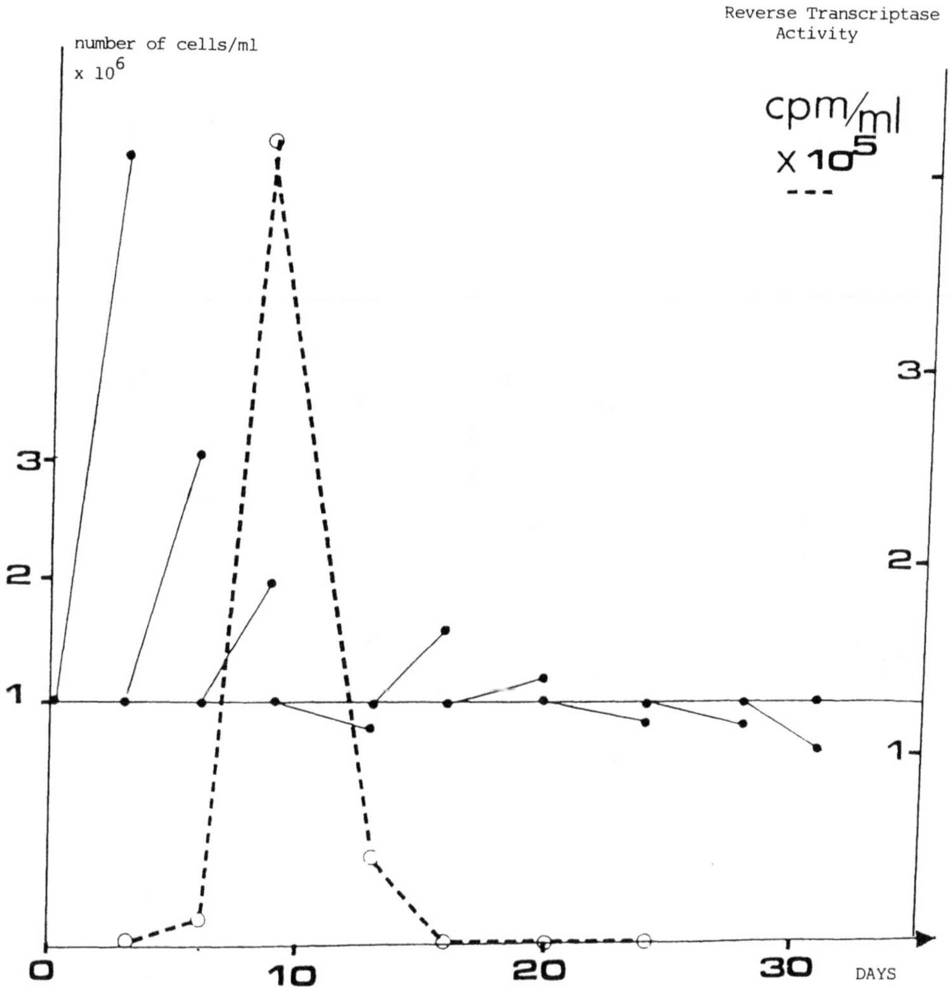

Figure 2. Growth of cells and virus production.

Infection of normal T-lymphocyte in vitro by HIV-I

(a) conditions for culture medium

To favour the attraction of virus on cells, a polycation like polybren is added to the culture medium. Polybren will cover the cell membrane positively and virus is usually charged negatively. The role of endogenous interferon on virus production of infected cells has already been demonstrated [2]. When a sheep anti-interferon serum is added to the medium, the endogenous interferon is neutralized and the virus production is enhanced (Fig. 3). Recently, the role of hormones, like hydrocortisone as enhancer of virus production has also been demonstrated [3].

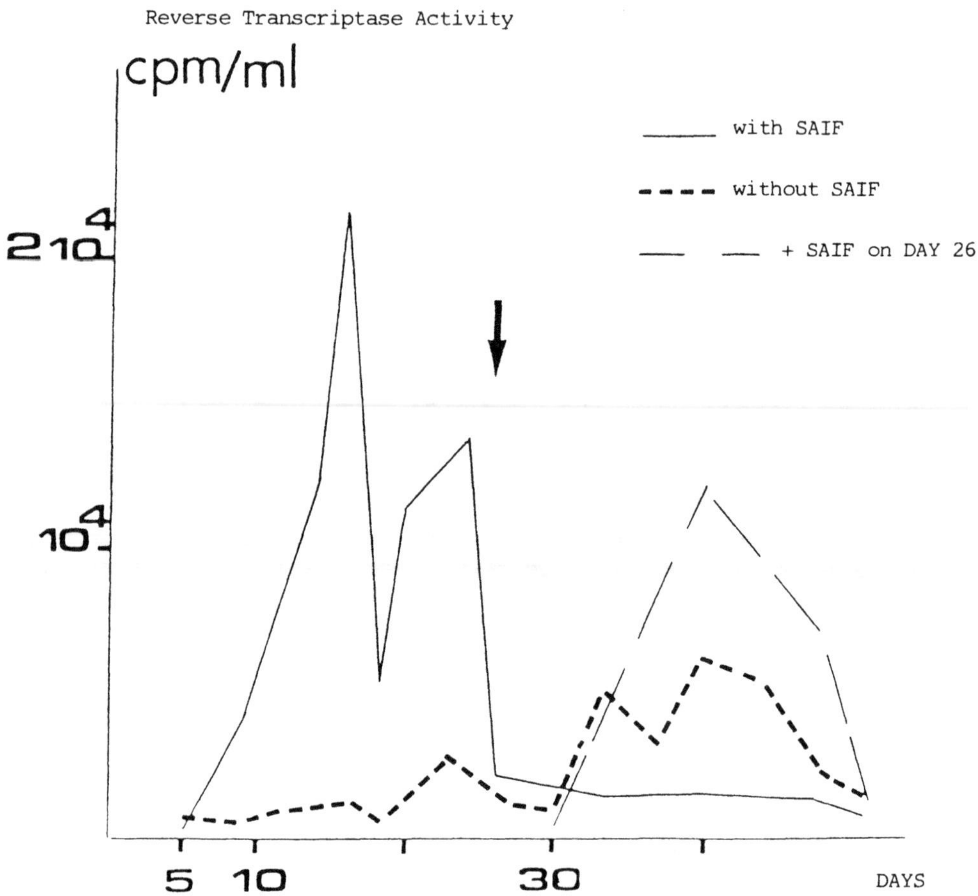

Figure 3. Role of anti-interferon serum on virus production.

(b) Detection of virus production

Normal T-lymphocytes can be infected either by free-virus or by cocultivation with irradiated infected cells (6000 rad). The virus production is measured by the enzymatic detection of a reverse transcriptase activity in 1 ml of ultracentrifuged supernatant. This enzyme is characteristic of retroviruses. Its detection is a very sensitive test [4]. Usually, virus production starts from day 7 to 10 after infection and is transient. Chronic infection with HIV-I cannot be established since this virus is non-transforming but cytopathic for cells (Fig. 2).

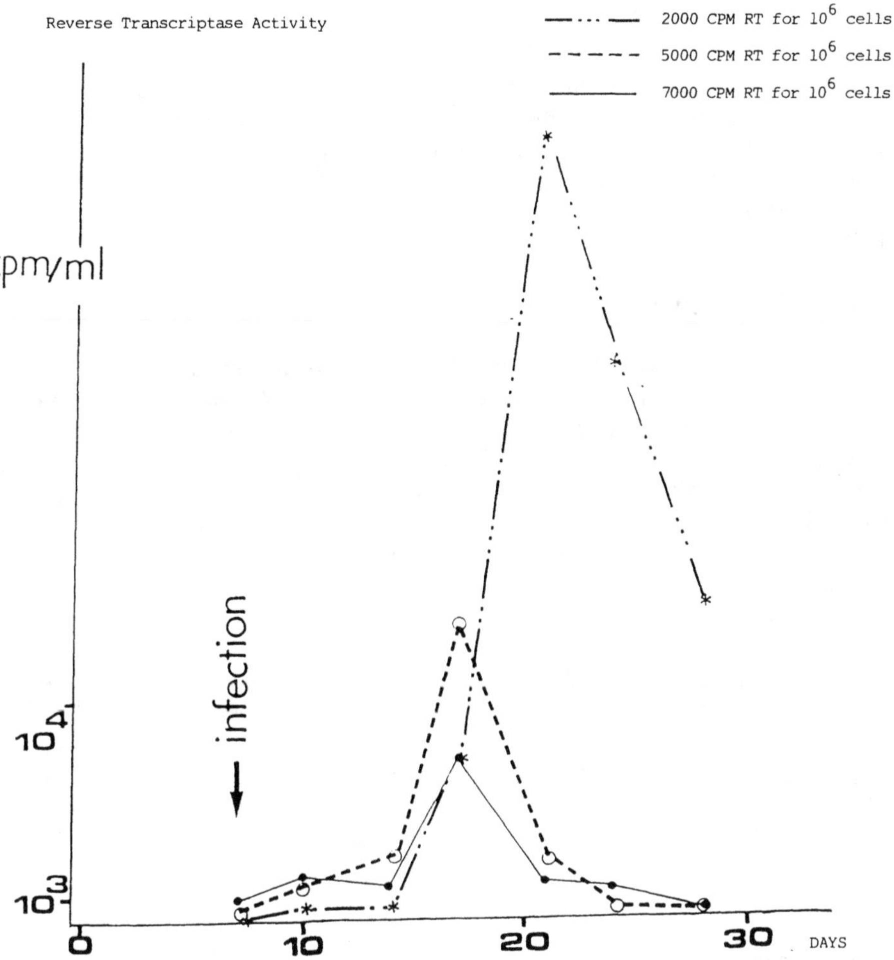

Figure 4. Virus production depends on the dose of virus for infection.

(c) Dose of virus for optimal virus production

As shown in Figure 4, virus production depends on the dose of virus used for infection. When a high titered supernatant was used for infection, the virus production was lower than the one obtained with a diluted supernatant. However, there is a dose limit of virus under which no virus production will occur. The cytopathic effect of HIV-I on susceptible cells can explain this inverted correlation between infection and production. With a low amount of viral particles, the infection can spread on more cells.

(d) Necessity of PHA stimulation for virus production

Non-stimulated T-lymphocytes can be infected by HIV-I but virus production will start only after a PHA stimulation. Virus can only be produced in culture medium by growing cells.

The HIV-I susceptible cells

The T-lymphocytes

Different data have shown that in peripheral blood only the T4+ T-lymphocytes were infected and produced HIV-I [5]. The T8 cells, separated from T4 are resistent to HIV-I infection. Blocking experiments with anti-T4 monoclonal antibody have demonstrated that the T4 molecule is involved in the HIV-I receptor [6]. But T4 could not be the receptor since recently, non-T4 cells were shown permissive for HIV-I.

The HIV-I cell lines

It is important to grow HIV-I in large quantities to prepare antigen for serologic tests. Normal T-lymphocytes were not useful for that purpose since they do not produce virus continuously. It has been possible to infect transformed T-lymphocytes like H9 and CEM [7]. These cell lines are premature T-lymphocytes with T4 marker. They were isolated from patients with leukemias. H9 and CEM produce HIV continuously but non-infected cells have to be mixed with the productive cells regularly to maintain a good virus production (cocultivation). The percentage of infected cells varies from 30 to 50 (by IF staining).

The B-lymphocytes

B-cell lines can be obtained by a transformation of normal B-lymphocytes by EBV (Epstein-Barr-Virus). After transformation, B-cells are permissive to the HIV-I and can produce HIV-I continuously if non-infected cells are added regularly to the culture [8]. Moreover, B-lymphocytes isolated from an EBV-positive AIDS patient grow indefinitely in vitro and produce HIV-I. These data show that non-T4 cells are also permissive to the AIDS virus.

Macrophages

Recently, Gallo's group has shown that macrophages are also permissive to HIV-I [9]. Normal macrophages were isolated from a donor and were infected in vitro by HIV-I. A low reverse transcriptase (RT) activity was detected in cell culture supernatant and it was possible to infect normal T-lymphocytes by cocultivation with the macrophages. Macrophages from AIDS patients spontaneously produced the virus. Thus, the role of macrophages as a reservoir for the AIDS virus has been postulated.

Bone marrow cells

It has been possible to infect bone marrow cells without T-markers after a depletion by anti-T3 and anti-T11 monoclonal antibodies. These pre-T-lymphocytes are permissive and produced HIV-I (data not published).

Superinfection of HTLV-I-infected cell lines

The HTLV-I cell lines

HTLV-I (human T leukemia virus) was the first retrovirus isolated from patients with ATL (adult T leukemias). HTLV-I is T-lymphotropic and transforms the cells. Several HTLV-I cell lines have been established. Since they are T-cell lines, it was possible to superinfect them with HIV-I. The results of superinfection depend on the HTLV-I cell line strain. For example, the C10 cells produce low level of HTLV-I. After superinfection with HIV-I, high levels of RT activity are detected in the supernatant, corresponding probably to a mixture of HTLV-I and HIV-I.

MT4 is another HTLV-I cell line; 8 days after superinfection with HIV-I, a radically cytopathic effect on MT4 can be observed, all the cells die while a high RT activity is detected in the supernatant [10].

Use of MT4 as target cells for the titration of HIV-I

Since no monolayer cell line was, so far, discovered to be permissive to HIV-I, no plaque assay is possible for titration of HIV-I. The only way of titration was the infection of normal T-lymphocytes with serial dilutions of a given infected sample, to determine the limit dilution with which a virus production is obtained. This is a time-consuming and expensive experiment. The observation of the radical cytopathic effect of HIV-I on MT4 leads to a test for titration of virus. For neutralization, a limit dilution of virus, still cytopathic is mixed with serial dilutions of tested sera. The residual virus is then titrated on MT4. Titers of 1/50 up to 1/1000 were found in asymptomatic blood donors, and no correlation was shown with the antibody titer by ELISA.

This test will be a useful tool for the screening of sera of vaccinated animals during the preparation of a vaccine against AIDS.

References

1. Mier JW, Gallo RC. Purification and some characteristics of human T-cell growth factor from phytohemagglutinin stimulated lymphocytes conditioned media. PNAS 1980;77:6134-8.
2. Barre-Sinoussi F, Montagnier L, Lidereau R, et al. Enhancement of retrovirus production by anti-interferon serum. Ann Microbiol 1979;130B:349.
3. Markham P, Salahuddin SZ, Veren K, Orndorff S, Gallo RC. Hydrocortisone and some other hormones enhance the expression of HTLV-III. Int J Cancer 1986;37:67-72.
4. Rey MA, Spire B, Dormont D, Barre-Sinoussi F, Montagnier L, Chermann JC. Characterization of the RNA dependent DNA polymerase of a new human T-lymphotropic retrovirus (LAV). Biochem Biophys Res Com 1984;121:126-33.
5. Klatzmann D, Barre-Sinoussi F, Nugeyre MT, et al. Selective tropism of lymphadenopathy associated virus (LAV) for helper/inducer T-lymphocytes. Science 1984;225:59-62.

6. Klatzmann D, Champagne E, Chameret S, et al. T-lymphocyte T4 molecule behaves as the receptor for human retrovirus LAV. Nature 1984;312:767-8.
7. Popovic M, Sarnghadaran MG, Read E, Gallo RC. Detection, isolation and continuous production of cytopathic retroviruses (HTLV-III) from patients with AIDS and pre-AIDS. Science 1984;224:497-500.
8. Montagnier L, Gruest J, Chamaret S, et al. Adaptation of LAV to replication in EBV-transformed B-lymphoblastoïd cell lines. Science 1984;225:63-6.
9. Salahuddin SZ, Rose RM, Groopman JE, Markham PD, Gallo RC. Human T-lymphotropic virus type III infection of human alveolar macrophages. Blood 1986;68:281-4.
10. Koyonagi Y, Harada S, Takahashi M, Uchino F, Yamamoto M. Selective cytotoxicity of AIDS virus infection towards HTLV-I transformed cell lines. Int J Cancer 1985;36:445-51.

DISCUSSION

C.P. Engelfriet and M. Körbling

A.E.G. Kr. von dem Borne (Amsterdam): Dr. Chermann, my question concerns your doubt that the T4 molecule is actually involved in the infection, the entrance of the virus in the cell. During the monoclonal antibody workshop in Oxford recently data were presented in which the T4 molecule has now been cloned and it has been shown that you can take whatever cell you want, put the T4 protein in the cell, get expression of T4 and make it infectable by HIV virus. Is that true?

J.C. Chermann (Paris): It is true that when you use a specific monoclonal antibody on T4 you block the penetration of the virus, which means that the receptor is associated with the T4. The receptor is associated with the T4 molecule, but it is not only the T4. If we deplete completely some T4 expressing cells like bone marrow precursor, we can infect them easily. We demonstrated that the Drosophyla cells could bind the virus. That means when using antibody against Drosophyla cell surface, we are able to block the penetration of the virus in T4 cells. We are convinced that T4 cells are susceptible to the virus as a subpopulation. The T4 population has a lot of functions and the T4 antigen is much more immunogenic than the receptors of the virus. The only way to discriminate between T4 susceptible cells is to use a fluorescent virus, which binds only a subpopulation of T4. That means that the receptor could be a part of the T4, but not only the T4.

C.Th. Smit Sibinga (Groningen): Mrs. Beelen, now that we have learned that the class II HLA antigens are of major importance for alloimmunization phenomena, specifically regarding the transfusion of platelets contaminated with white cells, what are your ideas about typing donors then. Would you prefer putting main emphasis on the typing of the class II antigens or rather continue in doing an entire typing – the class I as well as the class II antigens. Could we not restrict ourselves to the class II?

J.M. Beelen (Groningen): The induction of alloreactivity is most efficient in the presence of incompatible class II antigens. However, alloimmunization can also occur when the incompatible class I or thrombocyte-specific antigens are presented in the context of compatible class II antigens. The problem of sensitization in platelet transfusion is made up of two aspects: The prevention of sensitization and the donor selection required for the sensitized patients. The incidence of sensitization can be successfully reduced by the use of leukocyte-poor platelet suspensions. For several reasons this approach to prevent alloimmunization is more easy applicable than HLA-DR-matching. Antibodies against class I or against thrombocyte-specific antigens are the products of alloimmunization which are responsible for a poor platelet survival. Therefore, whenever we have not been able to prevent sensitization selection of donors compatible for class I antigens will be required. From this point of view class I-typing of Blood Bank donors is more relevant than class II-typing.

C.Th. Smit Sibinga: Dr. von dem Borne, one of the things we have been talking about in previous symposia is that platelet crossmatching is indeed becoming more and more important. However, it takes some time. When we are in a certain type of emergency to a bleeding problem in an alloimmunized or even refractory patient, and try to find a matched donor, it takes even more time. What I understood from dr. Sintnicolaas is that the possibility has now come to a forefront to have platelets present from a number of donors already typed, which you store. Then rapidly an ELISA crossmatch is done with cells of a number of donors and donor is selected instead of the other way round; the usual way to have a donor come in, draw some blood, do a crossmatch, have the donor wait, find out that it does not match, call another donor and go again losing an enormous amount of time. Do you see the procedure of dr. Sintnicolaas now as the way we should go for crossmatching in these patients.

A.E.G. Kr. von dem Borne: I think there are two strains of thoughts. The HLA typers of course, want files of donors, HLA typed and put into computers. They want the whole HLA selection procedure: Typing of the patient and typing of the donor, which is to my idea quite an expensive approach. The other approach, coming out of platelet serology as indicated by Sintnicolaas, is a workable approach. Also because now techniques for longer platelet storage have become available. One could envisage a platelet bank in which platelets with plasma of some a 100 or 200 donors are being stored, of which samples are sent to the platelet serology laboratory, which does the selection of negative donors in the way Sintnicolaas has shown us. It is very easy to store platelets in serology, you can simply put them in the wells, freeze them or even dry them and then get them out for serology testing and selection of the donor.

K. Sintnicolaas (Rotterdam): I would like to add that the crossmatch as we presented it here, is done on a limited number of patients. There are patients who are clearly refractory in whom we cannot detect antibodies and they do respond to HLA-matched platelets. So at this moment I think it is too early to say we can replace HLA-matching fully by only crossmatching.

A.E.G. Kr. von dem Borne: But that maybe a serological problem still. The fact that you find patients with a negative crossmatch and still no recovery could mean that, since you apply only anti-IgG, you have missed those of the IgM class or even of the IgA class. Moreover, you could include in your selection lymphocytes of the donors as well, for your matching procedure. So, I think that it is still possible to approach most refractoriness problems in the way you suggested and not going into the HLA-typed donors.

K. Sintnicolaas: I agree, but at this moment it is too early to say: We can now go exclusively that way.

S.J. Slichter (Seattle): The most practical approach to selecting compatible apheresis donors may be to combine both HLA selection with platelet crossmatching. It is conceivable that platelet samples could be frozen away on members of an HLA-typed volunteer donor apheresis panel. The initial selection would be based on running a computer generated match between the recipient and the panel members. Once the best HLA-matched donors were identified, the frozen platelet samples from these panel members could be pulled from the freezer and a platelet crossmatch test performed for the final selection.

www.ingramcontent.com/pod-product-compliance
Lightning Source LLC
LaVergne TN
LVHW011915200926
848484LV00002B/635
9780898389760